Person-Centred Practice in Nursing and Health Care

Theory and Practice

EDITED BY

Brendan McCormack

Professor and Head of the Division of Nursing
School of Health Sciences
Queen Margaret University
Scotland

Tanya McCance

Mona Grey Professor for Nursing R&D and Director of the Institute of Nursing & Health Research
Ulster University
Northern Ireland

SECOND EDITION

FOREWORD BY HESTER KLOPPER

WILEY Blackwell

Registered office: John Wiley & Sons, Ltd, The Atrium, Southern Gate, Chichester, West Sussex, PO19 8SQ, UK

Editorial offices: 9600 Garsington Road, Oxford, OX4 2DQ, UK
1606 Golden Aspen Drive, Suites 103 and 104, Ames, Iowa 50010, USA

For details of our global editorial offices, for customer services and for information about how to apply for permission to reuse the copyright material in this book please see our website at www.wiley.com/wiley-blackwell

Library of Congress Cataloging-in-Publication Data
Names: McCormack, Brendan, editor. | McCance, Tanya, editor. | McCormack,
  Brendan. Person-centred nursing. Preceded by (work):
Title: Person-centred practice in nursing and health care : theory and
  practice / editors, Professor Brendan McCormack, Professor Tanya McCance.
Description: Second edition. | Chichester, West Sussex ; Ames, Iowa : John
  Wiley & Sons Inc., 2016. | Preceded by Person-centred nursing : theory and
  practice / Brendan McCormack, Tanya McCance. 2010. | Includes
  bibliographical references and index.
Identifiers: LCCN 2016007088| ISBN 9781118990568 (pbk.) | ISBN 9781118990575
  (Adobe PDF) | ISBN 9781118990582 (ePub)
Subjects: | MESH: Holistic Nursing–methods | Nurse-Patient Relations |
  Patient Participation | Patient Satisfaction | Outcome Assessment (Health Care)
Classification: LCC R727.42 | NLM WY 86.5 | DDC 610.69/6–dc23 LC record available at
  http://lccn.loc.gov/2016007088

A catalogue record for this book is available from the British Library.

Set in 9.5/13pt, MeridienLTStd by SPi Global, Chennai, India.
Printed and bound in Malaysia by Vivar Printing Sdn Bhd

4   2017

Person-Centred Practice in Nursing and Health Care

Theory and Practice

We dedicate this book to our friends, colleagues, families and partners who supported us throughout. In particular we dedicate the work to Neil McCance (RIP) who sadly was unable to see a project he believed in so passionately come to fruition.

Contents

List of contributors

Barbara Bell
Chief Nurse Executive and Health Professions Officer
West Park Healthcare Centre, Toronto, Canada

Pauline Black
Lecturer in Nursing
School of Nursing, Ulster University, Northern Ireland, UK

Christine Boomer
Research Fellow
Ulster University/South Eastern Health and Social Care Trust,
Northern Ireland, UK

Marit Borg
Professor, Faculty of Health Sciences
The University College of South-East Norway, Drammen, Norway

Catherine Buckley
Practice Development Lecturer
St. Luke's Home Education Centre, Cork, Republic of Ireland

Shannon Burke
Advanced Practice Nurse
West Park Healthcare Centre, Toronto, Canada

Shaun Cardiff
Lecturer and Programme Leader
Fontys University of Applied Sciences, Eindhoven, The Netherlands

Neal Cook
Reader in Nursing
School of Nursing, Ulster University, Northern Ireland, UK

Barbara Cowie
Advanced Practice Nurse
West Park Healthcare Centre, Toronto, Canada

Penney Deratnay
Advanced Practice Nurse
West Park Healthcare Centre, Toronto, Canada

Belinda Dewar
Professor of Practice Improvement
Institute of Care and Practice Improvement, University of the West of Scotland,
Scotland, UK

Jan Dewing
Sue Pembrey Chair of Nursing and Director of The Centre for Person-centred Practice
Research
School of Health Sciences, Queen Margaret University, Edinburgh, Scotland, UK

Caroline Dickson
Senior Lecturer
School of Health Sciences, Queen Margaret University, Edinburgh, Scotland, UK

Jon Glasby
Director of the Health Services Management Centre (HSMC) and Professor of Health and
Social Care
University of Birmingham, Birmingham, UK

Karen Hammond
Practice Development Facilitator, Surgical Division
East Kent Hospitals University Foundation Trust, Kent, UK

Jennifer Haynes
Advanced Practice Nurse
West Park Healthcare Centre, Toronto, Canada

Nadine Janes
Adjunct Professor
Daphne Cockwell School of Nursing, Faculty of Community Services, Ryerson
University, Toronto, Canada

Bengt Karlsson
Professor, Faculty of Health Sciences
The University College of South-East Norway, Drammen, Norway

Antonia Lannie
Lecturer
School of Nursing and Midwifery, University of Dundee, Scotland, UK

Kim Manley
Professor, Practice Development Research and Innovation & Co-Director England Centre
for Practice Development
Canterbury Christ Church University, Canterbury, Kent, UK

Aisling McBride
PhD student
University of the West of Scotland
Hamilton, Scotland

Tanya McCance
Mona Grey Professor for Nursing R&D & Director of the Institute of Nursing & Health Research
Ulster University, Northern Ireland, UK

Brendan McCormack
Professor and Head of the Division of Nursing, School of Health Sciences
Queen Margaret University, Edinburgh, Scotland, UK

Deirdre O'Donnell
Associate Head of School, School of Nursing
Ulster University, Northern Ireland, UK

Lorna Peelo-Kilroe
Strategic Project Office for Person-Centred Culture Development
Health Service Executive Office of Nursing and Midwifery Services Director and Quality Improvement Division
Dublin, Republic of Ireland

Annette Solman
Adjunct Professor
The University of Technology Sydney, Australia

Cathy Sharp
Director, Research for Real
Edinburgh, Scotland, UK

Angie Titchen
Honorary Professor, Faculty of Life and Health Sciences
Ulster University, Northern Ireland, UK

Famke van Lieshout
Lecturer and Programme Leader
Fontys University of Applied Sciences, Eindhoven, The Netherlands

Val Wilson
Professor of Nursing Research & Practice Development
Sydney Children's Hospitals Network and University of Technology Sydney, Australia

Foreword

It is an honour to write the Foreword of the second edition of *Person-centred Practice in Nursing and Health Care: Theory and Practice*, edited by Brendan McCormack and Tanya McCance. Person-centred care was mainly linked to nursing for many years, but in recent developments we have seen that most health-care professionals are embracing the concept and principles. The World Health Organization has adopted a global strategy on people-centred and integrated health services. The evidence suggests that people-centred and integrated services are essential components of building universal health coverage and can improve health status (WHO 2015)[1]. It is evident that person-centred care is the ideal approach to practice, and the framework presented by McCormack and McCance is a valuable tool to guide theory and practice. The essence of person-centred care is having compassion, and McCormack and McCance unpack the concept in Chapter 1 and continue to describe the principles in Chapter 2 and a Person-centred Framework in Chapter 3. This provides a sound foundation for chapters that follow.

Every one you meet is fighting a battle you know nothing about. Be kind. Always

Although person-centredness evolved around the person, of note is that the person can be an individual, a family or the community. Exploring and describing the concept from various contexts provides clarity on the broad applicability of person-centred care. But in order to be person-centred, the provision of health-care services needs to change in order to be more flexible to meet the person's needs in a manner that is best for them. As Carl Rogers eloquently states, 'being listened to by someone who understands makes it possible for persons to listen more accurately to themselves, with greater empathy toward their own.' Collaboration and a partnership on the care implies working with the individuals and their families to find the best available option in the provision of their care. This implies active involvement in the decision-making process about care. All of these elements are extensively covered throughout the book. In Chapters 4 to 8, person-centred care is described and how it relates to policy, nursing strategy and policy, leadership, nursing education and research. To note is that in Chapter 6 Shaun Cardiff unpacks the impact of person-centred care from a leadership perspective, focusing on the contextual domain – what is true in one context may not be the case for another – and links the context to an organisational culture. A quote from the work of Peter Drucker speaks

---

[1] World Health Organization (2015) People-centred and integrated health services: an overview of the evidence. Interim Report. WHO.

specifically to this aspect: 'no institution can possibly survive if it needs geniuses or supermen to manage it. It must be organized in such a way as to be able to get along under a leadership composed of average human beings.' Average human beings can be the champions of spreading the word on person-centred care. In Chapter 9, Kim Manley adds a critical voice – one from practice – and in Chapter 11 Angie Titchen and Karen Hammond provide valuable insights on how to help practitioners to flourish.

The body of evidence is on the increase, demonstrating that person-centred care positively influences the quality of care delivered and improves patient outcomes. It is therefore of significance to get a depiction of how person-centred care can be operationalised in different populations. The book makes a meaningful contribution in this area. Chapter 13 focuses on the older person and residential long-term facilities, Chapter 14 on children, Chapter 15 on acute care, Chapter 16 on mental health, Chapter 17 on complex continuing care, Chapter 18 on community care and Chapter 19 on palliative care. Indeed, a comprehensive encounter of application of person-centred care.

In Chapter 20 the editors conclude with an insightful reflection and represent the person-centred framework. It is refreshing to read the critical thoughts on their body of work, and it gives direction to the use of the framework for the future. The authors have set themselves a goal with the book … that the book should be a journey. Indeed, this book is a journey, and I hope that each reader and user of this book will join in the journey to deliver person-centred care to improve the health of the world's population.

Professor Dr Hester Klopper
Immediate President of Sigma Theta Tau International (2013–15)

Acknowledgements

As the little prince dropped off to sleep, I took him in my arms and set out walking once more. I felt deeply moved, and stirred. It seemed to me, even, that there was nothing more fragile on all the Earth. In the moonlight I looked at his pale forehead, his closed eyes, his locks of hair that trembled in the wind, and I said to myself: 'What I see here is nothing but a shell. What is most important is invisible …

The Little Prince, *Antoine de Saint-Exupéry*

The 'invisible' elements of person-centredness and person-centred practice represent the deepest parts of our humanity and are often the less-tangible components of person-centred health care. It is these elements that have always interested us as practitioners, educators and researchers. We have been colleagues and friends on this journey of discovery for over 15 years, and each step we take leads us into new and interesting pastures – we each acknowledge that 'just when we think we have *got it* [person-centredness] we lose it again'! New questions and new insights challenge our existing understandings and take us on new journeys of discovery – to us, that is the joy of person-centredness and being a person-centred researcher.

We have not been alone in this experience and there are many people who have helped and encouraged us along the way; to these people we are eternally grateful – you know who you are and we thank you sincerely for your support, friendship, colleagueship, challenge and generosity. In particular we would like to thank Neil, Mark and Melissa (and their grandparents), Lorna, Michael, Aideen and Fionn for the love, support, encouragement and care you have shown to us in making this project happen and seeing it to fruition. We are grateful for the conditions you provided in enabling our writing and hopeful that you will forgive us for the lost hours away from you!

We are particularly grateful to all the authors who have contributed chapters to this edition. Since the original publication, *Person-Centred Nursing: Theory and Practice*, we have seen a burgeoning of work in this field and the globalisation of our Person-centred Nursing Framework, so that now we are genuinely able to write about it as a Person-centred Nursing Framework – used by a variety of nurses and other health-care practitioners in a variety of contexts around the world. A lot of this activity is reflected in the chapters of this book and we are very excited by it. We thank all these contributors for their commitment, dedication, passion and creativity – we have learned a lot from you.

Finally we would like to thank our colleagues at John Wiley & Sons, Ltd for encouraging us along the way and forgiving the missed deadlines. Your confidence in us has helped us stay the course.

Brendan McCormack and Tanya McCance

CHAPTER 1

Introduction

Brendan McCormack[1] & Tanya McCance[2]

[1] Queen Margaret University, Edinburgh, UK

[2] Ulster University, Northern Ireland, UK

Since publishing *Person-Centred Nursing: Theory and Practice* (McCormack & McCance 2010) the field of person-centredness in health care has grown significantly. In that short 5-year period, we have seen a burgeoning of interest in the topic, the development of a range of initiatives to promote person-centredness, and an increased volume of research exploring, understanding and evaluating person-centred practices. Person-centred care has a long association with nursing, with a focus on treating people as individuals; respecting their rights as a person; building mutual trust and understanding; and developing therapeutic relationships. However, this has now become a more inclusive health-care philosophy and strategic focus. It is for this reason that we have adopted a more broad-based health-care perspective in this book.

The promotion of 'person-centredness' is consistent with health-care policy direction internationally. There have been a number of challenges to the focus on person-centredness in nursing and health care and a view that other approaches such as relationship-centred care, compassionate care and even dignified care are more appropriate frameworks for expressing an inclusive family and community approach to what can generally be understood as holistic care practices. However, none of these have stood the test of time as 'alternatives' but instead are increasingly seen as components of person-centred nursing and health care, or as constructs that explain different dimensions of person-centredness. This goes some way to affirming the importance of person-centred approaches, not just as care practices in particular professional groups, but as a philosophical underpinning of health-care systems that places people at the centre.

This endorsement of people at the centre of care systems is particularly exemplified by the World Health Organization, which has set out a comprehensive framework of people-centred health services. They describe people-centred health services as

> ...an approach to care that consciously adopts the perspectives of individuals, families and communities, and sees them as participants as well as beneficiaries of trusted health systems that respond to their needs and preferences in humane and holistic ways. People-centred care requires that people have the education and support they need to

make decisions and participate in their own care. It is organized around the health needs and expectations of people rather than diseases.

World Health Organization (2015; p. 10)

This all-encompassing description of people-centredness calls for the delivery of health services that are organised, managed and delivered in a way that ensures people as individuals, communities and populations are at the heart of planning and policy making. It challenges health-care practitioners to think of the person first and then the disease. It requires governments to ensure that people have access to health-care services that reflect their needs, promote health, manage disease, support self-management of long-term conditions and in which people are educated about health in order to maximise well-being. The 'person' is at the heart of the WHO policy framework, and whilst it is a demanding 'ask' of nations all over the world to consider individual needs, many of which are at different stages of development of their health-care systems, the intention is that of a global movement in person-centredness.

The WHO has a global goal of humanising health care by ensuring that health care is rooted in universal principles of human rights and dignity, non-discrimination, participation and empowerment, access and equity, and a partnership of equals:

> The overall vision for people-centred health care is one in which individuals, families and communities are served by and are able to participate in trusted health systems that respond to their needs in humane and holistic ways …

World Health Organization (2007, p. 7)

Many countries are embracing this challenge, and health-care policy and strategy initiatives are focused on reorganising for people-centredness. The Health Foundation (2015a,2015b) has been central to many of these strategic developments and ensuring that, at least at the level of health systems, people are at the centre of care:

> We want a more person-centred healthcare system, where people are supported to make informed decisions about and to successfully manage their own health and care, and choose when to invite others to act on their behalf … We want healthcare services to understand and deliver care responsive to people's individual abilities, preferences, lifestyles and goals.

The Health Foundation (2015a)

The Health Foundation has produced a range of resources to enable an increased understanding of person-centred care and to support its development across the whole health-care system (The Health Foundation, 2015b). In the United Kingdom for example, person-centredness has been at the heart of health-care policy and strategy developments, through initiatives in England such as the 'personalisation agenda' (Department of Health, 2010), the '1000 Lives[+] campaign in Wales (http://www.1000livesplus.wales.nhs.uk/pp-driven-care) and the Person-centred Health and Care Collaborative in Scotland (http://www.qihub.scot.nhs.uk/person-centred/person-centred-health-and-care-collaborative-.aspx). In Northern Ireland, the Service Framework for Older

People is based on person-centred values and principles and has person-centred care at the heart of its quality framework.

In other countries such as Norway, Canada, the United States, Australia and Denmark, person-centredness forms the basis of health-care reform that is focused on humanising health-care systems and how care is provided – cf. Impact NSW (2008), Department of Health and Human Services (2012), Norwegian Ministry of Health and Care Services (2009), Alzheimer Society Canada (2014), and Healthcare Transformation and Integrated Care in Denmark (Henrikson 2015). These strategies and frameworks influence the delivery patterns of health care and ways in which practice is developed.

Despite all of these developments the focus continues to be on 'care' and less on how organisations create person-centred cultures. There is much still to be done in developing health-care cultures towards ones that truly place people at the centre of their care in order to achieve effective and meaningful outcomes. Richards et al. (2015, p. 3) suggest that it is 'time to get real about delivering person-centred care' and argue that it requires a sea change in the mindset of health professionals and patients/clients alike. Part of this need for change is a move away from the discourse of person-centred care to that of person-centred cultures. Over the past 10 years, nursing and health-care practice have been dominated by negative reports of poor, undignified, uncompassionate and at times inhumane care, particularly of older people, people living with learning/intellectual disabilities and other vulnerable adults. In all of the investigations into these breaches of what counts as acceptable care standards, the issue of care culture has been identified as a key issue. Whilst highlighting unacceptable practices, these reports all raised the significance of 'culture' and its influence on the experiences of care workers, service users and families. However, whilst culture has been highlighted, the proposed solutions reflect a continued managerialist-led agenda and a philosophy of 'training' of staff for change. However, increasing evidence (Davies 2002; Scott et al. 2003; Carlström & Inger 2012; McCance et al. 2013; Laird et al. 2015) demonstrates that bringing about culture change requires significant and deep change of patterns in organisational systems and approaches to change that are founded on humanistically derived principles of adult learning. Person-centredness can only happen if there are cultures in place in care settings that enable staff to experience person-centredness and work in a person-centred way. With a focus on culture, we adopt the following definition of person-centredness; the origins of this definition will be elucidated further in Chapter 3:

> … an approach to practice established through the formation and fostering of healthful relationships between all care providers, service users and others significant to them in their lives. It is underpinned by values of respect for persons, individual right to self-determination, mutual respect and understanding. It is enabled by cultures of empowerment that foster continuous approaches to practice development.

This definition is relationship-orientated, but includes *all* relationships in any health-care situation or context. The focus on healthfulness is consistent with contemporary theories of well-being and wellness as health goals, and reflects the diversity of relationships that people experience. Effective cultures have clearly articulated and shared values and so this definition is also clear about the kinds of values that are important in a person-centred culture. Finally, we argue through this definition that creating a person-centred culture is not a 'one-off' event that can be achieved through a short-term project or education/training programme. Instead it requires an ongoing and sustained commitment to culture enhancement through participatory, collaborative and inclusive approaches to development.

The WHO suggests that there are a range of issues to be addressed in order to make health-care systems more people-centred, including:

- Empowering and engaging people.
- Strengthening governance and accountability.
- Reorienting care models towards efficiency and effectiveness.
- Coordinating services around the needs of people, health-care provider integration and effective networks.
- Creating an enabling environment for change.

As well as using our definition of person-centredness as a 'rudder' to guide our thinking when planning this book, we also in this book address many of the issues identified by the WHO as significant in developing people-centred health-care systems. Chapter contributors focus on strategic and systems-level developments, management and leadership responsibilities, advancing models of care, as well as illustrating a variety of strategies that can be used to go 'deep' into the culture of teams and organisations in order to develop person-centred cultures.

A focus on developing person-centred cultures does not in any way negate the need to reaffirm the importance of the fundamentals of care, emphasised in publications over the past 10 years or so (e.g. Royal College of Nursing 2010), all of which highlight the challenges for nurses and midwives in providing sensitive and dignified care. The continued drive, however, within most health systems to demonstrate effectiveness and efficiency through performance management processes challenges developments in person-centred nursing and health care. A range of quality and clinical indicators have been developed, many of which pay little attention to how patients, clients and their families experience care but instead are focused on measuring performance and effectiveness (Maben et al. 2012). Whilst nurses have a significant contribution to make in determining positive patient experience, the evidence demonstrates that greater emphasis continues to be placed on quantified measurement of indicators rather than a focus on those that evaluate the impact of nursing and midwifery care, with a person-centred orientation (McCance et al. 2012). In this context, we argue that the time is ripe for promoting new ways of working that can deliver effective person-centred practices, using approaches that can demonstrate positive outcomes as a result, and working with indicators that show the emergence and sustaining of person-centred cultures of effectiveness.

Since 2001, we (B.M and T.M) have been working with the Person-centred Nursing Framework as our approach to articulating the dynamic nature of person-centredness, as well as its complexity at the levels of culture and systems. Since that time, this framework has grown and developed and has made a significant contribution to the landscape of person-centredness globally.

The Person-Centred Nursing Framework and its evolution

The Person-Centred Nursing Framework was originally developed by McCormack and McCance (2006) and was derived from previous empirical research focusing on person-centred practice with older people (McCormack 2001) and the experience of caring in nursing (McCance et al. 2001). The original framework comprised four constructs:

1 *Prerequisites*, which focus on the attributes of the nurses.
2 *Care environment*, which focuses on the context in which care is delivered.
3 *Person-centred processes*, which focus on delivering care through a range of activities.
4 *Outcomes*, the central component of the framework, are the results of effective person-centred nursing.

We suggested that in order to deliver positive outcomes for patients, families and staff, account must be taken of the prerequisites and the care environment, which are necessary for providing effective care through person-centred processes. In 2010, *Person-Centred Nursing: Theory and Practice* (McCormack & McCance 2010) provided a more comprehensive explanation of the four constructs that comprise the Person-Centred Nursing Framework and the core elements within each construct.

Since the publication of the framework, its reach has been worldwide, with it being translated into several different languages and tested in several different contexts and countries – for example, McCormack, B. and McCance, T. (2013) Personcentrad omvårdnad. In: J. Leksell and M. Lepp (eds) *Sjuksköterskans Kärnkompetenser*, Liber Publishers, Stockholm, pp. 81–110. The framework has been used as a guide for the structuring of implementation studies that have focused on the development of person-centred nursing in a variety of contexts. Through the use of the framework in this way, we have been able to identify and refine relationships between concepts as well as identify new areas of research. We have undertaken implementation studies in residential care settings for older people, in a variety of secondary and tertiary care settings, in community care and in palliative care (see McCormack et al. 2010; Yalden & McCormack 2010; McCance et al. 2011). In these studies, the framework has been used to promote an increased understanding of person-centred nursing with the aim of enabling practitioners to recognise key elements in their practice, generate meaning from data that can inform the development of person-centred nursing, and most importantly to focus the implementation and evaluation of developments in practice.

A number of instruments have been developed through these studies, all of which have enabled us to identify key processes in the development of person-centred nursing and resulting outcomes for service users, staff, teams and organisations. We have developed and tested the Person-centred Nursing Index, the Context Assessment Index and the Workplace Culture Critical Analysis Tool (Slater et al. 2009, 2010; McCormack et al. 2009a,2009b) and most recently, the Person-centred Practice Inventory (Slater et al. 2015). These instruments have been used in a variety of international studies that have shown outcomes from the implementation of person-centred nursing. The systematisation of other processes such as the collection of 'patient stories' has also emerged through this research (Laird et al. 2015).

We have also used the framework to influence policy, nationally and internationally. In Northern Ireland the framework has been used as the theory of choice to underpin the Chief Nursing Officer's Nursing Strategy (DHSSPSNI 2010). The Royal College of Nursing adopted the framework to inform its development of 'Principles of Nursing' and these are being implemented across the UK (Royal College of Nursing 2010). In the Republic of Ireland the framework has been used to develop a 'National Practice Development Strategy' commissioned by the Chief Nurse and which has been implemented throughout the Health Services Executive service areas. This has resulted in changes to how nursing professional development is organised, how care practices are developed and how patient care is delivered (e.g. care in residential long-term care settings; McCormack et al. 2009c, 2010). In Australia, a development programme in over 600 clinical areas that is facilitated by the Chief Nurse of New South Wales Health Department is based on the Person-centred Nursing Theoretical Framework (Wilson & Cross 2013). These high-profile implementation studies in Northern Ireland, The Republic of Ireland and in Australia are examples of national programmes of work that have been based on the Person-centred Nursing Framework. These programmes of implementation research have involved working collaboratively with large numbers of practitioners, patients/clients, families and service managers and have shown improved outcomes:

- in the ways in which nursing and health-care practices are delivered (such as pain management postoperatively in acute care, and the management of mealtimes in residential settings);
- in the way that the culture of participating practice settings has been improved to support more person-centred ways of working (such as improved leadership, better care coordination and more effective teamwork);
- in the care experiences of patients/clients (such as increased 'hope', more dignified care and more involvement in care); and
- in the way that staff experience person-centredness in the workplace (such as increased commitment, role clarification, more effective communication and more access to ongoing professional development).

It has also been exciting to observe the increasing number of universities that are adopting the framework as the framework of choice to underpin education curricula. The research underpins the curriculum for masters students in nursing at the University of Sydney and the undergraduate nursing curricula at the Ulster University Northern Ireland, and University College Dublin, Republic of Ireland. In New Zealand the Person-centred Nursing Theoretical Framework has been adapted to inform a new learning framework for continuing specialty nursing education over three District Health Boards in the Lower North Island. In Queen Margaret University, Edinburgh, the framework has been developed as the philosophical framework underpinning the new masters level Person-centred Nursing Framework (incorporating specialist routes in health visiting, school nursing and district nursing). Finally in Norway, the framework underpins the first ever doctoral education programme in Person-centred Healthcare at Buskerud and Vestfold University College.

In the context of doctoral education, we have had the privilege of supervising a range of doctoral students, many of whom are chapter authors in this book, and who have all based their work (conceptually and theoretically) on the Person-centred Nursing Framework. This work has been undertaken in a variety of settings, care contexts and countries. Not only have these doctoral candidates used the Person-centred Nursing Framework, but also they have tested and refined key elements, challenged underpinning concepts, informed key changes to the framework and advanced knowledge in the field. Many have developed new models and frameworks that extend our original thinking and that in themselves offer new perspectives into the development of person-centredness in different health-care contexts.

All of this work has enabled the continued testing of the framework in practice, the refinement of key elements of the framework as the evidence base increases and the evaluation of its effectiveness as a framework for developing person-centred cultures. Our work in this period has become increasingly multi-disciplinary and multi-professional in its focus and so too has our framework. In this book therefore we adopt a multi-disciplinary and multi-professional approach and present a new version of the framework, one that has been further refined and is reflective of this change of focus. Whilst the 2010 edition was written solely by the framework authors (McCormack and McCance), in this edition of the book we engage with a wide range of authors, all of whom are connected with the Person-centred Nursing Framework and all of whom are contributing to the advancement of the underpinning knowledge base and the ongoing development and refinement of the framework.

Structure of the book

This book is presented in four sections. Section 1 presents a synthesis of the philosophies, concepts and theories that underpin the 'Person-centred

Nursing Framework' and in addition, highlights particular refinements and new additions to the framework in order to move it from a nursing to a more generic health-care focus, and ultimately the first comprehensive presentation of 'The Person-centred Nursing Framework'.

Section 2 focuses on the infrastructure needed to support person-centred culture development and person-centred practices. It has a particular focus on strategy, leadership and research as key concerns in ensuring the embedding of person-centredness in health-care systems and organisations.

Section 3 specifically addresses the challenges associated with developing person-centred cultures and presents a number of chapters written by people who are all engaged in this kind of work. The section 'gets inside' culture and illustrates the depth-work that is needed, the strategies that can be used and the outcomes arising.

In Section 4 we invited a number of collaborators to present their research and development activities in which they make use of the Person-centred Nursing Framework to shape this work. They illustrate the framework being used as a methodology in itself, as a heuristic to guide decision-making and as a tool for practice development. These chapters focus on specific types of care and services but we hope that these can be viewed as illustrative as the principles used by these authors are transferrable across health-care contexts.

We have written this book with a broad target audience in mind, and have tried to ensure that it is accessible to nurses, health-care practitioners and decision-makers working at different levels and across a variety of contexts.

It has been our privilege to work in this field for more than 20 years, and this book reflects the range of activity we have been engaged in as individuals, colleagues and collaborators. The contributors to this book (and many who are not represented here) have in most cases shared that journey (or parts of it) with us. We are truly grateful for their collaboration, cooperation and friendship as well as the high challenge and support offered. It has been these relationships that have shaped what we now publish as the most recent version of the Person-centred Nursing Framework. We know the framework will continue to evolve and grow through these continued relationships, and that is a privilege that we are truly grateful for and which we hope is reflected in the contents of this book.

References

Alzheimer Society Canada (2014) *Culture Change towards Person Centred Care.* Retrieved from: http://www.alzheimer.ca/en/Living-with-dementia/Caring-for-someone/Long-term-care/culture-change-person-centred-care (accessed 4 February 2016).

Carlström, E.D. and Ekman, I. (2012) Organisational culture and change: implementing person-centred care. *Journal of Health Organization and Management*, **26**, 175–91.

Davies, H.T.O. (2002) Understanding organizational culture in reforming the National Health Service. *Journal of the Royal Society of Medicine*, **95**, 140–2.

Department of Health (2010) *Personalisation through Person-Centred Planning*, Department of Health England, London.

Department of Health and Human Services, Centers for Medicare and Medicaid Services [CMS] (2012) *Request to Convey Information: Partnership to Improve Dementia Care in Nursing Homes (S&C: 12-42-NH)*. Baltimore, MD: CMS. Retrieved from: http://www.cms.gov/Medicare/ Provider-Enrollment-and-Certification/SurveyCertificationGenInfo/Downloads/Survey- and-Cert-Letter-12-42-.pdf (accessed 25 January 2016).

DHSSPSNI (Department of Health, Social Services and Public Safety Northern Ireland) (2010) *A Partnership for Care – Northern Ireland Strategy for Nursing and Midwifery 2010-2015*, DHSSPSNI, Belfast.

Francis, R. (2013) *Report of the Mid-Staffordshire NHS Foundation Trust Public Inquiry*, The Stationery Office, London.

Henrikson HE. (2015) *Healthcare Transformation and Integrated Care in Denmark [slideshow]*. Available at: http://www.slideshare.net/curamroundtable/240315-integrated-care-in-denmark- wanscher02 (accessed 25 January 2016).

Impact NSW (2008) *Person Centred Practice – Guide to implementing person-centred practice in your health service*. Retrieved from: http://www.impactnsw.com/resources/tools/98-guide-to- implementing-person-centred-practice-in-your-health-service (accessed 25 January 2016).

Laird, E., McCance, T., McCormack, B., and Gribben, B. (2015) Patients' experiences of in- hospital care when nursing staff were engaged in a practice development programme to promote person-centredness: A narrative analysis study. *International Journal of Nursing Studies*, **52**, 1454–62.

Maben J, Peccei R, Adams M, Robert G, Richardson A, Murrells T. (2012) *Patients' experiences of care and the influence of staff motivation, affect and wellbeing*. Final report. National Institute for Health Research Service Delivery and Organisation programme.

McCance, T.V., McKenna, H.P., and Boore, J.R.P. (2001) Exploring caring using narrative methodology: an analysis of the approach. *Journal of Advanced Nursing*, **33**, 350–6.

McCance T, McCormack B, Dewing J. (2011) An exploration of person-centredness in practice. *Online Journal of Issues in Nursing*, **16**(2) manuscript 1. Available at: http://www.nursingworld .org/MainMenuCategories/ANAMarketplace/ANAPeriodicals/OJIN/TableofContents/Vol- 16-2011/No2-May-2011/Person-Centredness-in-Practice.html (accessed 25 January 2016).

McCance, T., Telford, L., Wilson, J., MacLeod, O., and Dowd, A. (2012) Identifying key performance indicators for nursing and midwifery care using a consensus approach. *Journal of Clinical Nursing*, **21**, 1145–54.

McCance T, Gribben B, McCormack B, Laird EA. (2013) Promoting person-centred practice within acute care: the impact of culture and context on a facilitated practice development programme. *International Practice Development Journal* **3**(1): art. 2. Available at: http://www .fons.org/library/journal/volume3-issue1/article2 (accessed 25 January 2016).

McCormack, B. (2001) Autonomy and the relationship between nurses and older people. *Ageing and Society*, **21**, 417–46.

McCormack, B. and McCance, T. (2006) Development of a framework for person-centred nursing. *Journal of Advanced Nursing*, **56** (5), 1–8.

McCormack, B. and McCance, T. (2010) *Person-Centred Nursing: Theory, Models and Methods*, Wiley-Blackwell Publishing, Oxford.

McCormack, B., Henderson, E., Wilson, V., and Wright, J. (2009a) The Workplace Culture Critical Analysis Tool. *Practice Development in Healthcare*, **8**, 28–43.

McCormack, B., McCarthy, G., Wright, J., Slater, P., and Coffey, A. (2009b) Development and testing of the Context Assessment Index. *Worldviews on Evidence Based Nursing*, **6**, 27–35.

McCormack, B., Dewing, J., Breslin, L. *et al.* (2009c) Practice development: realising active learning for sustainable change. *Contemporary Nurse*, **32**, 92–104.

McCormack, B., Dewing, J., Breslin, E. *et al.* (2010) Developing person-centred practice: nursing outcomes arising from changes to the care environment in residential settings for older people. *International Journal of Older People Nursing*, **5**, 93–107.

Norwegian Ministry of Health and Care Services (2009) Stortingsmelding nr. 47 (2008–2009), Samhandlingsreformen. Rett behandling – på rett sted – til rett tid. [Report No. 47 (2008–2009) to the Storting. The coordination reform.] Oslo: Helse- og omsorgsdepartementet [in Norwegian; summary in English].

Richards T, Coulter A, Wicks P. (2015) Time to deliver patient-centred care. *British Medical Journal* 350:h530 [editorial].

Royal College of Nursing (2010) *The Principles of Nursing Practice*, Royal College of Nursing, London.

Scott, T., Mannion, R., Davies, H.T.O., and Marshall, M.N. (2003) Implementing culture change in health care: theory and practice. *International Journal for Quality in Health Care*, **15**, 111–8.

Slater, P., Bunting, B., and McCormack, B. (2009) The development and pilot testing of an instrument to measure nurses' working environment: the Nursing Context Index. *Worldviews on Evidence-Based Nursing*, **6** (3), 173–82.

Slater, P., O'Halloran, P., Connolly, D., and McCormack, B. (2010) Testing the factor structure of the Nursing Work Index – *Revised. Worldviews on Evidence Based Nursing*, **7** (3), 123–34.

Slater P, McCance T, McCormack B. (2015) Exploring person-centred practice within acute hospital settings. *International Practice Development Journal* **5** (Suppl) [09]. Retrieved from: http://www.fons.org/Resources/Documents/Journal/Vol5Suppl/IPDJ_05%28suppl%29_09 .pdf (accessed 26 January 2016).

The Health Foundation (2015a) *Person-Centred Care*. Retrieved from: http://www.health.org.uk/areas-of-work/topics/person-centred-care/ (accessed 10 June 2015).

The Health Foundation (2015b) *Person-centred Care Resource Centre*. Retrieved from: http://personcentredcare.health.org.uk/ (accessed 10 June 2015).

The Vale of Leven Hospital Inquiry Report (2014) *Scottish Government*. Available at: http://www.valeoflevenhospitalinquiry.org/Report/j156505-00.html (accessed 26 January 2016).

Wilson V and Cross J. (2013) *Essentials of Care Research Report 2009-2012*. Nursing and Midwifery Office New South Wales Health, Australia. Available from: http://www.health.nsw.gov.au/nursing/projects/Pages/eoc.aspx (accessed 22 February 2016).

World Health Organization (2007) *People-Centred Health Care, A Policy Framework*. Retrieved from: http://www.wpro.who.int/health_services/people_at_the_centre_of_care/documents/ENG-PCIPolicyFramework.pdf (accessed 26 January 2016).

World Health Organization (2015) *WHO Global Strategy on People-centred and Integrated Health Services: Interim Report*. Retrieved from: http://apps.who.int/iris/bitstream/10665/155002/1/WHO_HIS_SDS_2015.6_eng.pdf?ua=1&ua=1 (accessed 4 February 2016).

Yalden, J. and McCormack, B. (2010) Constructions of dignity: a pre-requisite for flourishing in the workplace? *International Journal of Older People Nursing*, **5**, 137–47.

SECTION I
A framework for person-centred practice

CHAPTER 2

Underpinning principles of person-centred practice

Brendan McCormack[1] & Tanya McCance[2]

[1] Queen Margaret University, Edinburgh, UK
[2] Ulster University, Northern Ireland, UK

Introduction

In this chapter we aim to explore what is often considered to be the complex language of person-centredness and person-centred practice, and the connections and tensions between them. Whilst person-centredness may be an increasingly familiar term, the reality is that it is a complex one, with many and varied meanings and understandings. Part of the complexity of the term is its philosophical underpinnings, that is, the concept of being a 'person'. In philosophy, there are as many differing perspectives on the meaning of 'person' as there are applications in practice. These differing philosophical perspectives have shaped the way in which theoretical frameworks have developed and the way these frameworks are applied in practice. We will draw upon a variety of philosophical, theoretical and applied literature to articulate and critique the principles of person-centred practice. In addition, we will explore health, social care and nursing policy and strategy in order to locate person-centred practice in the wider health and social care landscape.

The core value of personhood

The word 'person' has been debated for as long as philosophical thought has existed. How we distinguish between persons and other species (such as non-human animals) is a key debate within this long tradition and one that underpins many moral and ethical frameworks. For example, animal-rights advocates and campaigners would argue vehemently that it is morally wrong for pharmaceuticals and cosmetics to be tested on animals before they are used with humans. Their argument would be predicated on the belief that humans and animals are equal and thus should be treated equally. For others, humans are considered to be a higher order species to animals and thus it is reasonable

Person-Centred Practice in Nursing and Health Care: Theory and Practice, Second Edition.
Edited by Brendan McCormack and Tanya McCance.
© 2017 John Wiley & Sons, Ltd. Published 2017 by John Wiley & Sons, Ltd.

to use animals in this way in order to benefit the greater good of persons. The position taken in such debates would in part be influenced by views about what it means to be a person. However, even within the 'human species' a 'person' may mean different things, so, for example, debates about abortion are influenced by different ideas about whether or not an embryo is a person; is a fetus a person or when does a fetus become a person? And, indeed, should a human being with certain kinds of brain damage/disorders (such as severe head injury or dementia) be bestowed with the status of 'person'?

For some philosophers (e.g. Frankfurt 1989) it is not enough to claim that human beings are persons on the basis of a collection of physical and psychological attributes because it is conceptually possible that members of another species could lay claim to personhood. If attributes such as sight, taste, smell, sexuality, memory, desires, motives and so forth were to be used as a means of distinguishing persons from non-persons, then we could easily provide a list of members of other species who would possess similar attributes. This argument was particularly highlighted in the debate about 'Tommy the Chimp' and the battle to have him recognised as a person. His owner in New York State has held Tommy in captivity for many years. A lawsuit submitted by a group called the 'Nonhuman Rights Project (NhRP)' seeks to have Tommy recognised as a person under law. The lawsuit does not argue that chimpanzees are human, but that they are entitled to the rights of 'personhood'. It cites research by great ape experts that has established they are 'autonomous, self-determined, self-aware, highly intelligent, emotionally complex' (http://www.bbc.co.uk/news/magazine-29542829). Tommy's case highlights the complexity of the idea of personhood, and whilst it may be an interesting case in terms of animal rights and the protection of the rights of animals (a worthwhile and important endeavour in itself), it also has implications for persons of the human kind! This collection of attributes of great apes is also found in humans and so if we wish to argue that there is a higher order of person, then we cannot rely on such attributes as these alone.

Further, if we argue that personhood is predicated merely on a set of physical and psychological attributes, then what happens to persons who may lose some of these attributes through disease and disability? For example, a person with dementia may experience deterioration of memory and motivation and loss of physical attributes (e.g. mobility, hand-eye coordination, etc.) and so could legitimately, on the basis of this argument, lose the status of person. Indeed even such higher order attributes as 'thought' and decision-making fail to distinguish persons from other creatures. Human beings are not alone in having desires and preferences. Members of other species share these attributes with human beings and some species could even be seen to base action on deliberation and even prior thought – as is argued in the case of Tommy the Chimp. Think about how a lion living in the wild plans the killing of his prey, an experience one of us (Brendan) had the privilege of seeing whilst on safari in South Africa. The lion Brendan observed seemed to engage in deliberation, 'thought' and sophisticated decision-making into setting up the conditions to enable a successful kill to occur. When the kill had occurred, he then appeared to 'manage' the way other members of his pride joined in the meal and protected the food from other species. Similarly, if we believe that the possession of a language distinguishes us as persons, then of course studies of animal communication patterns would suggest that different animal species have their own unique language. The loss of language (e.g. arising from certain brain injuries) could also mean the loss of the status of person.

So therefore distinguishing persons from non-persons on the basis of a hierarchy of attributes is problematic. Some authors, such as Post (2006) argue that a dominant focus in Western cultures on some attributes being more important than others has led to a position whereby cognitive attributes of persons are given greatest importance. We see this played out in all kinds of ways in daily life, in that the ability to connect our thinking with our behaviours is essential for day-to-day functioning. Thus the loss of these attributes can have significant impact on human beings and their personhood as it can result in reduced ability to engage in daily activities of living, loss of employment, an inability to converse with others, a loss of connection with community, disconnection with friends and family, and increased loneliness and isolation.

So how should we think about personhood in ways that help us to not privilege cognition and rationality and in ways that avoid hierarchies of attributes? Whilst there is no single answer to this question, it is probably not the most helpful thing to focus on what personhood is not, or as something we only recognise when it is lost or taken away.

Connecting with an innate sense of ourselves as human beings with feelings, emotions, thoughts and desires is an essential component of being a person and de facto having personhood. Leibing (2008) argues that personhood is that inner feeling we have that guides us as a person. It is the sum total of all these feelings, desires, motivations and values – or what Leibing refers to as 'that which really matters' (Leibing 2008, p. 180). This idea of personhood equating with that which really matters to us as persons, potentially enables us to rise above discussions of hierarchies and attribution and indeed arguments about the existence of 'the soul' (which many faith-based beliefs would equate with personhood). Instead it enables a connection with our unique humanness as persons – those inner perspectives that we hold in our body and that influence our being in the world. Leibing uses the term 'interiority' to describe this:

> The materialization of certain values in time—and the moral question of what matters to certain people
>
> *Leibing (2008, p. 180)*

What matters to us is possibly the closest we can get to having a neutral understanding of personhood and one that is connected with innate human characteristics. However, Leibing argues that in diseases such as Alzheimer's, this interiority of persons becomes flattened because of the medicalisation of persons and a dominant biomedical focus on disease processes. This argument is consistent with Sabat's (2002) view that personhood is connected with different understandings of 'the self'. Rejecting the idea of the 'loss of self' that is dominant in dementia discourse and that implies not just a flattening of personhood but its loss, with the consequence of being labelled as a 'non-person', Sabat (2002, p. 27) argues that we have three forms of self – Self 1, Self 2 and Self 3. Self 1 is 'the self of personal identity' evidenced through our use of personal pronouns: 'I', 'me', 'mine', 'myself', 'ours' (meaning mine and yours). This self relates to our individual and unique view of the world. It expresses how we relate to our being in the world and the words we use to describe this being. It is autobiographical in nature and forms the narrative of our lives. Through Self 1 we show how we take responsibility for ourselves and our being in the world. Sabat argues that a loss of words and language (such as happens with people living with dementia) does not mean a loss of self, and indeed this Self 1 remains intact. Self 2 comprises our physical and mental attributes – eye colour, height, weight, beliefs, religion, achievements, hobbies and so forth are all examples of Self 2, and again these remain relatively intact with the threat of disease and illness. Self 3 comprises the different social personas that we construct in different situations in which we live our lives. In different situations and contexts a person may display very different behaviours – a highly dedicated and professional nurse by day and a hard party-goer by night; a focused, targeted and 'hard-nosed' manager versus a loving, sensitive and intimate partner. Sabat argues that Self 3 is most vulnerable when threatened by disease and illness such as dementia, as it is dependent on a connection with at least one other person in our social world. Whilst this threat is obvious in a person living with dementia, we can also see the potential for loss of Self 3 in all kinds of illness situations where the autobiographical self is not paid attention to; that is, we are concerned with treatment and cure and not with the social construction of that illness and how it threatens our personhood – something that is core to the argument made for a recovery approach in mental health, by Borg and Karlsson in this book (see Chapter 16).

Of course these constructions of self can also be challenged and debated as there are a variety of ways in which Self 1–3 can change and or be altered. However, Sabat's ideas demonstrate how *interiority* (Leibing 2008) is an important basis for our external behaviours. Paying attention to Self 1 and 2 is therefore critical for the protection of personhood in situations where a person is vulnerable and in need of care. Sabat's expression of self resonates with Merleau-Ponty's (1989) argument about the primacy of a 'perceiving body' in the world. Merleau-Ponty argues against any idea of a mind-body split or that we are passive recipients of our history. Instead he suggests that our knowing is always subjective as we carry through the movement in our bodies, our pre-histories that we take up, inherit and transform through our being in the world. Therefore, Self 1 is ever-present, even in the absence of rational thought.

This 'interiority' positioning of persons and the different manifestations of 'self' contribute to the ways in which person-centredness is understood.

Person-centredness

An early definition of person-centredness is provided by Kitwood (1997), and continues to be widely used. He describes person-centredness as ' ... a standing or status that is bestowed upon one human being by others, in the context of relationship and social being. It implies recognition, respect and trust' (p. 8). Kitwood's definition is widely cited in the field of dementia care without what seems to us a recognition of the limitations of the definition in terms of what it means for persons. Kitwood's definition has conditions attached to it, namely, person-centredness is dependent on others recognising my status as a person and it only exists in relationship with others. Kitwood argues that persons don't exist in isolation, but instead we each have a 'context' in which our personhood is manifested. Kitwood's definition of personhood is informed by the work of Swiss psychologist Paul Tournier (1999) and the philosophies of Martin Buber (1984) and Carl Rogers (1961). A convincing argument is presented by Kitwood as to why people should be respected for their intrinsic worth even if they can no longer engage in rational reflection on action because of debilitating changes to the brain/mind. However, this view of person-centredness is also limited by its need for recognition by others in a relationship. Dewing (2008a) argues that Kitwood has influenced the way in which person-centred practice is generally conceptualised in care services, but the significance of his definition is rarely critiqued. Sabat's (2002) construct of Self 3 and its fragile nature, highlights the core problem with Kitwood's definition, because without meaningful connection with another person, the personhood of people in receipt of care is placed in a vulnerable state. This also challenges health and social care organisations to consider how staff are prepared to work in a person-centred way.

However, what is common among all the perspectives of personhood presented earlier is recognition of the importance of 'being', and of course person-centredness requires attention to be paid to our being as persons. Based on an extensive review of the literature, and using the definition provided by Kitwood as a starting point, McCormack (2004) argued that there are four core 'modes of being' at the heart of person-centredness:

- Being in relation
- Being in a social world
- Being in place
- Being with self.

Being in relation

Being in relation emphasises the importance of relationships and the interpersonal processes that enable the development of relationships that have therapeutic benefit. Indeed, models of nursing, irrespective of their philosophical underpinnings, have emphasised the importance of relationships (e.g. Peplau 1952; Boykin & Schoenhofer 1993; Watson 1999). Recent critiques in the gerontology literature, however, argue that the term 'person-centred' fails to recognise the importance of relationships. Nolan et al. (2004) argue that person-centredness focuses (in the care literature) on the primacy of the personhood of the person being cared for, at the expense of those doing the caring, and conclude that in gerontology, the term 'relationship-centred care' is more appropriate. Whilst the importance of relationships in person-centredness cannot be disputed, 'relationship' is only one component of personhood. In person-centred nursing, the relationship between nurses, persons being cared for and those significant to them in their lives is paramount, and it has been argued that sustaining a relationship that is nurturing to everyone requires valuing of self, moral integrity, reflective ability, knowing of self and others, and flexibility derived from reflection on values and their place in the relationship (Nolan et al. 2004; Dewing 2008b; McCormack et al. 2012; Yalden et al. 2013). Being in relation is also reflected in one of seven attributes of person-centredness identified by Slater's (2006) concept analysis – evidence of a therapeutic relationship between person and health-care provider. Slater (2006) describes this as a partnership between the person and carer that ensures the person's own decisions are valued, in a relationship that is based on mutual trust and mutuality, is non-judgemental and does not focus on the balance of power. This emphasis on relationships is also seen in the contemporary discourse of compassion, dignity and humanising health care (Hannah 2014). Hannah presents a convincing argument for the adoption of relationships based on 'kindness' as a starting point for respecting personhood in health-care encounters. She criticises the dominance of biomedicine as a frame of reference for categorising people and their health-care needs. Instead, she argues for an approach that starts from the point of relationships, that respects personhood and that builds on the strengths of individuals – something that is core to being person-centred. Hannah's emphasis on kindness in health-care relationships resonates with the work of the philosopher John McMurray (1995) who argued that we have a choice over how we relate to others – an impersonal way, a functional way or a personal way! McMurray contends that whilst this is a choice we can all make, it is only through the 'personal way' that we truly connect with others. Engaging personally enables us to be the person we can grow to be. According to McMurray, 'friendship' is the deepest form of personal relationship, and it is through friendship that we show love, kindness, compassion and care, or in other words, be person-centred!

Being in a social context

Earlier it was outlined how Merleau-Ponty considers persons to be interconnected with their social world, creating and recreating meaning through their being in the world. That being is presented and re-presented through narrative. There is an increasing literature in health care on the value of biography and narrative – see, for example, Chapter 13 by Catherine Buckley in this book.

Biographical and narrative approaches are not just about 'collecting stories' as a part of assessment, but as Post (2006) identified, are also manifestations of Self 1. Respect for the person's narrative reflects the Kantian ideal of respect for the intrinsic worth of a person (Kant 1785/2012). Narrative approaches enable a more accurate assessment of what is important to each person and in that context are able to understand the potential impact of care and treatment decisions. Narratives are holistic and provide a picture of the person's being in the world and their subjective interpretation of that being.

Being in place

The concept of 'place' and its impact on care experiences is increasingly recognised in nursing and health care. However, the impact of place on patients' experiences is still under-researched. Dementia care mapping has been well developed (Kitwood 1997; Brooker 2005, 2010) and it represents one of the only assessment and care planning approaches in gerontology that formally recognises the impact of the 'milieu of care' on the care experience. Paying attention to 'place' in care relationships is increasingly recognised as important (Andrews et al. 2013). Significant work has been undertaken in the field of palliative and end-of-life care, paying attention to the built environment and its impact on care experiences. The healing qualities of buildings, the enabling design of buildings and the qualities of the environment in which care is provided are all important considerations. Additionally, our emotional connections with places constitute an important consideration in care decisions – places have deep meanings, imbuing deep memories, and metaphorically as well as physically connecting us with our histories – a connection that is explicitly recognised in 'ageing in place' developments (Wiles et al. 2011). Andrews et al. (2013) further argue that spaces and places are relational. They suggest that places have deep connections with the 'self', and we make conscious or unconscious comparisons between spaces and places from the essences of memories of other places. Thus we embody spaces.

Being with self

The need to be recognised as a person is a fundamental human need. Recognition brings respect, upon which relationships are formed and through which our personhood is revealed. Drawing on Leibing's (2008) idea of personhood being 'that which really matters' then being able to reveal what really matters to us is a way of revealing our self with all its manifestations. Respecting what really matters essentially means respecting our values, and this is central to person-centred practice and core to the Person-centred Nursing Framework of McCormack and McCance (2010). Assisting a person to find meaning in care may help them to tolerate the incongruity of their situation and establish goals for the future. This reflects the stance of the philosopher John McMurray (1995), who argues for the primacy of 'self as agent', emphasising the importance of the person 'knowing self' in order to engage in an authentic relationship with others. McMurray highlights the importance of transparency of values reflecting behaviours and actions and ultimately in being authentic. This clearly highlights the importance of values clarification in relationships, in teams and in programmes of work that focus on developing (more) person-centredness. Health-care practitioners involved in care delivery need to be aware of 'self' and how their own values and beliefs can impact on decisions made about a person's care and treatment. This reinforces the centrality of shared decision-making in health care and the need for a 'negotiated' approach between practitioner and the person receiving care. Previously, McCormack (2001) argued for a 'negotiated autonomy' in care relationships and in any negotiated situation, being clear about values is critical.

Person-centred practice

Person-centred, patient-centred, client-centred and individualised are examples of terms often used interchangeably to express the idea of person-centred practice (McCormack et al. 2010). At the risk of complicating matters further, Nolan and colleagues have also introduced the concept of relationship-centred care, arguing for a move away from what they perceive as a focus on meeting individual needs, to focusing on interactions among all parties involved in care whose needs should be accounted for if good care is to result (Nolan et al. 2004). Several analyses have been conducted in an attempt to define the core attributes of person-centredness, although this activity is only a relatively recent development in the contemporary literature (McCormack 2004; Slater 2006; Leplege et al. 2007; Leibing 2008; McCormack & McCance 2010).

In contemporary health and social care, there is a tendency to talk about 'person-centred practice' as if it is universally understood and practised. Person-centred practice is regularly espoused in health strategy (as we highlighted in Chapter 1) and increasing numbers of countries have programmes in place for the development of person-centred services and practices. It is not unusual for 'innovations' in person-centredness to equate to an array of 'quick-fixes' that are more to do with ensuring consistency of decision-making, maximising efficiency and effectiveness, and ensuring individual choice than a genuine connection with personhood as a basis for health and social care practice. Person-centred practice without a focus on personhood fails to connect with the core humanity of persons and is just another quality improvement activity. Therefore we define person-centred practice as:

> …an approach to practice established through the formation and fostering of healthful relationships between all care providers, service users and others significant to them in their lives. It is underpinned by values of respect for persons, individual right to self-determination, mutual respect and understanding. It is enabled by cultures of empowerment that foster continuous approaches to practice development.

The central building block of this definition is respect for personhood manifested through mutual respect, self-determination and understanding. So much of health-care practice requires a connection with the body and so respect for the body during practice is a showing of respect for personhood. Merleau-Ponty (Dillon 1988) argues that the person 'is the body' and that we exist through bodily engagement with the world. Thus, the body is 'our expression in the world, the visible form of our intentions' (Baldwin 2004, p. 36). Mental and physical properties are inseparable, each intertwined with the other creating a seamless whole (Edwards 2001). Thus our existence is constituted by our 'being in the world', by the relationship between 'our body and the world, between ourselves and our body'. Edwards (2001) argues that thinking about persons from the perspective of 'body' enables us to think about illness and disability in different ways and in the case of (for example) people with severe physical or mental disabilities, makes a significant contribution to understanding how the personhood of such a person can be retained, by paying attention to bodily responses in the absences of rational reflective abilities.

Drawing on Merleau-Ponty's ideas, Dewing (2007) demonstrates that there are four fundamental life-world themes (or existentials) that constitute lived experience. These existentials provide helpful 'discovery guides' for reflecting on personhood and lived experiences. The four existentials are: lived body (corporeality), lived human relation (relationality), lived space (spatiality) and lived time (temporality). By implication of Merleau-Ponty's idea of them being existentials, they cannot be separated from each other and each existential is embedded and interwoven with the other. Fundamental to Merleau-Ponty's theses is that the person is the body, which is the embodiment of mind and body as one. This is the opposite of the Cartesian worldview where mind and body are separate and mind takes precedence over the body. Merleau-Ponty (1989, p. 12) summarises this as: 'our relation to the world is not that of a thinker to an object of thought'. Further, the body inhabits space and because of this it is also within time. For Merleau-Ponty space is not an abstract entity that merely maps itself onto the body. Instead the body actively occupies space through perception, intentional movement and activity (1962, p. 136). Space does not exist outside the body as space is experienced from within the body. Neither does the mind map itself onto the body. Consequently the body is not moved by the mind. Further, bodily movement can be best or only fully understood at a preconscious level because it is the body not the mind that is in space and time. Thus, in the explication of this theory, the lived body (with flesh and depth) and existential space and time must be constantly accounted for. Not to take account of spatiality, temporality, or the various dimensions of perception would be inadequate and would decontextualise and dehumanise lived experience.

Merleau-Ponty's ideas on embodiment, especially in the context of people with impaired cognition, offer a radically different and even hopeful construction of the body as an agent that is trying to act appropriately based on perception, even where the brain and/or mind may be said not to be cognitively intact. In the context of person-centred practice, body-work that in a nursing context focuses on engaging in what are referred to as 'the fundamentals of care' becomes the route through which nurses connect with the personhood of the person in receipt of care and to understanding individual care needs. Reflecting the importance of this body-work, recent developments in nursing performance indicators argue for this work to be seen as the core of what we consider important in nursing and what we 'measure' in terms of nursing effectiveness (McCance et al. 2011; Maben et al. 2012). Previously, McCance (2003) argued that it is through the delivery of physical care that nurses connect with persons, and these activities are not merely tasks but are instead the window through which connectedness begins with the other person. Martinsen (2006) suggests that this connection with another person means that we take away something of the person when we have connected with them in a meaningful way: 'we all have something of each other's lives in the palms of our hands' (p. 71). Martinsen's view places responsibility on individual practitioners to treat each encounter with another person as unique, an encounter that can transform an individual's being in the world through authentic connections. Being authentic requires us to consider such factors as the meaning of individual relationships, emotional engagement, knowledge and decision-making capacity in determining our 'being in the world'. A person's authenticity is composed of 'signs' (Heidegger 1927/1990, p. 108):

> Among signs there are symptoms, warning signals, signs of things that have happened already, signs by which things are recognized; these have different ways of indicating, regardless of what may be serving as such a sign.

'Signs' represent our lives, that is, beliefs, values and life experiences. We can treat these either as detached things that have little significance, or we can view them as being central to our lives. It is not enough just to take note of another's beliefs, values, views and experiences. They must be integrated into the being in the world for that individual. Being conscious of another's beliefs and values does not provide a prescription for action, but instead provides guidance towards the most appropriate approach for action based on the individual's life experience. In recognition of this interconnectedness, the individuality of all parties is made explicit in the relationship. Such an approach requires commitment on the part of persons to want to engage in such a relationship and to accept it.

Taking note of 'signs' enables a person to place actions in context, or as MacIntyre (1992, p. 210) suggests, 'the act of utterance becomes intelligible by finding its place in a narrative'. In other words, for an individual's values to have meaning they need to be placed in the context of their lives, as we only become aware of our values when they are challenged either positively or negatively (Heidegger 1927/1990, p. 112). Without clarifying the meaning of a value in its original context, then it may be difficult to move it from something that is available to us, to something that guides action. If a value cannot be clarified, that doesn't mean it doesn't exist but other values may be needed to access it. For example, even if a person values the right to determine decisions for him/herself, it may not be possible for another person to understand the importance of that value to him/her until other values have been clarified, such as those the person holds about (for example) the importance of fairness and justice in society.

From the perspective of caring, taking note of 'signs' enables the facilitation of decision-making from the patient's perspective, that is, facilitating their authenticity. Heidegger argues that when the maintenance of another's authenticity is not a priority in caring practices then there is a danger of stepping into the place of the other and solving the problems or meeting the needs on behalf of the other. Heidegger calls such practice 'defective solicitude', for one becomes dominant and the other is made dependent, thus reducing the other to a thing. In a 'freedom-gaining' relationship (Barker 1991), one looks ahead with the other to help him or her understand what lies ahead and to develop appropriate coping mechanisms. There are times when such a partnership may not be possible and one may have to 'leap ahead' of the other in order to facilitate the other's authenticity. The goal remains that of helping the other recognise what he/she needs for him or herself and to develop a mechanism for the other to cope successfully on their own. One steps back to enable the other to deploy his or her strategies, but steps forward to support in times of weakness, leaving the other free to determine his or her own fate (Barker 1991, p. 191; Heidegger 1927/1990, p. 159). This concept of authenticity concurs with philosophies of 'personhood' within a nurse-patient relationship that requires involvement, risk taking, stepping back to create space and stepping forwards in times of vulnerability.

Viewing person-centred practice from the perspective of authenticity starts from the position that everyone has 'inborn potential', but that individuals learn how to exercise that potential through socialisation. All adults have the same inborn potential but that potential is fully realised or not through processes of socialisation. Various internal and external constraints may be in place that prevent an individual's full potential from being realised, and thus people may need assistance in determining the most appropriate course of action. This approach demands that the practitioner's role should focus on facilitating an individual's authenticity, so that their full potential can be realised and their capacity to exercise autonomous action maximised through the erosion of constraining factors.

Essential principles for person-centred practice

The person-centred practice literature is replete with advice, tools and processes that are essential for the adoption of person-centredness in practice, and we have referred to some of these in Chapter 1. Each of these offers particular approaches to engaging with health and social care activities in a person-centred way.

However, it is our contention that person-centredness is best operationalised at the level of 'principle', because how it operates is highly dependent on the implementation context, and no single tool, process or method is going to fit every context!

It is also evident in the literature that 'practice patterns' influence the way that person-centredness is experienced by staff and service users. Some patterns are overt, such as those explicitly articulated in care pathways. Others are more implicit to established ways of being of individual practitioners, and it is these implicit patterns that differentiate espoused standards of practice and that are experienced by patients and service users. A lot of the work of practice development is what we would call 'unearthing the architecture of practice patterns', and in Chapter 10, Jan Dewing and Brendan McCormack illustrate how different patterns create different energies that can either enhance or inhibit innovation. Emancipatory practice development has as its core purpose the development of person-centred cultures through narrowing the gap between espoused values and those practised (see Chapter 9). Closing that gap requires an analysis of practice context in order to determine characteristics of the setting that help or hinder the development of a person-centred culture. Over many years of engagement in emancipatory practice development, our evidence (e.g. Andvig & Biong 2014; Parlour et al. 2014) shows the need to understand how established patterns of practice are consistent or not with espoused person-centred values. Without systematically facilitated critical creative reflection on practice and the use of multiple sources of evidence that shine a light on the dark, unconscious and embodied established ways of knowing, being and doing, then no amount of tools or processes will create more person-centredness.

The architect, Christopher Alexander (1977) coined the phrase 'patterns language' – a method of describing good design practices within a field of expertise. Alexander described it as a language, because he believed that understanding these deeper patterns that are embedded in good design exposes the deeper wisdom of practice. This idea of deeper wisdom is important to the development of person-centredness, as it is often the case that many person-centred initiatives and projects overly focus on the use of tools that capture the artefacts (Schein 2004) of person-centredness, but which don't articulate the expertise needed to connect with it at an authentic level. Alexander argued that it becomes a language because of the interconnected expressions that are used by members of the field of practice to describe the expertise embedded in the design. This is also evident in health-care practice where patterns are often not given a voice and their language is manifested through the embodied knowing of practitioners. Like all languages, it comprises vocabulary, syntax and grammar:

- *Vocabulary:* Named and described solutions to a problem in a field of interest. For example, in person-centredness, named solutions could include assessment tools and processes, decision-making tools, feedback mechanisms, actions to ensure safety (such as 'red trays' for people who need help with nutrition).

- *Syntax:* A description of how a particular solution fits in a larger, more complex system, thus linking individual solutions in particular contexts with larger more comprehensive systems. This linkage is important for person-centred practice because we have previously argued that patients largely experience 'person-centred moments' rather than 'person-centred care' (McCance et al. 2013). We argued that the existence of moments of person-centredness arose because of a lack of linkage between individual moments of care and the whole model of care experienced by patients and staff. Thinking about syntax requires organisations to explore individually effective practices and how they connect with other practices in order to create a person-centred system.

- *Grammar:* Describes how the solution solves a problem or produces a benefit. For example, an organisation committed to the continuous development of person-centredness would have a system in place to review the effectiveness of solutions used to solve particular problems and a methodology in place to help translate those solutions into everyday practices across an organisation/health-care system. Such system-wide solutions can be documented in a logical way so that they can be repeated time and time again.

In recognising the importance of patterns, Alexander identified 15 'properties of nature' that through his research he considered to be essential in good design, that is, design that complemented and resonated with the natural environment whilst at the same time creating 'mental jolts' to make us think differently about design and what it is for. In the same way, we can never be complacent about person-centredness and its properties – what is an effective pattern one day can be an ineffective pattern the next, if not continuously reflected upon, adjusted and refined. In addition, as illustrated by The Health Foundation, person-centredness is not a fixed or static unidimensional concept, but instead is multifaceted, multidimensional and dynamic. In Figure 2.1 we depict Alexander's (1977) '15 properties of nature' and suggest that these properties exist like satellites rotating around an individual's personhood, and the way in which they are languaged (particularly the interlinking of vocabulary and syntax) determines the extent to which person-centredness is realised. These properties are ever-present in the patterns of person-centredness that exist in health and social care systems (Box 2.1).

In Table 2.1 we set out each of these properties and suggest ways in which they are patterned in the context of person-centredness in an organisation. We hope that by working your way through this table, you can identify ways to address different patterns in your organisation and potential ways of changing or further developing these patterns in order to achieve a more person-centred culture.

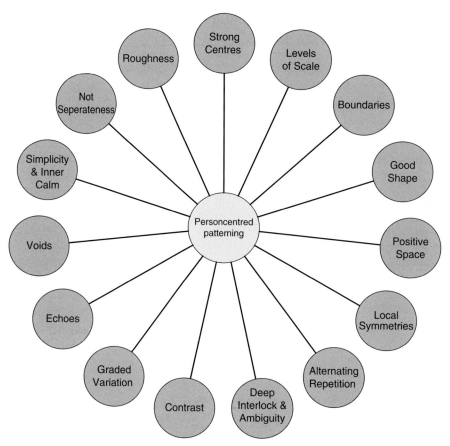

Figure 2.1 The 15 properties of person-centred practice. Source: Alexander (1977).
Reproduced with permission of OUP.

Box 2.1 The 15 properties in action: an illustrative case study.

Willow Lands University Hospital is a large tertiary referral centre in a metropolitan city in
the UK. The hospital has 1100 inpatient beds and a full range of emergency, outpatient and
ambulatory care services. It employs approximately 7000 staff and is recognised internationally for its innovative research and practice in a number of specialties, particularly cardiac
services. Over a 5-year period, the hospital has been focused on transforming its culture to
one that has person-centred principles embedded at all levels of the organisation. Significant
restructuring and reorganisation has taken place and the chief executive has actively led programmes of work to embed the espoused values of the organisation into every aspect of work
undertaken. Willow Lands consistently gets 'excellent' external review/accreditation reports
for the quality of the services offered. Service-user and staff feedback is also consistently
positive and the organisation has no difficulty in recruiting excellent staff.

Table 2.1 The 15 properties of person-centred practice in action

Property	Vocabulary	Syntax	Grammar	Pattern
Strong centres *Person-centred values at the centre of decision-making*	Recruitment of staff using a values-based approach	Unit leaders committed to the development of shared values	An organisation has a system in place to receive qualitative feedback from staff and patients in order to determine consistency between espoused values and patient experience	Each year the organisation holds an engagement event where the learning from the individual unit values are shared with other teams. Using a reflective and creative approach, teams consider how other teams' values reflect theirs and aspects of practice that could be improved in order to further enhance the operationalisation of their espoused values
Levels of scale *Paying attention to all parts of the system that contribute to creating person-centredness*	Not overlooking 'the little things' and considering how these so-called little things fit within the larger care delivery system	The use of tools that enable every 'voice' to be heard. Tools such as practice development tools, engagement tools, continuous quality improvement processes and feedback tools	The practice development framework of the organisation interlinks with the service improvement system and together key learnings are identified from 'small' developments in individual teams and units	Every month, volunteers on wards that provide services to older people are brought together with the practice development facilitators. The volunteers are asked to share their experiences of helping patients with their food and drink and to share their stories. Using 'Claims, Concerns & Issues (Guba & Lincoln 1989) and emotional touchpoints (Dewar et al. 2009) the facilitators identify key issues that need to be considered in order to change some of the practices in the units
Boundaries *A boundary helps focus attention on the centre*	Knowing the boundaries of individual competence and building a team where individuals complement each other's areas of expertise	Processes in place for the continuous evaluation of professional attributes of individual practitioners	Mapping of staff effectiveness against service-user feedback and ensuring that development programmes are in place to enhance effectiveness	The organization has been committed to matching its CPD programmes with its performance review policy, service-user feedback, audit programmes and quality monitoring systems. Each year the patterns of activity across teams are reviewed and new programmes developed, as well as the removal of unnecessary programmes

(continued overleaf)

Table 2.1 (*continued*)

Property	Vocabulary	Syntax	Grammar	Pattern
Good shape *A good shape has a strong centre and a logical form that supports different connections*	Ensuring the well-being of service users and staff through offering a range of health-supporting services	Stress management is considered an important part of wellness in the service, so staff are taught mindfulness techniques, simple massage and relaxation for their own self-management and for use with service users	Mindfulness and other stress reduction strategies are integrated into the staff support programme and made available to all staff. Service users and their care partners can access stress-management and well-being services	The organisation, in recognising the international evidence about the importance of 'wellness strategies', has made a strategic commitment to ensuring that the maintenance and enhancement of staff health is a priority for effective patient outcome. The organisation supports a range of health and well-being programmes, many of which are free to staff and service users and others are subsidized
Positive space *Every part of a space makes a positive contribution to wholeness*	Ensuring that the environment in which care is delivered and received is conducive to healing	The quality of the physical environment is considered important in contributing to a good experience of care	Regular environmental observations are undertaken in order to determine the quality of the physical environment and continuous improvements made to enhance care experiences	In recognition of the important contribution that the physical environment makes to healing and the creation of an effective person-centred culture, the organisation has committed to an arts and environment programme, has employed an arts coordinator and has signed up to the values of 'Planetree' (http://planetree.org/). In addition, each month the Executive Team reviews feedback from service users and staff that relates to the quality of the environment and a continuous programme of 'environmental enhancement' is in place
Local symmetries *A balanced contribution of elements that together strengthen the whole*	Workload planning models that are appropriate to the client group and that reflect the mix of knowledge, skills and expertise needed to deliver effective person-centred care	Skill-mix in teams is not considered to be static but is thought of as something that needs to continuously respond to changing patient need	A workload model is in place that is based on person-centred principles, reflects the expertise needed in different clinical situations and that prioritises patient-focused outcomes	The organisation uses a model for determining the number of staff needed in different clinical contexts that is focused on maximising the expertise available, ensuring that the outcomes of its person-centred care strategy can be delivered and that maintains staff well-being. The model is dynamic as it is regularly adjusted according to vacancy rates, feedback from leaders and from service users. The organisation recognises the importance of having human resource policies in place that reflect a person-centred approach

Alternating repetition *The common traits shared among a group because of their proximity to one another, with each intensifying the other*	All care needs are considered significant no matter how small	Individualised care planning and prioritisation of 'what matters' to the patient	A patient assessment process is in place that has biographical assessment as the central building block of all other assessment. Active engagement with patients and their care partners is a priority in all assessment	Quality improvement strategies that focus on the 'fundamentals of care' with patients and families are in place. The practice development team works in collaboration with the nurse leaders and the service improvement teams to ensure that the fundamentals of care are given top priority in development programmes. Continuous processes of evaluation and feedback are in place so that teams own the developments and are committed to continuous improvement
Deep interlock and ambiguity *Objects that have a high degree of life hook into their surroundings and are embedded in their natural surroundings so that it is difficult to disentangle the two*	Sharing of decision-making in teams that values the contributions of all staff and that views collaborative decision-making with patients and families as essential to effective care	Based on individualised and biographical assessments, shared decision-making forums are established among teams. Tools to enhance sharing of information are used to ensure that all voices are heard	A number of complementary strategies are in place to enable participation in decision-making – including, end-of-shift handover, reflective review of care plans, staff huddles, case reviews and periodic review of individual cases	Shared governance is a well-established process for engaging all stakeholders in decision-making. Organisational structures are altered to reduce hierarchical decision-making and to increase key stakeholder participation in decisions. A number of 'councils' are in place to discuss key parts of organisational performance and these connect with the executive structure to inform strategy, effectiveness reviews and ongoing quality improvement programmes
Contrast *Embracing the differences between opposites. Differences strengthen the centre*	Feedback processes that embrace all perspectives and that are focused on learning and developing	Service-user feedback is actively sought as well as feedback from staff about their experiences of being person-centred	A number of feedback processes are in place as it is recognised that no single method is good enough. Volunteers are used to interview patients and families, electronic systems of feedback are in place as well as a number of forums for face-to-face discussion	The Executive Board recognises that feedback is the platform upon which continuous quality is maintained. The Chief Executive role models this by prioritising activities that result in her/him gaining feedback each week from a variety of stakeholders. Key learning is collated from all the feedback obtained and mapped against a framework of person-centredness by the practice development and improvement team. This feedback, learning and actions taken are reported through the organisation's governance processes and communicated through its various multi-media systems

(continued overleaf)

Table 2.1 *(continued)*

Property	Vocabulary	Syntax	Grammar	Pattern
Graded variation *All living things tend to have a certain softness. Individual qualities change slowly and blend with each other*	Facilitated approaches to learning in and from practice	Facilitated approaches to learning are embedded in leadership practices as well as the CPD framework	Facilitation happens at different levels of the organisation. There is an embedded programme of facilitator development in place and staff in key roles are encouraged to participate in these programmes and to engage in facilitated learning activities	The Executive Board believes in a 'joined-up approach' to achieving quality patient/family care outcomes, continuous quality improvement and the continuous development of practice. To that end, they have integrated the clinical education, service improvement and practice development teams to form a single 'person-centred practice facilitation' team. The training, CPD and innovation budgets have also been combined and integrated to support the work of the team. The team runs a variety of facilitator development programmes, practice development schools, service-improvement training modules and one-off training events. It is all supported by a variety of reflective practice approaches (group supervision, action learning, etc.). They use a variety of data to evaluate effectiveness as well as determine ongoing priorities
Roughness *Embracing what doesn't naturally fit*	Paying attention to what matters most and letting go of what matters less	Regular review of care pathways resulting in continuous refinement of patient journeys	Quality monitoring data are proactively used in decision-making forums in order to ensure that services offered are the most efficient and effective for patients and families as well as being consistent with evidence of the most expert professional practice	The organisation has worked in partnership with the national quality and standards regulatory agency, so that there is an empowering, enabling and partnership approach adopted to quality monitoring and review. Whilst the organisation is still subjected to the same programme of announced and unannounced reviews by the agency, the data are reported and used internally to the organisation in a proactive and enabling way and centred within a culture of learning. The agency staff work with the organisation to find creative solutions and to advise regarding innovations and safety. The organisation consistently achieves excellent quality reports

Echoes *Individual elements reflect each other and together form a wholeness*	Providing holistic care	Ensuring that all staff have the necessary knowledge, skill, expertise, resources and support to provide holistic care at all times	Person-centred care is seen as the same thing as holistic care and is never compromised for the sake of expediency. All other parts of the system work towards enabling staff to provide, and patients/families to experience the best possible person-centred care	Real-time monitoring of patient journeys is a key component of the organisation's strategy for ensuring that person-centred care is provided and that patients/families experience more than 'person-centred moments'. The integrated 'person-centred practice' facilitation team facilitates observations of practice; patient, family and staff feedback; and maps key decisions on the patient's journey. Practice development programmes that incorporate 'small cycles of change' and feedback loops are put in place to deal with care discontinuities and enable a holistic experience
Voids *Creating spaces for stillness and calm in order to enable strength*	Staff well-being is critical to positive patient/family outcomes and experiences	Creating opportunities for all staff to stay well	Staff well-being strategies are in place and actively promoted and facilitated. A number of wellness programmes are available for staff to participate in. Extended periods of sickness among staff are treated as an organisational learning issue	Consistent with the focus on person-centredness in the organisation, the Human Resources Department has rebranded as the 'Personal Effectiveness Enhancement' team. They have worked collaboratively with staff teams to revise their policies and procedures to reflect this change in culture. For example, the sick-leave policy has been changed to the 'staying-well policy' and whilst it still contains the statutory and legal requirements of such a policy, its values are based on enabling wellness

(continued overleaf)

Table 2.1 (*continued*)

Property	Vocabulary	Syntax	Grammar	Pattern
Simplicity and inner calm *Stripping away those things that confuse or are unnecessary*	Creation of a healthful culture	Paying attention to all parts of the organisation and ensuring that each element contributes to the health and well-being of all stakeholders	Creating and sustaining a healthful culture is an important part of the work of the organisation. Drawing on national and international initiatives to benchmark the health of the organisation is integral to this work	The organisation has embraced a set of person-centred 'indicators of success'. These indicators focus equally on the quality of care experienced by patients/families and the quality of work life of staff teams. All strategies, policies, processes and key relationships are reviewed against these indicators and development programmes put in place as necessary. In addition, successes are regularly celebrated and rewarded, communicated through social media and integrated into future work programmes. Staff satisfaction and retention is high and patient/family feedback is constructive and helpful
Not separateness *The degree of connection an element has with all that is around it*	Staff who are engaged	Ensuring that processes are in place to maximise the engagement of staff with their work	Understanding that an engaged employee experiences a blend of job satisfaction, organisational commitment, job involvement and feelings of empowerment. This is not achieved through strategies that serve to emotionally manipulate an employee into giving more of themselves, but instead it is achieved by espoused organisational values being experienced in daily work-life by employees	The Chief Executive (CEO) holds 'engagement' as a critical indicator of organisational effectiveness and success. Despite high levels of commitment and low staff turnover rates, the CEO knows that engagement is a two-way process between an organisation and its staff. She/he is aware that an engaged organisation is one that has strong and authentic values, has clear evidence of trust at all levels, and is fair and strives to create a culture of mutual respect. She/he therefore, with the Executive Team, uses all the available strategies to ensure that commitments are shared, values are lived and promises are fulfilled. The organisation's person-centred framework is active at individual, team, unit and organisational levels

Conclusions

In this chapter we have presented some conceptual and philosophical perspectives on personhood and person-centredness as well as set out some essential principles for operationalising person-centred practices and creating a person-centred culture. We have offered different perspectives of personhood. These are not mutually exclusive perspectives and, indeed, when one explores them through the unifying concept of 'authenticity' then the areas of overlap are obvious. In the real world of course we do not think about our own and others' being in this fragmented way and indeed to do so would lead to faulty decision-making and the potential erosion of a person's personhood as it would create 'blindspots' in our reflection and decision-making. Whilst authenticity can be seen to be a unifying concept in enabling more effective decision-making, we need to be acutely aware of the fact that many people are unable to represent their authentic self autonomously and so need help from others in situations where their authenticity may be under threat. If we are going to be in a position to facilitate the authenticity of others who need our help most, then we need to ensure that we are in the best possible state to do so. When we are truly connected in a person-centred relationship we share our deepest sense of 'self', enabling others to know who we are as persons, what values are important to us, the dreams, hopes and desires we hold in our lives, and the kind of life that we strive to live. Through our discussions, reflections, debates, arguments and agreements one's 'self' is shaped and reshaped, ordered and reordered, prioritised and reprioritised as one's life progresses. Taking such a dynamic into a professional relationship and as a health-care practitioner facilitating the care of another person, that life plan translates into (for example) a formal comprehensive assessment that includes biography and narrative. Knowing the person in this way is essential to person-centred practice. However, our lives are dominated by patterns – some good and others not so good, some helpful and others not so, some explicit and others implicit. These patterns shape our very existence and the quality of the relationships we experience. We have therefore proposed a set of 'pattern-based principles' to guide person-centredness at individual, team and organisational levels and to connect with the Person-centred Nursing Framework.

References

Alexander, C. (1977) *A Pattern Language: Towns, Buildings, Construction*, Oxford University Press.

Andrews, G., Evans, J., and Wiles, J.L. (2013) Re-spacing and re-placing gerontology: relationality and affect. *Ageing and Society*, **33**, 1339–73.

Andvig E and Biong S. (2014) Recovery oriented conversations in a milieu therapeutic setting. *International Practice Development Journal* **4**(1): art. 6. Available from: http://www.fons.org/library/journal/volume4-issue1/article6 (accessed 26 January 2016).

Baldwin, T. (ed) (2004) *Maurice Merleau-Ponty: Basic Writings*, Routledge, London.

Barker, E.M. (1991) Rethinking family loyalties, in *Aging and Ethics* (ed N.S. Jecker), Humana Press, Clifton, NJ, pp. 187–98.

Boykin, A. and Schoenhofer, S. (1993) *Nursing as Caring: A Model for Transforming Practice*, National League for Nursing Press, New York.

Brooker, D. (2005) Dementia care mapping: a review of the research literature. *The Gerontologist*, **45** (Special Issue I), 11–18.

Brooker D. (2010) Dementia care mapping. In: Abou-Saleh MT, Katona C, Kumar A (eds), *Principles and Practice of Geriatric Psychiatry*, 3rd edn. Chichester, UK: John Wiley & Sons, Ltd, pp. 157–61.

Buber, M. (1984) *I and Thou*, T & T Clark, Edinburgh.

Dewar, B., Mackay, R., Smith, S., Pullin, S., and Tocher, R. (2009) Use of emotional touchpoints as a method of tapping into the experience of receiving compassionate care in a hospital setting. *Journal of Research in Nursing*, **15**, 29–41.

Dewing J. (2007) An exploration of wandering in older persons with a dementia through radical reflection and participation. PhD thesis, University of Manchester.

Dewing, J. (2008a) Personhood and dementia: revisiting Tom Kitwood's ideas. *International Journal of Older People Nursing*, **3**, 3–13.

Dewing, J. (2008b) Process consent and research with older persons living with dementia. *Association of Research Ethics Journal*, **4** (2), 59–64.

Dillon, M.C. (1988) *Merleau-Ponty's Ontology*, 2nd edn, Northwestern University Press, Evanston, IL.

Edwards, S.D. (2001) *Philosophy of Nursing: An Introduction*, Palgrave, Basingstoke, UK.

Frankfurt, H.G. (1989) Freedom of the will and the concept of a person, in *The Inner Citadel: Essays on Individual Autonomy* (ed J. Christman), Oxford University Press, Oxford.

Guba, E.G. and Lincoln, Y.S. (1989) *Fourth Generation Evaluation*, Sage Publications.

Hannah, M. (2014) *Humanising Healthcare: Patterns of Hope for a System Under Strain*, Triarchy Publishers, Axminster, UK.

Heidegger M. (1927/1990) *Being and Time* (trans. Macquarrie J and Robinson E, 1962). Oxford: Basil Blackwell.

Kant I. (1785/2012) *Groundwork of the Metaphysics of Morals* (trans. Abbott TK). New York: Start Publishing LLC.

Kitwood, T. (1997) *Dementia Reconsidered: The Person Comes First*, Open University Press, Milton Keynes.

Leibing, A. (2008) Entangled matters – Alzheimer's, interiority, and the 'unflattening' of the world. *Culture, Medicine and Psychiatry*, **32**, 177–93.

Leplege, A., Gzil, F., Cammelli, M., Lefeve, C., Pachoud, B., and Ville, I. (2007) Person-centredness: conceptual and historical perspectives. *Disability and Rehabilitation*, **29**, 1555–65.

Maben J, Peccei R, Adams M, Robert G, Richardson A, Murrells T. (2012) Patients' experiences of care and the influence of staff motivation, affect and wellbeing. Final report. *NIHR Service Delivery and Organisation programme*. National Institute for Health Research.

MacIntyre, A. (1992) *After Virtue – A Study in Moral Theory*, Duckworth, London.

Martinsen, K. (2006) Care and Vulnerability *[English translation]*, Akribe, Oslo.

McCance, T.V. (2003) Caring in nursing practice: the development of a conceptual framework. *Research and Theory for Nursing Practice: An International Journal*, **17**, 101–16.

McCance, T., Telford, L., Wilson, J., MacLeod, O., and Dowd, A. (2011) Identifying key performance indicators for nursing and midwifery care using a consensus approach. *Journal of Clinical Nursing*, **21**, 1145–54.

McCance T, Gribben B, McCormack B, Laird EA. (2013) Promoting person-centred practice within acute care: the impact of culture and context on a facilitated practice development programme. *International Practice Development Journal* **3**(1): art. 2. Available from: http://www.fons.org/library/journal/volume3-issue1/article2 (accessed 26 January 2016).

McCormack, B. (2001) *Negotiating Partnerships with Older People – A Person-Centred Approach*, Ashgate, Basingstoke.

McCormack, B. (2004) Person-centredness in gerontological nursing: an overview of the literature. *International Journal of Older People Nursing (in association with the Journal of Clinical Nursing)*, **13** (3A), 31–8.

McCormack, B. and McCance, T. (2010) *Person-Centred Nursing: Theory, Models and Methods*, Wiley-Blackwell Publishing, Oxford.

McCormack, B., Karlsson, B., Dewing, J., and Lerdal, A. (2010) Exploring person-centredness: a qualitative meta-synthesis of four studies and their contribution to advancing our understanding of person-centred nursing. *Scandinavian Journal of Caring Sciences*, **24**, 620–34.

McCormack, B., Roberts, T., Meyer, J., Morgan, D., and Boscart, V. (2012) Appreciating the 'person' in long-term care. *International Journal of Older People Nursing*, **7**, 284–94.

McMurray, J. (1995) *The Self as Agent: The Form of the Personal*, Faber & Faber, London.

Merleau-Ponty, M. (1989) *Phenomenology of Perception* (trans. C. Smith C, with revisions by F. Williams and D. Gurriere). London: Routledge.

Merleau-Ponty M. (1962) *The Phenomenology of Perception* (trans. C. Smith). London: Routledge & Kegan Paul.

Nolan, M., Davies, S., Brown, J., Keady, J., and Nolan, J. (2004) Beyond 'person-centred' care: a new vision for gerontological nursing. *Journal of Clinical Nursing*, **13** (3a), 45–53.

Parlour, R., Slater, P., McCormack, B., Gallen, A., and Kavanagh, P. (2014) The relationship between positive patient experience in acute hospitals and person-centred care. *International Journal of Research in Nursing*, **5**, 25–34.

Peplau, H.E. (1952) *Interpersonal Relations in Nursing*, Putnam & Sons, Philadelphia.

Post, S. (2006) Respectare: moral respect for the lives of the deeply forgetful, in *Dementia: Mind, Meaning and the Person* (eds J.C. Hughes, S.J. Louw, and S.R. Sabat), Oxford University Press, Oxford, pp. 223–34.

Rogers, C. (1961) *On Becoming a Person*, Houghton Mifflin Co., Boston.

Sabat, S. (2002) Surviving manifestations of selfhood in Alzheimer's disease: a case study. *Dementia*, **1**, 25–36.

Schein, E.H. (2004) *Organizational Culture and Leadership*, 3rd edn, Jossey-Bass, San Franscisco.

Slater, L. (2006) Person-centredness: a concept analysis. *Contemporary Nurse*, **23**, 135–44.

Tournier, P. (1999) *Meaning of Persons*, SCM Press Ltd., London.

Watson, J. (1999) *Nursing: Human Science and Human Care – A Theory of Nursing*, National League of Nursing Press, New York.

Wiles J, Leibing A, Guberman N, Reeve J, Allen R. (2011) *The meaning of "Ageing in Place" to older people*. The Gerontologist. Available from: http://gerontologist.oxfordjournals.org/content/early/2011/10/07/geront.gnr098.full.pdf+h (accessed 26 January 2016).

Yalden, J., McCormack, B., O'Connor, M., and Hardy, S. (2013) Transforming end of life care using practice development: an arts-informed approach in residential aged care. *International Journal of Practice Development*, **3** (2), 1–18.

CHAPTER 3

The Person-centred Practice Framework

Tanya McCance[1] & Brendan McCormack[2]

[1] *Ulster University, Northern Ireland, UK*
[2] *Queen Margaret University, Edinburgh, UK*

Introduction

In this chapter the person-centred nursing theoretical framework developed by us (McCormack & McCance 2006, 2010) will be updated, taking account of a multi-disciplinary and interprofessional context. The framework comprises four key domains: prerequisites for person-centred practice; the care environment; person-centred processes; and person-centred outcomes. In the previous edition of this book (McCormack & McCance 2010) we provided a comprehensive exploration of each construct within the four domains of the Person-centred Nursing Framework, placing it in the context of existing theoretical and research literature. We would encourage our readers to refer to this original source for the detailed description and to gain an understanding of the origins of the framework, which is founded on the concepts of caring and person-centredness. It is our intention in this chapter to relate the continued development of the framework to contemporary perspectives on caring, compassion, dignity and flourishing and to illustrate their relevance to changing models of health and social care.

Development of the framework: the story so far ...

The development of the Person-centred Nursing Framework has spanned nearly a decade and during that time it has been used in a variety of different ways, across a range of contexts. The framework is underpinned by empirical research, was developed as part of a large-scale research study, and continues to be tested and refined through an ongoing programme of applied research (http://www .science.ulster.ac.uk/inhr/pcp/index.php). At this stage it is important to reaffirm the key constructs of the framework that have remained stable, but also highlight how the framework has evolved over time.

Development of a framework for person-centred nursing (McCormack & McCance 2006)

The original framework published in 2006, presented in Figure 3.1, was developed for use in the intervention stage of a large quasi-experimental research study, which focused on measuring the effectiveness of the implementation of person-centred nursing in a tertiary hospital setting (McCormack et al. 2008). The framework was derived from McCormack's conceptual framework (McCormack 2003) focusing on person-centred practice with older people, and McCance's framework focusing on patients' and nurses' experience of caring in nursing (McCance 2003). The process for developing the framework is described in this original paper, but the key message that has stood the test of time is the shared philosophical underpinnings that formed the sound basis for the development of the Person-centred Nursing Framework. The philosophy underpinning the framework is embedded in the concept of being a 'person' as

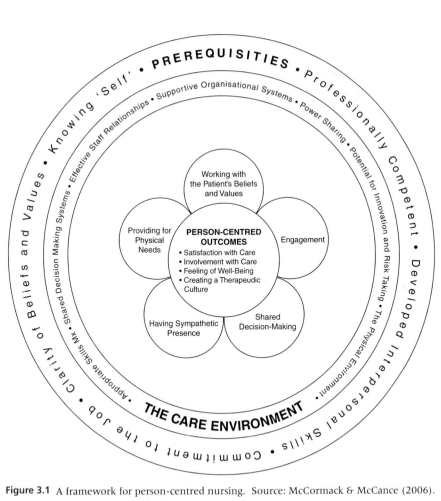

Figure 3.1 A framework for person-centred nursing. Source: McCormack & McCance (2006). Reproduced with permission of Wiley.

discussed in Chapter 2, and is consistent with a philosophy of human science, which focuses on what it means to be human. Human science principles that form the foundation of the Framework include human freedom, choice and responsibility; holism (non-reducible persons interconnected with others and nature); different forms of knowing (empirics, aesthetics, ethics and intuition); and the importance of time and space, and relationships (Watson 1985).

The original framework essentially comprised four domains:

1 *Prerequisites*, which focus on the attributes of the nurse and include: being professionally competent, having developed interpersonal skills, being committed to the job, being able to demonstrate clarity of beliefs and values, and knowing self.

2 *Care environment*, which focuses on the context in which care is delivered and includes: an appropriate skill mix; systems that facilitate shared decision-making; effective staff relationships; supportive organisational systems, the sharing of power, and the potential for innovation and risk-taking.

3 *Person-centred processes*, which focus on delivering care to the patient through a range of activities and include: working with patients' beliefs and values, engagement, having a sympathetic presence, sharing decision-making and providing for physical needs.

4 *Expected outcomes*, which are the results of effective person-centred nursing and include: satisfaction with care, involvement in care, feeling of well-being, and creating a therapeutic environment.

The relationship between the constructs of the framework was represented pictorially, in that to reach the centre of the framework, the attributes of staff must first be considered, as a prerequisite to managing the care environment, in order to provide effective care through the care processes. This ordering ultimately leads to the achievement of the outcomes – the central component of the framework. It is also acknowledged that there are relationships between the constructs.

The period of time following the publication of the original framework was characterised by wide exposure to the framework, mainly within nursing but on an international stage. This main focus was to generate much needed critical dialogue and debate about its applicability to practice. A significant driver at this early stage was the integration of the framework into Practice Development, which is described as an approach to improving practice that has the development of effective person-centred cultures as its core purpose (McCormack et al. 2013). The relationship between the framework and practice development is given full attention in Section 3 of this book. The key message at this time was the utility of the framework as a means of operationalising person-centredness in practice, recognising that at a level of principle the idea of person-centredness is well understood, but the issue is often recognising it in practice. The framework became increasingly recognised as a tool that shone a light on practice and brought a shared understanding and a common language to person-centredness in nursing.

Person-centred nursing: theory and practice (McCormack & McCance 2010)

The publication of the Person-centred Nursing Framework in the first edition of this book in 2010, which is presented in Figure 3.2, consolidated the four domains and many of the constructs within the framework, and the relations between them. At this stage only a few changes were made to the original framework as a result of critical dialogue and feedback:

- the addition of the *physical environment* as a component within the care environment in recognition of the impact of our physical surroundings on person-centred practice; and

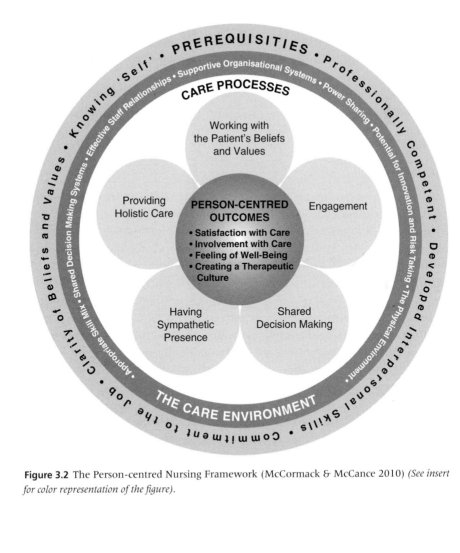

Figure 3.2 The Person-centred Nursing Framework (McCormack & McCance 2010) *(See insert for color representation of the figure).*

- amendment to the component *providing for physical needs* to read *providing holistic care*, in recognition of the range of interventions undertaken by nurses that are not always physical in nature.

Following this publication, the framework continued to be used as a tool for practice and to be tested through ongoing research (e.g. Lynch et al. 2011; McCance et al. 2013; Buckley et al. 2014). More interestingly, however, it began to have influence across other areas such as strategy and policy within nursing, and in health care more broadly (e.g. DHSSPSNI 2010, 2013; Royal College of Nursing 2010). Nursing education and leadership development were other areas that began to demonstrate the usefulness of the framework in different contexts. These developments are the focus of Section 4 of this book.

The Person-centred Nursing Framework: a middle range theory

From the outset, the Person-centred Nursing Framework was described as a mid-range theory (McCormack & McCance 2006). Its place on the continuum of theory development was made explicit by McCormack and McCance (2010) drawing on the seminal work of Fawcett (1995), who describes a hierarchy of nursing knowledge that has five components. At the highest level of abstraction is the metaparadigm that represents a broad consensus for nursing, which provides general parameters for the field, and next to this are philosophies, which provide a statement of beliefs and values. Conceptual models are at the next level and provide a particular frame of reference that says something about 'how to observe and interpret the phenomena of interest to the discipline' (Fawcett 1995, p. 3). Theories are the third component in the hierarchy; these are less abstract than conceptual models. They can be further described as grand theories or middle-range theories, with the latter being narrower in scope and 'made up of concepts and propositions that are empirically measurable' (Fawcett 1995, p. 25). Fawcett distinguishes between conceptual models and mid-range theories, in that mid-range theories articulate one or more relatively concrete and specific concepts that are derived from a conceptual model. Furthermore, the propositions that describe these concepts propose specific relationships between them. The final component in the hierarchy of nursing knowledge is empirical indicators, which provide the means of measuring concepts within a middle-range theory. The Person-centred Nursing Framework has been described as a middle range theory in that it has been derived from two abstract conceptual frameworks, comprises concepts that are relatively specific, and outlines relationships between the concepts. Recent advancements have been made to develop empirical indicators to measure concepts within the framework, with further work ongoing (Slater et al. 2015).

More recently, the Person-centred Nursing Framework has become a recognised model of nursing (McCormack & McCance 2015). The essence of nursing depicted within the framework reflects the ideals of humanistic caring, where there is a moral component and practice has at its basis a therapeutic intent, which is translated through relationships that are built upon effective interpersonal processes. Hence, the definition of nursing used within the framework is as follows:

> Person-centred nursing is an approach to practice established through the formation and fostering of therapeutic relationships between all care providers, service users and others significant to them in their lives. It is underpinned by values of respect for persons, individual right to self-determination, mutual respect and understanding. It is enabled by cultures of empowerment that foster continuous approaches to practice development.

The framework highlights the complexity of person-centred nursing, and through the articulation of the key constructs, emphasises the contextual, attitudinal and moral dimensions of humanistic caring practices. There is, however, a growing interest and relevance of the Person-centred Nursing Framework to multi-disciplinary and interprofessional team working, which we hope will characterise further development of the framework as we move forwards into the future, and is the context in which we present the next iteration of the Person-centred Nursing Framework within this book.

From person-centred nursing to the Person-centred *Practice* Framework

When looking to the future, it is our aim to situate the Person-centred Nursing Framework within a broader context to illustrate its applicability to a wide range of health-care workers. This section presents the framework as it currently stands, which is presented in Figure 3.3. As a starting point it is important to emphasise that the four domains and many of the constructs within the Person-centred Nursing Framework have remained stable over time. Furthermore the relationship between the domains has also been validated through use of the framework in practice and research, supporting the assumption that the prerequisites must first be considered, then the care environment, both of which are necessary in providing effective care through the care processes in order to deliver person-centred outcomes. There have, however, been further changes made to constructs within the framework since the 2010 publication, which will be highlighted in the remainder of this chapter.

Prerequisites
The *prerequisites* focus on the attributes of staff and are considered the key building blocks in the development of health-care professionals who can deliver effective person-centred care. Attributes include: being professionally competent, having developed interpersonal skills, being committed to the job, being able to demonstrate clarity of beliefs and values, and knowing self. There is no hierarchy in relation to these attributes, with all considered of equal

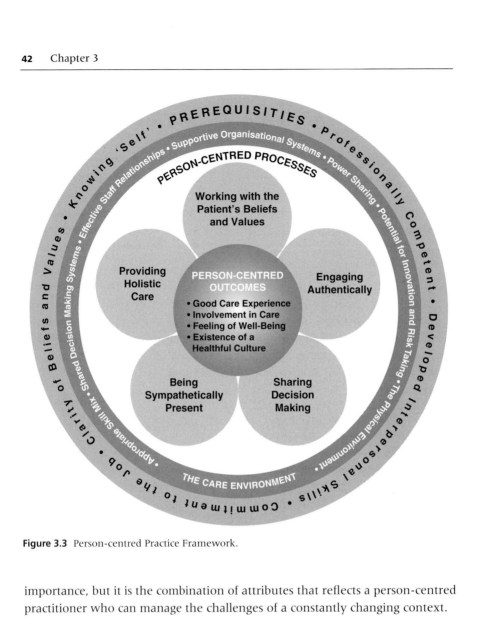

Figure 3.3 Person-centred Practice Framework.

importance, but it is the combination of attributes that reflects a person-centred practitioner who can manage the challenges of a constantly changing context.

Professionally competent

> The knowledge, skills and attitudes of the practitioner to negotiate care options, and effectively provide holistic care.

In the context of person-centredness, competence is more than simply undertaking a task or demonstrating a desired behaviour, but is more reflective of a holistic approach that encompasses knowledge, skills and attitudes. When discussing the concept of competence there are three main approaches adopted in the literature: a task-based or behaviourist approach; a general attributes approach; and the holistic approach (Hager et al. 1994). The holistic approach is consistent with the underpinning values of person-centredness and places emphasis on bringing together individual abilities derived from a combination of attributes and tasks to be performed within particular situations, that also incorporates professional judgement. Sundberg (2001), when discussing a holistic approach to competency development, provides a pragmatic view of competence as:

- *knowledge* – what you learn in education;
- *experience* – what you gather in your job, at your workplace and in social life;
- *abilities* to use your knowledge and experience (p. 104).

He argues that we are not able to develop another person's competence, considering this to be in the hands of the individual, but what we can do is 'set the scene, provide the tools and act like catalysts' (p. 104).

The appropriate and relevant competencies for practitioners are reflected in many competency frameworks reported in the literature, the most important being those produced by the regulatory bodies who govern the professions. The implicit assumption within the Person-centred Nursing Framework is that the minimum standards for registration will be met by a professional. The prominence of person-centredness as a concept within competency frameworks and in the delivery of curricula is growing. The challenge in professional education, however, is not dissimilar to the dilemma in practice – we use the term freely but it tends to reflect an understanding of person-centredness at a level of principle, without the follow-through that enables it to be operationalised in practice. This issue is illustrated in Chapter 7 of this book by O'Donnell et al. In this chapter they describe the findings of a meta-synthesis of person-centredness in nursing curricula that was led by O'Donnell and colleagues at Ulster University. They concluded that despite the merits of person-centred practice being widely espoused in contemporary health-care literature, there was limited evidence of approaches to explicitly facilitate this in the construction and/or delivery of nursing curricula. There are, however, advancements in this area, with person-centredness becoming a core concept within curricula alongside innovative approaches to curriculum development becoming more evident as illustrated by the example provided in Chapter 7.

Developing person-centred practitioners doesn't stop at the point of registration. Following registration there is a requirement on practitioners to continue to learn and develop, and to acquire skills that enable them to become more expert in practice. The challenge, however, in the development of expertise is the influence of workplace culture. Culture shapes the values shared by teams in the workplace and this also applies to the competencies that are considered most important within a team. An illustration of this can be drawn from emergency care, where value is placed on a medical-technical competence over caring (McConnell et al. 2015). Patient safety is also high on the agenda across the globe, and approaches to demonstrate improvement in clinical indicators that contribute to the endpoints of morbidity and mortality are continuously being promoted in health care. Some of the most saddening and shocking stories within health care, however, are often less about technical competence and minimising physical harm and more about the dehumanising experience of health care.

The highly publicised Francis Report (Francis 2013), followed by the Berwick Inquiry (Berwick 2013), provided stark evidence of this within a UK context. Furthermore, the call for more compassionate care is a global message (e.g. WHO 2007; Lown et al. 2011; Dewing et al. 2014a), emphasising the need to develop practitioners who are committed to a holistic approach to practice that takes account of the needs of patients as people.

Developed interpersonal skills

> The ability of the practitioner to communicate at a variety of levels with others, using effective verbal and non-verbal interactions that show personal concern for their situation and a commitment to finding mutual solutions.

Person-centredness is built on positive relationships and is dependent on a strong interpersonal skill base. Effective communication requires a combination of good verbal and non-verbal skills. Verbal communication deals with what is said (speech), and what is heard (listening), whilst non-verbal communication is concerned with body language such as posture, proximity, touch, movements, facial expressions, eye contact, gestures and other behaviours, which can add another layer of communication to verbal messages. There are many professional texts available that focus on these fundamental communication skills; however, we would argue that person-centred communication is more than the sum of its parts and that each interaction is dependent on the people involved. In essence we communicate with individuals based on what we know about them as people. This will influence what we say, how we say it, the language used and the use of specific strategies. Getting this right is really important because the impact of poor communication can be profound and often increases the vulnerability experienced by patients and their families.

At one level, a warm friendly practitioner is indicative of good interpersonal skills, and the impact of this on patients and families, and indeed other team members, should not be underestimated. The appropriate use of humour can also build rapport (Tanay et al. 2013; Tremayne 2014). There is, however, a need to move beyond simply building rapport to developing trusting partnerships that will ensure holistic needs are identified, making shared decision-making a real possibility. As professionals we can be warm and friendly, but if we don't have the courage to step into the world space of another person and engage in the important conversations, then our impact will only ever be superficial. This requires professionals to develop advanced communication skills that enable them to engage in courageous conversations in order to get to the heart of what is important to the person. As previously argued by McCormack & McCance (2010), the development of effective interpersonal ability is linked to the notion of emotional intelligence as described by Goleman (1999). Emotional intelligence uses emotions intelligently and is a combination of knowing 'self' and knowing 'others' in the context of emotional beings; that is, *how I and others that I relate to respond emotionally.* It is through an understanding of 'self' as an emotional being that we can respond effectively to the emotional behaviours of others, and this aligns closely to the attribute of 'knowing self' within the Person-centred Nursing Framework.

Knowing self

> The way an individual makes sense of his/her knowing, being and becoming as a person-centred practitioner through reflection, self-awareness, and engagement with others.

As professionals we are also persons with our own life history and experiences, which shape how we develop relationships and how we engage at an emotional level. We grow as persons during our lifetime through engagement with the social world, and it is this that informs our personal meanings, beliefs and values and determines 'who I am'. In the context of the Person-centred Nursing Framework, this implies that the way an individual sees himself/herself, and the way they construct their world, can influence how they practise as a professional and how they engage with others. The development of self-awareness, however, is not a skill that can be taught, but comes with lifelong learning and personal growth that is based on self-reflection. Facilitated self-reflection is one mechanism for increasing our self-awareness and understanding our behaviours. Schon (1983) suggests that the capacity to reflect on action so as to engage in a process of continuous learning is one of the defining characteristics of professional practice and is aligned to the notion of competence described previously. Being able to reflect in action (while doing something) and on action (after you have done it) has become an important feature of professional training programmes in many disciplines. In becoming a person-centred practitioner we also have to be open to giving and receiving feedback and being able to work with that feedback through critical reflection. Increasing personal self-awareness, however, can be difficult as it can push us to face the things we don't like about ourselves and also can bring to the fore painful experiences from the past that colour how we act in the present.

Clarity of beliefs and values

> Awareness of the impact of beliefs and values on care provided by practitioners/received by service users and the commitment to reconciling beliefs and values in ways that facilitate person-centredness.

The Person-centred Nursing Framework identifies clarity of beliefs and values as one of the prerequisites that enable practitioners to work with the care environment. According to Manley (2004), 'values determine what people think *ought* to be done' (p. 55, italics in original) and these are closely linked with moral and ethical codes. Beliefs on the other hand are 'what people think is true or not true' (p. 55). Beliefs and values are interrelated in that 'it is difficult to separate values from their believed effect' (p. 55). Finally, basic assumptions involve beliefs, interpretation of beliefs plus values and emotions and are understood as accepted truths that are held unconsciously and are taken for granted (Brown 1998). Very often we live in a world of assumption without even realising it. The ideal situation is for practitioners to develop and agree a set of professional values that are shared by everyone and then lived out in everyday practice. This, however, is the greatest challenge because often the espoused values of the team (i.e. the values we talk about) do not match the behaviours seen in practice. The development of person-centred cultures is built on the premise that everyone is committed to closing the gap between values that are talked about and how those values are demonstrated (or not, as often can be the case) in behaviours observed in practice. The aspiration is an effective workplace culture where specific values are shared in the workplace, for example person-centredness, lifelong learning, high challenge and high support, and are realised in practice through the development of a shared vision and mission, with individual and collective responsibility to maintain this standard (Manley et al. 2011). Practice development is the improvement methodology that offers a suite of tools and approaches that enables teams to work towards these goals (McCormack et al. 2013; Dewing et al. 2014b).

Commitment to the job

Demonstrated commitment of individuals and team members to patients, families and communities through intentional engagement that focuses on providing holistic evidence-informed care.

Being committed to the job at its most fundamental level reflects dedication and a sense that the nurse wants to provide care that is best for patients and their families. Commitment at individual level reflects the nurse who demonstrates a high level of commitment to patients and families by going the extra mile. Commitment to the job, however, is more than going the extra mile. It is also linked to the idea of intentionality defined as 'the fact of being deliberate or purposive' (www.oxforddictionaries.com). The concept of intentionality is discussed in the caring literature by several nurse theorists. Watson (1985) defines caring as 'a value and an attitude that has to become a will, an intention or a commitment that manifests itself in concrete acts' (p. 32). Furthermore, she believes that 'our intentionalities inform our choices and actions, helping us to be sensitive and mindful about what is most important in our lives and work' (p. 17). Commitment to the job in this sense is more than simply acts of kindness but about taking mindful action that is informed by different types of evidence.

Commitment at an individual level, however, can be hard to sustain if it is at odds with the philosophy within the team. When this situation arises the committed practitioner finds they are constantly swimming against the tide and becomes disillusioned and dissatisfied with the standard of care within the team. The contemporary leadership literature emphasises the importance of transformational leadership, described by Kouzes and Posner (2002) as 'enabling others to act', by embracing approaches that foster collaboration, building trust and providing visible support. Individuals and teams, however, also work within organisations, highlighting commitment at an organisational level. Furthermore, it is suggested from the literature that organisational commitment is influenced by organisational culture, and understanding organisational culture is important because 'it influences how we understand organisational life and the meaning we place on activities' (Manley 2011; Napier et al. 2014). This emphasises the relationship between commitment to the job and clarity of beliefs and values not just at an individual level, but at team and organisational levels.

The care environment

In the previous section the attributes of staff were discussed and described as prerequisites for person-centred practice. We would argue, however, that irrespective of the characteristics of staff, unless the care environment is conducive to person-centred ways of working then the true potential of teams cannot be fully realised. This reflects a complexity within the care environment that focuses on the context in which care is delivered. Increasingly, context is recognised as having a significant impact on clinical and team effectiveness. There is an increasing literature in the field of knowledge translation and knowledge utilisation focusing on: exploring the meaning of context; identifying the key elements of context and their enabling or hindering qualities (for evidence/knowledge use); and developing approaches to measuring the impact of context on clinical and team effectiveness, including impact on patient outcomes (Rycroft-Malone 2004; McCormack et al. 2009; Rycroft-Malone et al. 2013). What is increasingly recognised is that context is a complex phenomenon, and whilst it may be easy to state what it is (in our case context refers to the care environment) it is less easy to delineate its characteristics and qualities. To some extent this difficulty reflects the relationship between context and culture, an area that is explored in greater depth in Section 2 of this book. The position taken in relation to the framework is that context is synonymous with the care environment, and contained within the care environment are multi-faceted characteristics and qualities of the environment (people, processes and structures) that impact on the effectiveness of person-centred practice. To this end, seven characteristics of the care environment are described within the framework including:

- appropriate skill mix;
- systems that facilitate shared decision making;
- the sharing of power;
- effective staff relationships;
- organisational systems that are supportive;

- potential for innovation and risk-taking;
- the physical environment.

Furthermore, we would contend that the constructs that comprise the care environment have a significant impact on the operationalisation of person-centred practice and have the greatest potential to limit or enhance the facilitation of person-centred processes (McCormack et al. 2011).

Appropriate skill mix

> Skill mix is most often considered in a nursing context and means the ratio of registered nurses (RNs) and non-registered nurses in a ward/unit nursing team. In a multi-disciplinary context it means the range of staff with the requisite knowledge and skills to provide a quality service.

According to Buchan and Calman (2005) 'skill mix' is a relatively broad term that can refer to 'the mix of staff in the workforce or the demarcation of roles and activities among different categories of staff' (p. 4). It is also acknowledged that most of the policy attention on using skill-mix changes to improve health system performance has been on the mix between physicians and nurses. Furthermore, debates about skill mix have existed throughout the history of nursing, and refer to the ratio of registered (RNs) and non-registered nurses in a nursing team. There is, however, increased interest in focusing more broadly on health workforce redesign, and as highlighted in a recent international update by Antunes and Moreira (2013) this is often driven by an attempt to find a policy solution for a range of health system-related problems, such as response to shortages of staff; cost containment; and facilitating the interface between organisations. Approaches to optimising the available workforce and achieving the right number and mix of staff needed to provide high quality care are, however, challenging and complex, with a lack of robust evidence on which to base policy decisions (Dubois & Singh 2009; Antunes & Moreira 2013).

An issue that is central to the debate on skill mix is the value placed on different kinds of work undertaken by health-care staff. Nursing work has been characterised in a variety of ways – for example, technical versus non-technical; direct versus indirect; skilled versus unskilled; acute versus non-acute, and urgent versus non-urgent. The majority of these categorisations are morally loaded terms suggesting a hierarchy of 'value or worth' placed on different activities. The challenge, however, is that greater value is often placed on tangible, observable and objectively measurable activities. The inherent risk in taking such an approach is the reduction of nursing and indeed other roles within the multi-professional team into a series of tasks to be completed. This is contrary to the evidence from service users who, when asked for feedback on the quality of services, usually focus on the more 'relationship'-oriented experiences, the provision of comfort and aesthetic experiences, with the technical aspects of their care often 'taken for granted' (Edwards et al. 2004; McCormack et al.

2008; Laird et al. 2015). Engaging in person-centred ways of working within multi-professional teams requires a different sort of investment that can take account of the intrinsic value of persons in the care experience that needs to be factored into the ongoing debates about skill mix.

Shared decision-making systems

> Organisational commitment to collaborative, inclusive and participative ways of engaging within and between teams.

We have consistently reiterated the importance of person-centredness being about both patients/service users and staff. In this context it is essential that staff experience ways of engaging that facilitate active participation in decisions being made that directly impact on their working environment. Central to this way of working is the development of an effective team. It could be argued that the attributes of an effective workplace culture identified by Manley et al. (2011) are the building blocks to developing an effective team. These attributes include:

- specific values are explicitly shared in the workplace and all these values are realised in practice with an individual and collective responsibility;
- adaptability, innovation and creativity characterise practice;
- appropriate change is driven by the needs of patients/service users/communities; and
- there are formal systems to enable continuous evaluation of learning, evaluation of performance and shared governance.

Furthermore, the development of an effective person-centred and evidence-informed workplace requires the continued commitment to the development of a learning culture at work. Learning cultures are productive cultures, characterised by their ability to tolerate productive tensions, learn from mistakes, support and enable innovation, maximise individual potential and understand the interrelationship between team/system processes and the effectiveness of outcomes achieved (Titchen & Binnie 1995; Kaye & Jordan-Evans 2005). A learning culture is a culture where nurses view their work as exciting and revitalising, offering them the prospect for both personal and professional growth. Creating an environment in which learning occurs takes account of the ward/unit atmosphere, the context within which practice takes place (acute, community, etc.) and the process used to enable learning to occur. Senge (2006) suggests that sustained learning only occurs in a supportive context and where learning is viewed as an integrated component of practice. In 2007, McCormack et al. undertook a realist synthesis of the evidence underpinning practice development. They concluded that a central principle of practice development methodology was that of CIP, that is, individual, team and organisational commitment to Collaborative, Inclusive and Participative ways of working (McCormack et al. 2007). The articulation of CIP principles is consistent with

Senge's (2006) ideas of 'being' in relationship with others, in ways that value the hearing of all voices and the engagement of all in decision-making.

Effective staff relationships

> Interpersonal connections that are productive in the achievement of holistic person-centred care.

In the dialogue surrounding person-centredness there is a propensity, often at a subconscious level, to think in terms of patient and family, often forgetting that we are also talking about relationships within the team. The simple premise within the framework is that we should pay attention, not just to how we develop positive relationships with our patients and service users, but also how we care for our professional relationships. Furthermore, professional interaction should be subject to the same standards of respect and value for persons as applied to those patients under our care. We cannot deny the existence of negative cultures within health and care systems that are characterised by behaviours that fly in the face of person-centredness and that will undoubtedly have an impact, be it direct or indirect, on the care experience for patients and their families. This is reflected in the work of Brown and McCormack (2011), who when exploring context in relation to pain management with older people identified three key themes (psychological safety, leadership, oppression) and four subthemes (power, horizontal violence, distorted perceptions, autonomy) that are significant in the development of a positive relationship and that influenced effective nursing practice. It is important to highlight the connection of these constructs with others within the prerequisites domain, such as our interpersonal abilities, clarity of beliefs and values, and knowing self.

Power sharing

> Non-dominant, non-hierarchical relationships that do not exploit individuals, but instead are concerned with achieving the best mutually agreed outcomes through agreed values, goals, wishes and desires.

Closely linked to the development of effective staff relationships is the issue of power sharing. Whatever approach to ongoing team development is chosen, the issue of power in teams is an inevitable issue and one that is important to consider when thinking about the development of shared decision-making and person-centred practice. Furthermore, it is often in the context of teams that we think about power and its impact on decision-making. Stereotypical hierarchical relationships still exist within organisational systems; this situation requires practitioners to challenge existing practices that cause domination, so we can move away from a reliance on hierarchical power/domination and understand the critical role of knowledge as power. Also, central to this is clarity of role and an appreciation of the contribution of different team members in the overall care experience.

The issue of power sharing in the context of nursing was discussed in detail by McCormack and McCance (2010), but the focus in moving forwards needs to be how we consider the issue of power in our professional relationships with patients and the relationships within the multi-professional team. There is no doubt that for person-centred practice to exist, there is a need for a work organisation method that enables staff to exercise power whilst simultaneously being able to negotiate the nature of that power in relationships with others (including patients and families). Person-centred practice makes explicit the need for autonomy, equality in relationships, and the centrality of beliefs and values in guiding decision-making. Contemporary work into the development of 'models of care' that have the patient at the centre and health-care professionals positioned to facilitate autonomous decision-making, can be seen as attempts to reorientate the design of health-care services towards ones that are based on patient, family and staff experiences.

The physical environment

Health-care environments that balance aesthetics with function by paying attention to design, dignity, privacy, sanctuary, choice/control, safety and universal access with the intention of improving patient, family and staff operational performance and outcomes (adapted from Hospice Friendly Hospitals 2008).

There is now a wide evidence base demonstrating the importance of the physical environment to care and healing. The reality, however, is that the majority of health-care settings continue to be clinical, drab, depressing and soulless. Most hospitals and health-care facilities have been designed with 'clinical efficiency' in mind and not person-centredness. One example is the increase in single rooms, a development that has largely been driven by a safety agenda and based on the assumption that single rooms will reduce the incidence of hospital acquired infection (Cepeda et al. 2005; Bracca et al. 2007). The underpinning evidence, however, remains weak in terms of clinical outcomes. There is also a line of argument that single rooms improve patient satisfaction, and whilst this might be the case in relation to aspects of experience such as noise and privacy and dignity (van de Glind et al. 2007), it does not take account of the presence and visibility of health-care staff, aspects that we know are important to person-centred practice. The aesthetic environment is also a key consideration. Considerable developments have taken place in ensuring the environments are aesthetically pleasing and promote healing, nurturing, care, belonging and sensory engagement. The connection of the arts and humanities with health has been a major development in contemporary health care and is a significant movement internationally. The strategic placement of art (pictures, sculptures and installations) for sensory and emotional stimulation; the use of different light, sounds and smells to promote relaxation and as therapeutic engagement; and the integration of performance art with health-care practice have all become more commonplace.

Whatever the intent, be it therapeutic or social engagement, it is clear that in contemporary health and social care systems, aesthetics matter and the arts play a significant role in creating aesthetically pleasing spaces. The structures and aesthetic qualities of the care environment are interconnected with an individual's sense of self, sense of being and sense of connection with the world, and as such are key considerations in the delivery of person-centredness. Whilst there is a shift to ensuring that new health-care facility designs adopt a person-centred approach, not all patients and staff can expect to work in facilities that are designed with person-centredness explicitly in mind. Hence there is a need to consider how existing environments can be enhanced to facilitate effective person-centred practice.

Supportive organisational systems

> Organisational systems that promote initiative, creativity, freedom and safety of persons, underpinned by a governance framework that emphasises culture, relationships, values, communication, professional autonomy and accountability.

Whilst supportive systems at the team level are essential it is important to recognise that teams exist within a wider organisational context, which can have a significant impact on team functioning. The ongoing research into 'magnet hospitals' has begun to illustrate the organisational conditions that are necessary for staff to feel empowered. Magnet hospitals have been associated with organisational attributes that have been positively linked to nursing staff outcomes (Aiken & Sloan 1997a,b; Aiken et al. 1997). Magnet hospitals have specific organisational attributes that enable effectiveness of practice and patient outcome. Their success is associated with three areas that would have relevance for multi-professional teams:

- Administration – decentralised structures, flexible working, participatory and supportive management style, adequate staffing, the use of specialists, and well-prepared and qualified [nurse] executives.
- Professional practice – professional practice models of delivery, associated autonomy and responsibility, availability of specialist advice and emphasis on teaching.
- Professional development – planned orientation of staff, emphasis on in-service/continuing education, competency-based clinical ladders and management development.

The findings from research by Aiken and colleagues reinforce the need for staff to be recognised, supported and involved in decision-making about patient care and hospital governance through professional autonomy, an environment supportive of professional practice and development, and strong supportive leadership (Gleason-Scott et al. 1999).

Potential for innovation and risk-taking

> The exercising of professional accountability in decision-making that reflects a balance between the best available evidence, professional judgement, local information and patient/family preferences.

In a nursing context, professional autonomy is ranked as one of the most important factors contributing to nurses' job satisfaction (Stamp & Piedmonte 1986). The researchers define autonomy as 'the amount of job independence, initiative, and freedom either permitted or required in daily work activities' (1986, p. 60). From the original research undertaken by McCormack (2001), which underpins the Person-centred Nursing Framework, autonomy is presented as 'interconnectedness', an idea that is well established in the literature (e.g. Gilligan 1982; Gadow 1990; Agich 1993; Tronto 1993). It is based on the premise that people are sometimes autonomous, sometimes dependent and sometimes provide care to those who are dependent (Tronto 1993) and therefore are best described as 'interdependent'. Tronto argues that individualistic notions of 'autonomy as independence' places autonomy and dependence at either end of a continuum, but in reality, dependency in some aspects of life does not lead to dependency in all aspects of life. McCormack (2001) further argues that nurses need to engage with four processes in an interconnected relationship with patients in order to facilitate adaptation and decision-making. These four processes form the foundation for innovation and risk-taking and can equally be applied in a multi-professional context. The four processes include:

1 The facilitation of decision-making through information sharing and the integration of new information into established perspectives and care practices.
2 The recognition of the importance of individual values for decision-making and of knowing how each person's values influence decisions made.
3 The making explicit of intentions and motivations for action and the boundaries within which care decisions are set.
4 The creation of a culture of care that values the views of the patient as a legitimate basis for decision-making whilst recognizing that the [older] person does not always need to be the final arbiter of decisions.

Central to these processes is our understanding of best available evidence, and we look to the seminal work of Rycroft-Malone and colleagues to offer guidance on what constitutes evidence and what should be used to influence decision-making.

Person-centred processes

Person-centred processes focus on delivering care through a range of activities that operationalise person-centred practice; these include: working with patients' beliefs and values; engaging authentically; being sympathetically present; sharing decision-making; and providing holistic care. This is the component of the framework that specifically focuses on the patient, describing person-centred practice in the context of care delivery. It is important at the outset to acknowledge that the person-centred processes are synergistic and often interwoven in the delivery of care.

Working with patients' beliefs and values

> Having a clear picture of what the patient values about his/her life and how he/she makes sense of what is happening from their individual perspective, psychosocial context and social role.

Working with patients' beliefs and values reinforces one of the fundamental principles of person-centred nursing, which places importance on developing a clear picture of what the patient values about his/her life and how he/she makes sense of what is happening. Reality refers to the everyday world and is imbued with personal meanings, beliefs and values that are essential to the way the person 'sees' themselves and the way their world is constructed. Knowing about another's values and beliefs requires caring about the other in a way that appreciates an understanding of each patient as an individual human being. A person's life history shapes who they are today with events influencing and directing the choices they make and the kind of life they want to live. It is this history that gives meaning to the values of the individual, providing an enhanced understanding of what is important to the patient in order to be able to integrate personalised information into a plan of care.

A person-centred assessment is key to obtaining information that builds up a picture of a patient as an individual with a unique life story. This is an area that is also closely connected to the assessment process, and to the thorny issue of documentation and what constitutes the patient record. Professionals approach assessment with specific goals in mind in terms of information required, and it is this that often directs the dialogue with the patient as opposed to engaging in a process that facilitates the gathering of information that begins to build up a picture of that patient as a person. We would argue, however, that information gleaned about a patient is not about a good assessment, but rather is an ongoing process, and it is through authentic engagement that the patient as a person will emerge. Whilst this sounds a lot like 'mom and apple pie' the reality of everyday practice can often work against engaging with patients and their families in this way, frequently resulting in a poor care experience.

Sharing decision-making

> The facilitation of involvement in decision-making by patients and others significant to them by considering values, experiences, concerns and future aspirations.

This element of the framework focuses on professionals facilitating patient participation in decision-making through providing information and integrating newly formed perspectives into established practices. It is closely linked to working with patients' beliefs and values and must involve a process of negotiation that takes account of individual values to form a legitimate basis for decision-making, the success of which rests on successful processes of communication (McCormack & McCance 2006). There is a large and diverse literature about decision-making in professional practice; however, the focus within the framework is on how professionals can facilitate participation in shared decision-making that is underpinned by the principles of person-centredness. In the previous chapter we identified that the right to 'self-determination' is a valued human right. If we do value self-determination, then it follows that we have the right to participate in decision-making about treatment, care options and processes.

Person-centred decision-making holds central the knowledge and experience that each person brings to the care situation and that is necessary for decisions that will best serve the patient's well-being. At the heart of this style of practice is the therapeutic relationship that exists between professional and patient, which acknowledges and values each person's individual perception of their health-care experience. The aim is to transform the person's experience and enable them to consider a variety of perspectives that can help shape perceptions and understandings. The role of the person-centred practitioner is to *be there*, offering personal support and practical expertise, while enabling the patient to follow the path of their own choosing and in their own way

McCormack (2003), in his original research, identifies mutuality as central to the process of shared decision-making, which recognises the others' values as being of equal importance in decision-making. A good therapeutic relationship establishes a personal-professional connection based on mutual respect and honesty (Genevay & Katz 1990). It involves 'being with' and 'doing with', through the active participation of the patient in order to activate the potential within themselves. If a practitioner can trust in the relationship she/he has with a patient, then it is alright to be led by the patient, not in a passive sense of being led, but in a dynamic sense where the cues and nuances of the patient's behaviour direct the focus of the action that needs to be taken. The patient is thus given a real part to play in helping the practitioner to discover new ways of working and a real partnership is established. There are of course other times when firmness in approach has to be taken and sometimes without this firmness the person would feel insecure and at risk. However, as long as the reasons for this are negotiated into the plan of care, partnership can still be maintained. Through mutuality, those who care and those who are cared for don't have to relate to each other as strong and weak, but both can grow in each other's capacity to learn from each other as equals.

Engaging authentically

> The connectedness of the practitioner with a patient and others significant to them, determined by knowledge of the person, clarity of beliefs and values, knowledge of self and professional expertise.

Engagement is a way of working that reflects the connectedness of a practitioner with her/his patient. If we accept that each care situation is approached as a unique interaction and that the focus is on the interaction with *that* person at *that* time, based on their own values and beliefs, we can assume the practitioner is engaging authentically with the patient. The ability to engage and be truly connected with patients is, however, dependent on the practitioner's abilities, as reflected in the prerequisites discussed previously. Knowledge of the person, clarity of beliefs and values, knowledge of self and professional expertise are fundamental to this way of working. As the framework suggests, however, components within the care environment can have a significant bearing on the nurse's ability to engage with patients in the way that has been described, and this further reinforces the need for the nurse to have skills that enables her/him to manage the care environment to maximise benefits for patients.

With this in mind McCormack (2003) presents different levels of engagement (connectedness) – full engagement, partial disengagement and complete disengagement. *Full engagement* is present when the patient and nurse are connected in the relationship and a care partnership exists. Collaborative decision-making takes place and the values of both nurse and patient are present at an unconscious level in the giving and receiving of care. A nurse may be aware of political, environmental and cultural pressures that affect the way they give care, but she/he interprets and prioritises the salient features of such pressures and integrates these into her/his practice. A dilemma, however, may arise in the care relationship that affects the way the nurse and patient are able to work together. As a result *partial disengagement* occurs while the nurse takes stock of the situation and formulates the problem. At this point the interconnected working between the nurse and patient is interrupted, and whatever the cause, the relationship between the nurse and patient is altered and the nurse may lose the maximum grasp that was available while engaged with the patient (Benner & Wrubel 1989). Such disengagement then requires a period of contemplation and, for a period of time, *complete disengagement* occurs. In this stance the nurse contemplates the available options from a more objective stance and reassesses the values that underpin the relationship and decision-making. At this point the nurse needs to decide on appropriate action to reconnect the relationship. Support mechanisms that facilitate reflective practice (Johns 2005; Freshwater 2002) can help achieve this goal. While the nurse continues to work with the patient in seeking the most satisfactory resolution, the connectedness in the relationship is broken until such time as a resolution can be found that is coherent with the values of the patient.

A skilled practitioner will be able to adopt these three different stances at different times with the patient. Each stance may be short lived, but what is important is for the practitioner to be able to move between these positions in order to stand back from the relationship with the patient, contemplate options and establish the most appropriate resolution. Having a clear picture of what patients value about their lives and how they make sense of what is happening to them is needed, which provides a standard against which the practitioner can compare current decisions and behaviours of each patient.

Being sympathetically present

> An engagement that recognises the uniqueness and value of the individual, by appropriately responding to cues that maximise coping resources through the recognition of important agendas in their life.

This component of the framework has generated much discussion due to the use of the term 'sympathetic'. The argument frequently presented is why not use the term empathy, often considered to be more appropriate within a health-care context. Our counterargument has been consistent over time and is well rehearsed in the 2010 edition of the book, but essentially rejects the ability of anyone to be able to fully comprehend another individual's particular experience. The experience of bereavement is a good example that really does place these terms apart. Empathising with a bereaved person, even if you have experienced a similar life event, leaves you no closer to understanding what that experience truly feels like for that individual. Our use of the term 'sympathetic presence' has been chosen carefully to describe a way of being with patients that recognises the uniqueness and value of the individual and reflects the quality of the relationship between practitioner and patient, and in many respects is the fabric that weaves together other person-centred processes. To have a practitioner show, through acceptance of the person, a sympathetic understanding of the patient's losses and present limitations, is to establish a therapeutic relationship, which is directed at gaining an effective outcome from care that is centred on the person's needs and life perspectives. The ability to project a sympathetic presence is therefore dependent on knowing the patients and having insight into their beliefs and values, as discussed previously in this chapter.

The everyday challenge for practitioners is how we convey a sense of sympathetic presence. There can be a strongly held perception that person-centred care is mostly about talking to, and spending time with the patient. We would argue, however, that it is the ability of a practitioner to be available to each patient in that moment. Benner (1984) captures the essence of this when she describes presencing as the art of 'being with' a person without the need to be 'doing to' the person. Every time a patient is approached by a practitioner for whatever reason, be it to administer medication, to perform a procedure, or to ask a specific question, it is an opportunity to be person-centred. There is, however, an argument that being present in this way will uncover issues that need addressing, and this can be challenging for a range of reasons. It might be because the practitioner doesn't feel confident or lacks the competence to deal effectively with the patient's needs, or indeed it could be a consequence of the environment and the other priorities that are bearing down on the practitioner at that time.

Providing holistic care

> The provision of treatment and care that pays attention to the whole person through the integration of physiological, psychological, sociocultural, developmental and spiritual dimensions of persons.

The Person-centred Nursing Framework embraces a broader notion of health that reflects living a positive life, one that embraces all dimensions of being. Considering a social model of health, we have focused on the work of Seedhouse (1986), who refers to a set of conditions that enables a person to work to reach his or her potential and describes health in relation to 'foundations for achievement'. The foundations that make up health, according to Seedhouse, include the basic needs of food, drink, shelter, warmth and so on; access to the widest possible information and the skills and confidence to assimilate this information; and the recognition that an individual is never totally isolated from other people and the external environment and cannot be fully understood separated from the influence of his or her environment. In this context, we encourage a more holistic multi-dimensional approach to identifying patient need derived from a conceptual model developed by Betty Neuman (1995) within mental health nursing:

> The *physiological variable* refers to bodily structure and function; the *psychological variable*, to mental processes and relationships; the *sociocultural variable*, to social and cultural functions; the *developmental variable* to the developmental processes of life; and the *spiritual variable*, to the influence of spiritual beliefs.
>
> Neuman (1995, p. 225; italics in original)

There is, however, still an acceptance that irrespective of the person-centred processes discussed above, important aspects of holistic care are often achieved during the process of delivering routine technical and physical aspects of care. The challenge is ensuring that practitioners pay attention to the whole person in a way that can deliver an overall therapeutic benefit.

Person-centred outcomes

Person-centred outcomes are the central construct within the framework and represent the results expected from effective person-centred practice. It is worthy of note that this is the domain within the framework that has changed most significantly since the 2010 publication, which reflects advances in evaluation of practice development work. The outcomes include a good experience of care (previously satisfaction with care), involvement in care, feeling of well-being, and existence of a healthful culture (previously creating a therapeutic environment).

Good care experience

A good care experience reflects the evaluation a patient, or indeed a nurse, places on their care episode. The decision to refine this outcome measure was based on research outputs but also on strategy and policy directions that were focusing on patient experience. Whilst accepting that *satisfaction with care* is a well-established outcome measure in nursing and health care, it is also one of the most challenging outcomes to evaluate, a point well rehearsed in the 2010 edition. The challenges discussed still stand, but the most pertinent point to reinforce is the evaluation of patient satisfaction, which is often undertaken at organisational level using surveys, which lack depth, fail to capture individual perspectives of satisfaction and can often lack conceptual rigour (Edwards et al. 2004). Patient experience, on the other hand, provides very different feedback and is defined as 'feedback from patients on "what actually happened" in the course of receiving care or treatment, both the objective facts and their subjective views of it' (http://www.healthcaregovernance.org.au/docs/the-intelligent-board-patient-experience-2010.pdf). Innovative and creative ways to capture patient experience are also evolving, with the data produced arguably more compelling when it comes to making changes in practice (Laird et al. 2015). Furthermore, a good care experience is more inclusive of staff who also want to experience good care. We already know from the evidence that being enabled to deliver person-centred care has benefits for staff and consequently enhances retention and job satisfaction (Slater et al. 2009, 2010; Brown & McCormack 2011; Hahtela et al. 2015).

Involvement in care

Feeling involved in care is a key part of contemporary health-care strategy and policy, and there is an explicit expectation that patients will be active participants in their own care. Examples such as 'the expert patient initiative' are predicated on the assumption that people will be active participants in their care and work in partnership with health-care professionals. Thus evaluating the extent to which people feel involved in their care would seem to be a key focus of person-centred outcome evaluation. In addition, from a staff perspective, being involved in the decision-making process is a key focus of many models of care that aim to ensure that care decisions are made by practitioners working directly with patients.

Feeling of well-being

Having a feeling of well-being underpins the aims of many caring theories, rehabilitation models and care practices. McCance (2003) clearly articulated how positive care experiences engendered feelings of well-being among patients and are indicative of the patient feeling valued. Similarly, practitioners need to feel valued for their work, and this is also considered a key aspect of outcome evaluation in person-centred practice. This is also supported by more recent work undertaken by Titchen and McCormack (2010), who suggest that human flourishing is the overall outcome arising from working in a person-centred way. They argue that when practitioners integrate the creative energies of different forms of knowledge and intelligences, growthful experiences for all (e.g. staff, service users, families) are enabled.

Existence of a healthful culture

A healthful culture is described as one in which decision-making is shared, staff relationships are collaborative, leadership is transformational and innovative practices are supported; it is the ultimate outcome for teams working to develop a workplace that is person-centred. This is a key factor in the delivery of person-centred care, and the extent to which the environment supports and maintains person-centred principles has been shown to be critical to person-centred practice. The move away from the term 'therapeutic' is consistent with the broader notion being used in the context of the framework, which focuses on living a positive life embracing all dimensions of our being. The term 'therapeutic' was used to reflect the positive nature of expected outcomes, but analysis of the term would suggest a 'health' benefit, thus not accurately reflecting the potential outcomes for all who are engaged in the care process. The use of the term 'healthful' reflects good health achievement more broadly. This is reinforced in a study by Laird et al. (2015), whose findings reflected care environments that emphasise more than care and treatment, but offer insights in terms of the social and cultural context. This broader notion of health is also more relevant from the perspective of staff, where a healthful culture is one in which they are supported and enabled to deliver person-centred care in line with their values. We already know from the evidence that being enabled to deliver person-centred care has benefits for staff and consequently enhances retention and job satisfaction (Kings Fund 2010). These outcomes again reflect a broader notion of health that reflects different dimensions of our life including the experiences we have in our work life. For these reasons, we have broadened our definition of person-centredness:

> … an approach to practice established through the formation and fostering of healthful relationships between all care providers, service users and others significant to them in their lives. It is underpinned by values of respect for persons, individual right to self-determination, mutual respect and understanding. It is enabled by cultures of empowerment that foster continuous approaches to practice development.

The outcomes identified within the framework provide a clear focus for evaluation of person-centred practice. Outcomes can be demonstrated from the perspectives of both staff and patients/families. In our programme of work we have used multiple approaches to evaluation and embraced a wide range of methods. A detailed critique of outcome evaluation is provided in the 2010 edition, with suggested frameworks aimed at supporting practitioners to evidence their practice. This is, however, an area that continues to develop with emergence of innovative ways to approach evaluation of person-centred outcomes.

Summary

This chapter presents the Person-centered Practice Framework, a conceptual model that has been developed from practice, for use in practice. The development of the model is presented, describing changes made over time, based on its use in practice and research. The framework highlights the complexity of person-centred practice, and through the articulation of the key constructs, emphasises the contextual, attitudinal and moral dimensions of humanistic caring practices. The relationship between the constructs describes the need for competent practitioners, who have the ability to manage the numerous contextual and attitudinal factors that exist within care environments, to engage in processes that keep the person at the centre of caring interactions. The outcomes arising from the development of person-centred practice demonstrate the potential to enhance the care experience for both patients and staff. Whilst the framework originated within nursing and was developed largely within a nursing context, its use can now be evidenced across the wider health-care workforce and its impact within multi-professional environments is the focus for the future.

References

Agich, G.J. (1993) *Autonomy and Long-Term Care*, Oxford University Press, Oxford.

Aiken, L.H. and Sloane, D.M. (1997a) Effects of organizational innovations in AIDS care on burnout among urban hospital nurses. *Work and Occupations*, **24** (4), 453–77.

Aiken, L.H. and Sloane, D.M. (1997b) Effects of specialization and client differentiation on the status of nurses: The case of AIDS. *Journal of Health and Social Behavior*, **38** (3), 203–22.

Aiken, L.H., Sloane, D.M., and Lake, E.T. (1997) Satisfaction with inpatient acquired immunodeficiency syndrome care – A national comparison of dedicated and scattered-bed units. *Medical Care*, **35** (9), 948–62.

Antunes, A. and Moreira, P. (2013) Skill mix in healthcare: An international update for the management debate. *International Journal of Healthcare Management*, **6** (1), 12–17. doi: 10.1179/2047970012Z.00000000028

Benner, P. (1984) *From Novice to Expert: Excellence and Power in Clinical Nursing Practice*, Addison-Wesley Publishing Co.

Benner, P. and Wrubel, J. (1989) *The Primacy of Caring: Stress and Coping in Health and Illness*, Addison-Wesley Publishing Company, Wokingham.

Brown, A. (1998) *Organisational Culture*, 2nd edn, Pitman Publishing, London.

Berwick, D.M. (2013) *A promise to learn – a commitment to act*, Improving the safety of patients in England. London, Department of Health.

Bracco, D., Dubois, M.J., Bouali, R., and Eggimann, P. (2007) Single rooms may help to prevent nosocomial bloodstream infection and cross-transmission of methicillin-resistant Staphylococcus aureus in intensive care units. *Intensive Care Medicine*, **33**, 836–40.

Brown, D. and McCormack, B. (2011) Developing the practice context to enable more effective pain management with older people: an action research approach. *Implementation Science*, **6** (9). doi: 10.1186/1748-5908-6-9

Buchan J and Calman L. (2005) *Skill-Mix and Policy Change in the Health Workforce: Nurses in Advanced Roles.* OECD Health Working Papers, No. 17, OECD Publishing. Available from: 10.1787/743610272486 (accessed 28 January 2016).

Buckley, C., McCormack, B., and Ryan, A. (2014) Valuing narrative in the care of older people. *Journal of Clinical Nursing*, **23**, 2565–77.

Cepeda, J.A., Whitehouse, T., Cooper, B. *et al.* (2005) Isolation of patients in single rooms or cohorts to reduce spread of MRSA in intensive-care unit: prospective two centre study. *Lancet*, **365**, 295–304.

Dewing, W.N., Evans, D., Bradley, H., and Ullrich, S. (2014a) Person-centred care in the Indonesian health-care system. *International Journal of Nursing Practice*, **20**, 616–22.

Dewing, J., McCormack, B., and Titchen, A. (2014b) *Practice Development Workbook for Nursing, Health and Social Care Teams*, Wiley-Blackwell, Oxford.

DHSSPSNI (Department of Health, Social Services and Public Safety Northern Ireland) (2010) *A Partnership for Care – Northern Ireland Strategy for Nursing and Midwifery 2010-2015.* Belfast: DHSSPSNI. Available from: www.dhsspsni.gov.uk (accessed 9 August 2015).

DHSSPSNI (Department of Health, Social Services and Public Safety Northern Ireland) (2013) *Service Framework for Older People.* Belfast: Department of Health, Social Services and Public Safety. Available at: http://www.scie-socialcareonline.org.uk/service-framework-for-older-people/r/a11G000000CTDW7IAP (accessed 22 February 2016).

Dubois, C.A. and Singh, D. (2009) From staff-mix to skill-mix and beyond: towards a systematic approach to health workforce management. *Human Resources for Health*, **7** (87), 1–20.

Edwards, C., Staniszweska, S., and Crichton, N. (2004) Investigation of the ways in which patients' reports of their satisfaction with healthcare are constructed. *Sociology of Health & Illness*, **26**, 159–83.

Fawcett, J. (1995) *Analysis and Evaluation of Conceptual Models of Nursing*, 3rd edn, F.A. Davis Co., Philadelphia.

Francis, R. (2013) *The Mid-Staffordshire NHS Foundation Trust Public Enquiry*, The Stationery Office, London.

Freshwater, D. (2002) *Therapeutic Nursing: Improving Patient Care through Self Awareness and Reflection*, Sage, London.

Gadow, S. (1990) Existential advocacy: philosophical foundations of nursing, in *Ethics in Nursing: An Anthology* (eds T. Pence and J. Cantrell), National League for Nursing, New York.

Genevay, B. and Katz, R.S. (1990) *Countertransference and Older Clients*, Sage, London.

Gilligan, C. (1982) *In a Different Voice: Psychological Theory and Women's Development*, Harvard University Press, Cambridge, MA.

Gleason-Scott, J., Sochalski, J., and Aiken, L. (1999) Review of magnet hospitals research. *Journal of Nursing Administration*, **29** (1), 9–19.

Goleman, D. (1999) *Working with Emotional Intelligence*, Bloomsbury, London.

Hager, P., Gonzi, A., and Athamasou, J. (1994) General issues about assessment of competence. *Assessment and Evaluation in Higher Education*, **19**, 3–16.

Hahtela, N., Paavilainen, E., McCormack, B., Slater, P., Helminen, M., and Suominen, T. (2015) Influence of workplace culture on nursing-sensitive nurse outcomes in municipal primary health care. *Journal of Nursing Management*, **23**, 931–9.

Hospice Friendly Hospitals Programme (2008) *Design and Dignity Guidelines for Physical Environments of Hospitals Supporting End-of-Life Care.* Dublin: The Irish Hospice Foundation. Available at: www.hospicefriendlyhospitals.net

Johns, C. (2005) Appreciating (guided) reflection as a process of self-inquiry and transformation toward realizing desirable practice. *International Journal of Human Caring*, **9** (2), 139.

Kaye, B.L. and Jordan-Evans, S. (2005) *Love 'Em or Lose 'Em: Getting Good People to Stay*, Berrett-Koehler Publishers, San Francisco.

Kings Fund (2010) *The Intelligence Board: Patient Experience*, Kings Fund, London.

Kouzes, J. and Posner, B. (2002) *The Leadership Challenge*, 3rd edn, Jossey-Bass, San Francisco.

Laird, E.A., McCance, T.V., McCormack, B., and Gribben, B. (2015) Patients' experiences of in-hospital care when nursing staff were engaged in a practice development programme to promote person-centredness: A narrative analysis study. *International Journal of Nursing Studies*, **52**, 1454–62.

Lown, B.A., Rosen, J., and Marttila, J. (2011) An agenda for improving compassionate care: A survey shows about half of patients say such care is missing. *Health Affairs*, **30**, 1772–8.

Lynch, B., McCormack, B., and McCance, T. (2011) Development of a model of situational leadership in residential care for older people. *Journal of Nursing Management*, **19**, 1058–69.

Manley, K. (2004) Transformational culture: a culture of effectiveness, in *Practice Development in Nursing* (eds B. McCormack, K. Manley, and R. Garbett), Blackwell Publishing, Oxford, pp. 51–82.

Manley K, Sanders K, Cardiff S, Webster J. (2011) Effective workplace culture: the attributes, enabling factors and consequences of a new concept. *International Practice Development Journal* **1**(2): art. 1, 1–29.

McCance, T.V. (2003) Caring in nursing practice: the development of a conceptual framework. *Research and Theory for Nursing Practice: An International Journal*, **17**, 101–116.

McCance T, Gribben B, McCormack B, Laird E. (2013) Promoting person-centred practice within acute care: The impact of culture and context on a facilitated practice development programme. *International Practice Development Journal* **3**(1): manuscript 2.

McConnell, D., McCance, T., and Melby, V. (2015) Exploring person-centredness in emergency departments: A literature review. *International Emergency Nursing*. doi: 10.1016/j.ienj.2015.10.001

McCormack, B. (2001) *Negotiating Partnerships with Older People: A Person-centred Approach*, Ashgate, Basingstoke.

McCormack, B. (2003) A conceptual framework for person-centred practice with older people. *International Journal of Nursing Practice*, **9**, 202–9.

McCormack, B. and McCance, T.V. (2006) Developing a conceptual framework for person-centred nursing. *Journal of Advanced Nursing*, **56**, 472–9.

McCormack, B. and McCance, T.V. (2010) *Person-Centred Nursing; Theory and Practice*, Wiley-Blackwell, Chichester.

McCormack B and McCance T. (2015) United Kingdom: Person-centred Nursing Model. In: Fitzpatrick JJ and Whall AL (eds), *Conceptual Models of Nursing: Analysis and Application*. Pearson Education.

McCormack, B., Wright, J., Dewar, B., Harvey, G., and Ballintine, K. (2007) A realist synthesis of evidence relating to practice development: interviews and synthesis of data. *Practice Development in Health Care*, **6**, 56–75.

McCormack, B., McCance, T., Slater, P., McCormick, J., McArdle, C., and Dewing, J. (2008) Person-centred outcomes and cultural change, in *International Practice Development in Nursing and Healthcare* (eds K. Manley, B. McCormack, and V. Wilson), Blackwell Publishing, Ltd., Oxford, pp. 189–214.

McCormack, B., McCarthy, G., Wright, J., and Coffey, A. (2009) Development and testing of the Context Assessment Index (CAI). *Worldviews on Evidence-Based Nursing*, **6**, 27–35.

McCormack B, Dewing J, Breslin L et al. (2010) The Implementation of a Model of Person-Centred Practice in Older Person Settings. Final Report. Dublin: Office of the Nursing Services Director, Health Services Executive.

McCormack B, Dewing J, McCance T. (2011) Developing person-centred care: addressing contextual challenges through practice development. *Online Journal of Issues in Nursing* **16**(2): manuscript 3.

McCormack, B., Manley, K., and Titchen, A. (eds) (2013) *Practice Development in Nursing and Healthcare*, Wiley-Blackwell, Oxford.

Napier, A.D., Ancarno, C., Butler, B. *et al.* (2014) Culture and health – The Lancet commissions. *The Lancet*, **384**, 1607–39.

Neuman, B. (1995) Neuman's Systems Model, in *Analysis and Evaluation of Conceptual Models of Nursing* (ed J. Fawcett), F.A. Davis Co., Philadelphia, pp. 217–76.

Royal College of Nursing (2010) *The Principles of Nursing Practice*, Royal College of Nursing, London.

Rycroft-Malone, J. (2004) PARIHS Framework: A framework for guiding the implementation of evidence based practice. *Journal of Nursing Care Quality*, **19**, 297–304.

Rycroft-Malone, J., Seers, K., Chandler, J. *et al.* (2013) Role of evidence, context, and facilitation in an implementation trial: implication for the development of the PARIHS Framework. *Implementation Science*, **8** (28). doi: 10.1186/1748-5908-8-28

Schon, D.A. (1983) *The Reflective Practitioner: How Professionals Think in Action*, Basic Books, New York.

Seedhouse, D. (1986) *Health: The Foundations for Achievement*, John Wiley & Sons, Ltd., Chichester.

Senge, P. (2006) *The Fifth Discipline*, Random House Business Books, London.

Slater, P., Bunting, B., and McCormack, B. (2009) The development and pilot testing of an instrument to measure nurses' working environment: The Nursing Context Index. *Worldviews on Evidence-Based Nursing*, **6**, 173–82.

Slater, P., O'Halloran, P., Connolly, D., and McCormack, B. (2010) Testing the Factor Structure of the Nursing Work Index – Revised. *Worldviews on Evidence Based Nursing*, **7** (3), 123–34.

Slater P, McCance T, McCormack B. (2015) Exploring person-centred practice within acute hospital settings. *International Practice Development Journal* **5** (Suppl) [09]. Available at: http://www.fons.org/Resources/Documents/Journal/Vol5Suppl/IPDJ_05%28suppl%29_09.pdf (accessed 28 January 2016).

Stamp, P.L. and Piedmonte, E.B. (1986) *Nurses and Work Satisfaction an Index of Measurement*, DC Heath, Lexington, MA.

Sundberg, L. (2001) A holistic approach to competence development. *Systems Research and Behavioural Science*, **18**, 103–14.

Tanay, M.A.L., Roberts, J., and Ream, E. (2013) Humour in adult cancer care: a concept analysis. *Journal of Advanced Nursing*, **69**, 2131–40.

Titchen, A. and Binnie, A. (1995) The art of clinical supervision. *Journal of Clinical Nursing*, **4**, 327–34.

Titchen, A. and McCormack, B. (2010) Dancing with stones: critical creativity as methodology for human flourishing. *Educational Action Research*, **18**, 531–54.

Tremayne, P. (2014) Using humour to enhance the nurse-patient relationship. *Nursing Standard*, **28** (30), 37–40.

Tronto, J.C. (1993) *Moral Boundaries: A Political Argument for an Ethic of Care*, Routledge, London.

van de Glind, I., de Roode, S., and Goossensen, A. (2007) Do patients in hospital benefit from single rooms: A literature review. *Health Policy*, **84**, 153–61.

Watson, J. (1985) *Nursing: Human Science and Human Care – A Theory of Nursing*, National League of Nursing Press, New York.

WHO (World Health Organization) (2007) *People-centred Healthcare: A Policy Framework*, WHO, Geneva.

The building blocks to enable person-centredness

CHAPTER 4

Person-centred approaches: a policy perspective

Jon Glasby

University of Birmingham, UK

As all the different contributions to this edited collection attest, person-centred approaches have long been a core feature of nursing and of health care more generally. However, such concepts have not always been centre stage in terms of policy, sometimes giving the impression that what happens in front-line practice is a long way from what gets talked about nationally. For all the reasons set out in the introduction to this book, however, the notion of person-centred care is now being picked up, explored and hopefully prioritised in a series of different policy debates – all of which are influenced by (but which in turn will help influence) practice. Designed as something of an overview of these issues, this chapter focuses on three such developments, each of which tends to be viewed in isolation, but which (it is argued here) are all essential to any serious exploration of what being 'person-centred' means. These are:

- the focus on integrated care;
- the importance of delivering compassionate care;
- the need to make services more personal to the individual receiving them.

While the bulk of this chapter focuses on these issues in a UK context (and many of the specific policies named are actually from England), similar priorities typically exist internationally – see, for example, Vidhya Alakeson's (2007, 2010) work on personalisation in a US context, or the work of bodies such as the International Foundation for Integrated Care around national and international attempts to develop more joined-up services (http://integratedcarefoundation .org/). Thus, this chapter is a case study of the UK National Health Service (NHS) context, but one that would identify themes relevant to and recognisable by an international audience.

In one sense, the three policy priorities above might be conceived of as operating at different levels: how *national systems/structures* deliver care in a joined-up way; how *local organisations* deliver compassionate care; and how *individual practitioners* tailor the support they give to individual circumstances. This is similar to a framework initially identified by Glasby (2003) in the context of hospital

Person-Centred Practice in Nursing and Health Care: Theory and Practice, Second Edition.
Edited by Brendan McCormack and Tanya McCance.
© 2017 John Wiley & Sons, Ltd. Published 2017 by John Wiley & Sons, Ltd.

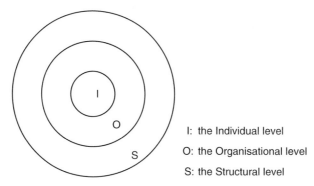

I: the Individual level

O: the Organisational level

S: the Structural level

Figure 4.1 Different levels of intervention. Source: Glasby (2003). Reproduced with permission of Taylor & Francis.

discharge inter-agency working, which sought to identify the different types of focus there may need to be if more coordinated care is to be achieved (Figure 4.1). While some actions might be needed at the level of *structures* or *systems* (the 'S' level), others might depend on *local organisations* (the 'O' level) or *individual practitioners* (the 'I' level). To be truly effective, action might be needed at all three levels at once, as each interacts with and is influenced by the other. Thus, the way in which individual workers practise is important, but is shaped by a local organisational context and by the way in which services more generally are structured. Equally, the national structure of health and social care depends in part on the characteristics, behaviours and culture of a series of local organisations, which ultimately depend on the people working in those organisations. In this sense, each level of the framework is mutually reinforcing, and only a multi-faceted response will be sufficient. Thus, this chapter argues that the apparently simple concept of 'person-centred' care is actually very complex – and that an equally multi-faceted, multi-level response will be required if person-centred practice is to become a reality and to become the norm. This might then help to develop the initial framework of person-centred practice set out in this book (see Chapter 3), potentially adding a consideration of broader policy and the wider context to more individual and organisational dimensions.

Integrated care (structural/systems level)

Any complex system needs to reflect on the best way of organising its work, and there will always be a potential balance to be struck between a specialist approach (requiring very detailed and specific technical expertise) and a more generic approach (which might be able to respond to a broader range of needs in a more holistic manner). However, in services as complex as health and social care, there is a danger that the way in which we organise our work can become very rigid and compartmentalised, failing to do justice to the richness of people's lives (not just the complex nature of specific health problems, but also the ways in which multiple, cross-cutting needs can interact and create additional complexity). A classic example of this is the current focus on 'integrated care' or joint working, where policy makers over time have sought to find ways of encouraging a series of different health and social services to work together more effectively in situations where people using services have multiple needs. While the 'New Labour' government (1997–2010) tended to talk about 'partnership working', more recent policy refers more to 'integrated care' – but the aspirations are arguably the same. Whether we describe this as 'seamless services', 'collaboration', 'joint working' or 'person-centred care', the aim is for services that could help an individual to work together to meet need in a holistic way (rather than the individual having to divide up their life in different ways to fit the needs and requirements of individual agencies). As an example, National Voices (a national coalition of health and social care charities in England) has worked with a number of patient groups to create a series of so-called 'I statements' (things that people using services want to experience when different services need to work together to meet needs; see Box 4.1).

Box 4.1 National Voices 'I statements'.

Person centred coordinated care means that: '*I can plan my care with people who work together to understand me and my carer(s), allow me control, and bring together services to achieve the outcomes important to me.*'

(National Voices 2013)

This desire for greater coordination of care and support takes a number of forms, but a key fault line in the English system is the now notorious divide between health and social care (see Glasby & Dickinson 2014 for an overview). Ever since the foundation of the NHS, our system has been based on the assumption that it is possible (and may be even desirable) to distinguish between people who are 'sick' (who we see as having 'health needs' met free at the point of delivery by the NHS) and people who are merely 'frail' or 'disabled' (who we see as having 'social care needs' met by local government and where people are means-tested and charged for their care). Whether or not such a distinction ever made sense, this division feels increasingly inappropriate given more recent demographic changes and in an era of long-term conditions. Certainly, it is hard to imagine anyone inventing a 'health and social care divide' if they were starting with a blank sheet of paper, and there have been numerous policy initiatives from successive governments to encourage more effective collaboration across this structural division. However, once such a distinction is embedded in service structures it spawns a series of different ways of working, so that health and social care today have different legal frameworks and budgets, different IT systems, different geographical boundaries, different cultures and different ways of training and educating practitioners. This has led one commentator to argue that 'you can't integrate a square peg into a round hole' (one of the 'five laws of integration' identified by Leutz 1999). And yet this is precisely what front-line practitioners (nurses included) are asked to do – part of the task is to try to join up services that haven't been designed with integration in mind.

Against this background, health-care practitioners seeking to work in a person-centred manner are likely to have experienced the knock-on effects of some of the policies set out in Box 4.2 – and are also likely to be working in much more multi-disciplinary settings than ever before (whether part of a nursing team and working in depth with a wide range of colleagues from different professional backgrounds through to being part of fully integrated health and social care teams, with a single line manager, a single assessment process, data sharing agreements, a shared office, etc.). This might bring new opportunities and new challenges, but also means that the ability to work collaboratively, to build relationships and to compare and contrast different ways of seeing the world and doing things will be even more important in future than previously. As suggested above, these are also longstanding debates in other health systems, with a range of different models emerging in different settings in order to try to tackle the same underlying problems of complexity and fragmentation (see, e.g., Glasby and Dickinson 2009).

Box 4.2 Policy initiatives to encourage more integrated care (very selected).

Over time, new policies at national (England) and local level have included developments such as:
- Co-location of staff.
- The creation of multi-disciplinary teams.
- Single assessment.
- New care/case management roles with a focus on care coordination.
- Greater emphasis on data sharing and use of IT.
- The creation of pooled health and social care budgets.
- Joint appointments.
- Joint commissioning.
- The development of services such as intermediate care to prevent older people being admitted to hospital where appropriate and to facilitate swift discharge.
- The creation of a single health and social care inspectorate.
- The transfer of some public health responsibilities to local government.
- The creation of new Health and Well-being Boards to oversee joint working at local level.
- The creation of integrated health and social care organisations.
- National integrated care organisation pilots and 'integrated care pioneers' (to learn more about and share what works).

Compassionate care (organisational level)

In addition to the current emphasis on 'integrated care', there is also significant emphasis being placed on the need to deliver more compassionate care. That this even needed saying will come as a surprise to many – but the ramifications of the Francis Inquiry (Francis 2013) into events in Mid-Staffordshire and other recent care scandals have provoked a broader debate about current practice and about the priorities of health policy (see Chapter 1 in this book for further discussion). Again, this is not uncommon internationally, with high-profile scandals often prompting a period of significant soul-searching and media debate. However, at this moment in time, the recent UK focus has been around the growing sense that too much emphasis has been placed on very narrow measures of performance (both financial and waiting time targets), with insufficient attention on the quality of care actually being delivered. When care scandals have occurred, it has often been nurses and their work that have been directly in the firing line, with other professions and workers seeming to attract less vitriol and criticism from the media.

When care scandals occur, members of the public frequently wonder how such terrible things could occur and how people who have chosen to work in a caring profession could end up being responsible for such awful situations and events. However, the work of Yvonne Sawbridge and Alistair Hewison (2011, 2012, 2013, 2014) has provided a series of important insights into these issues – arguing that health care is a form of 'emotional labour'. While this might be unfamiliar language to some, it draws attention to the fact that care is frequently very difficult, very distressing and can often be very disgusting (involving tasks and topics that we rarely discuss in broader society). Doing care work day in and day out is phenomenally challenging, and doing it well requires amazing levels of resilience and support. All of us have an 'emotional bank account' that is constantly depleted by the things we see and have to do – and each of us has to find ways of keeping that emotional bank account topped up. If we're not careful, we can easily reach a situation where we feel stressed and burned out; where we get a sense of compassion fatigue; and where we fail to deliver the kind of care we would want to receive ourselves if we were using services. In a worst case scenario, we can experience what is sometimes described as a 'corruption of care', where the aim ceases to be looking after people who need our help, and becomes more about getting through the working day in a way that still leaves us sane at the end of it (see Martin 1984, for a summary of the lessons from long-stay hospital scandals – an extreme example of a 'corruption of care' in practice).

In contrast, Sawbridge and Hewison argue for the need for health-care organisations to pay as much attention to the ways in which they support staff to deliver high-quality, dignified, person-centred care as they do to issues such as finances or waiting times. Building on this, work is underway on a number of projects, including action learning sets with nurse leaders to explore new ways of supporting staff to joint work with the Samaritans to draw out lessons for the NHS from the way in which the Samaritans support their volunteers. A helpful summary is also provided by Jocelyn Cornwell (2011) in a Health Foundation blog on care and compassion in the NHS:

> Staff don't need more blame and condemnation; they need active, sustained supervision and support. In the high-volume, high-pressure, complex environment of modern health care it is very difficult to remain sensitive and caring towards every single patient all of the time. We ask ourselves how it is possible that anyone, let alone a nurse, could ignore a dying man's request for water? What we should also ask is whether it is humanly possible for anyone to look after very sick, very frail, possibly incontinent, possibly confused patients without excellent induction, training, supervision and support.
>
> *Cornwell (2011)*

Personalisation (individual level)

Although newer to the NHS, the personalisation agenda has been a key feature of adult social care since the mid-2000s (and many of the concepts involved go back many years to the mid-1980s and early 1990s). Like other themes in this chapter, it is also arguably part of an international trend towards greater choice and control and greater self-direction of services received (see, e.g., Alakeson 2010). While 'personalisation' is often poorly defined and hotly debated (see Needham & Glasby 2014, for a summary), two of the key UK mechanisms include:

- *Direct payments*: Invented by disabled people in order to give people greater choice and control over their services and hence over their lives, direct payments were introduced in the UK in the early 1980s, with groups of disabled people lobbying their councils for greater control over the money being spent on their behalf. This was recognised in 1996 with the Community Care (Direct Payments) Act after a longstanding struggle by disabled campaigners. With a direct payment, money is transferred to the disabled person to hire their own personal assistants and/or to commission a private or a voluntary agency to provide care, with the disabled person becoming either an employer or the micro-commissioner of their own care. A crucial aspect of direct payments has been the availability of support, with disabled people's Centres for Independent Living providing significant practical and peer support.
- *Personal budgets*: Developing initially in learning disability services, a personal budget involves being clear with the person from day 1 how much money is available to spend on meeting their needs, then allowing them greater control over how this money is spent. This could be via public, private or voluntary services, via a mix of all three or via something that does not look like traditional services at all. By being fully transparent about the money, both service user and the social worker know how much they have to play with when trying to meet need and, in theory, can be much more creative and innovative. Successive governments have pledged that all adult social care will be delivered via a personal budget (except in an emergency), with more recent pronouncements

suggesting that the default position should be a direct payment (unless there is a good reason why not).

More recently, such approaches have spread to the NHS, with the advent of personal health budgets (Forder et al. 2012; Alakeson 2014). Although these are likely to be very new to an NHS audience, they are potentially very powerful ways of working – and might involve the worker and the person receiving care coming together as a partnership of equals (with one person a technical expert, but the other an expert in what works for them/what they would like their life to be like). While this would not be appropriate for many areas of the NHS, it could be particularly important in areas where:

- It could make a real difference if people (service users and staff) knew in advance how much money was available to spend on meeting a given need.
- The need could be met much more fully if the person and the worker had the genuine capacity to be creative and innovative.
- The way a need is met is likely to be highly personal (and where the process is almost as important as the outcome).

Applying such criteria in practice might lead to experiments around new, more person-centred ways of working in services for people with long-term conditions, in continuing health care, in mental health rehabilitation and crisis services, in services for disabled children, in end-of-life care, and so on (see Box 4.3 for a case study). Ultimately, some would argue that a true test of whether care is sufficiently person-centred is the extent to which patients and those who know them well/really care about them feel that they can control what happens to them – and are fully involved as partners in care at all stages of the process.

Box 4.3 Personal health budgets in action: Thomas's story (see http://www.peoplehub.org.uk/thomas-story/)

Our son, Thomas, has profound and multiple learning disabilities. The traditional system of support through a care provider failed to meet his needs. The stress and impact on day to day family life was, at times, unbearable. This all changed when we chose to take greater responsibility for Thomas's care through a personal budget, which enabled us to make important decisions and choose how Thomas was cared for and who supports him. Having this choice and control is vital to keep Thomas safe, healthy and happy.

Thomas has Lennox–Gastaut syndrome (a form of severe epilepsy that begins in childhood and is characterised by multiple types of seizures and intellectual disability). Early prognosis and treatment was problematic and inconsistent, with no clear picture from clinicians and other experts of what the future would hold for Thomas. This inevitably caused significant stress and anxiety and we were given very little choice or information as to how Thomas could be supported or how his complex medical needs could be met. As Thomas's epilepsy was difficult to control at home, we felt he may be better supported at a specialist centre for people with epilepsy. This residential placement was based over a hundred miles away from his family home and proved to be disastrous. Thomas was neglected, his medication was not administered or managed properly and the care he received was shocking. Thomas's agreed care plan was not followed. As a result, Thomas became withdrawn and was unhappy.

His weight dropped rapidly causing serious concerns for his health. With the support of our GP and Social Worker, Thomas returned home and we decided, the only way to keep Thomas safe was to take control over his care. This was met through a local authority funded direct payment. Under this arrangement we employed and trained Thomas's carers, who followed his Care Plan, with our support. We also managed the care on a day to day basis, through a circle of support, including input from school, neurologist, GPs and other clinicians.

This new way of working transformed Thomas's life for the better. His weight improved and he became healthier and much happier. We demonstrated that we did know Thomas better than anyone else, and as experts by experience, we were able to ensure that Thomas could live the life he wants to live and is able to make changes when required. We received local authority direct payments for 9 years, until Thomas was 18. At this time he was assessed and qualified for fully funded continuing health care. However, the choice and control Thomas had previously benefitted from was no longer available to him. The NHS had just completed a 3-year pilot for Personal Health Budgets (PHBs), which would allow Thomas to continue to benefit from choice and control over his health and well-being; however, at that time they were unable to offer this option. This meant we had to submit a proposal and detailed care plan to demonstrate how Thomas's needs could be met through greater personalisation than the traditional model of agency support deployed by the NHS for people who qualified for continuing health care. We contacted the National Peer Network for PHBs, who provided invaluable support and practical advice and information from people who had lived experience of PHBs. By working with the Peer Group Network, we were able to produce a detailed proposal and care plan, which contained processes and protocols and, importantly, measureable outcomes and clear roles and responsibilities for commissioners, Thomas' representatives, third party provider and care staff to ensure Thomas is safe and receives the best possible care. Our proposals were fully supported by Healthwatch (http://www.healthwatch.co.uk/) and approved by the local NHS team. Thomas's PHB was in place on 1 April 2013.

To ensure we focus our time and effort on Thomas, we use a Third Party to help us manage Thomas's budget and to provide additional support with HR and training for a larger care team. This arrangement is working well and, importantly, ensures we can demonstrate to the local NHS that Thomas is safe and that his money is used efficiently in a targeted way to support delivery of his care plan. We are now working locally and nationally to promote PHBs, and other families are now starting to benefit from this new, and better way of delivering quality care to some of the most vulnerable people in society.

Summary

Anyone using health services themselves or worried about a loved one with health needs would want the care that is provided to be person-centred. And yet, frontline staff trying to deliver more person-centred care in practice do so in an environment that is heavily influenced by the organisational and policy context (and where many of the trends influencing UK health care are international in nature). While the framework of person-centred practice set out in this edited collection is extremely helpful, it arguably underplays these significant contextual factors.

Being person-centred sounds easy, but of course it isn't. In recent years, national and local policy has become more accustomed to talking about the importance of person-centred care – with the emphasis on integrated care, the focus on compassionate care and the personalisation agenda three prominent examples. Although each of these approaches the issue of 'person-centredness' in different ways and at different levels of intervention, they nevertheless all feel important. Hardly surprisingly, people want care that is joined-up around their needs, that is delivered compassionately and that is tailored to their individual circumstances – and the task of policy makers, senior leaders and frontline staff is to find a way to deliver this in practice. While this might seem self-evident and straightforward to many members of the public, nurses and other health-care professionals working in the emotionally charged and organisationally complex arena of health care know that it is much harder than it may first appear. Adopting and slightly adapting a quote initially associated with Professor Peter Beresford, a mental health service user campaigner and social policy academic: 'this isn't rocket science – it is much more subtle and complicated than that'.

Further reading and resources

For further reading around integrated care, see Glasby and Dickinson's (2014) *Partnership Working in Health and Social Care: What is Integrated Care and How Can We Deliver It?* (2nd edn; Bristol: The Policy Press). Helpful overviews are also provided by Cameron et al.'s (2012) review of the literature on the outcomes of partnership working and an evaluation of New Labour's integrated care organisation pilots (Rand Europe/Ernst and Young 2012). Useful journals include the UK's *Journal of Integrated Care* and the *International Journal of Integrated Care* (the latter is available free online via www.ijic.org).

For care as a form of emotional labour, see the work of Yvonne Sawbridge and Alistair Hewison (2011, 2012, 2013, 2014).

For personalisation, see key summaries by Glasby and Littlechild (2015) and by Needham and Glasby (2014). An introduction to personal health budgets is provided by Alakeson (2014), and details of the government's national evaluation are reported by Forder et al. (2012). Further policy papers, concepts and research are available from the Centre for Welfare Reform (www.centreforwelfarereform.org.uk), while personal stories of people receiving personal health budgets are available via https://www.england.nhs.uk/healthbudgets/understanding/lives-stories/patient-stories/.

References

Alakeson, V. (2007) *The Case for Extending Self-Direction in the NHS*, Social Market Foundation, London.

Alakeson, V. (2010) *International Developments in Self-Directed Care*, The Commonwealth Fund, New York.

Alakeson, V. (2014) *Delivering Personal Health Budgets: A Guide to Policy and Practice*, The Policy Press, Bristol.

Cameron, A., Lart, R., Bostock, L., and Coomber, C. (2012) Factors that promote and hinder joint and integrated working between health and social care services, in *SCIE Research briefing 41*, Social Care Institute for Excellence, London.

Cornwell J. (2011) Care and compassion in the NHS. *The Health Foundation*. Available at: http://www.health.org.uk/blog/care-and-compassion-in-the-nhs/ (accessed 28 January 2016).

Forder J, Jones K, Glendinning C et al. (2012) Evaluation of the personal health budget pilot programme. Discussion paper 2840_2. London, Department of Health.

Francis, R. (2013) *Report of the Mid-Staffordshire NHS Foundation Trust Public Inquiry*, The Stationery Office, London.

Glasby, J. (2003) *Hospital Discharge: Integrating Health and Social Care*, Radcliffe Medical Press, Abingdon.

Glasby, J. and Dickinson, H. (eds) (2009) *International Perspectives on Health and Social Care: Partnership Working in Action*, Wiley-Blackwell, Oxford.

Glasby, J. and Dickinson, H. (2014) *Partnership Working in Health and Social Care: What is Integrated Care and How Can We Deliver It?* 2nd edn, The Policy Press, Bristol.

Glasby, J. and Littlechild, R. (2015) *Direct Payments and Personal Budgets: Putting Personalisation into Practice*, 3rd edn, The Policy Press, Bristol.

Leutz, W. (1999) Five laws for integrating medical and social services: lessons from the United States and the United Kingdom. *Milbank Memorial Fund Quarterly*, **77**, 77–110.

Martin, J.P. (1984) *Hospitals in Trouble*, Basil Blackwell, Oxford.

National Voices (2013) A Narrative for Person-Centred Coordinated Care. Available at: http://www.england.nhs.uk/wp-content/uploads/2013/05/nv-narrative-cc.pdf (accessed 28 January 2016).

Needham, C. and Glasby, J. (eds) (2014) *Debates in Personalisation*, The Policy Press, Bristol.

RAND Europe/Ernst and Young (2012) *National Evaluation of the Department of Health's Integrated Care Pilots*. Cambridge, UK: RAND Europe.

Sawbridge Y and Hewison A. (2011) Time to care? Responding to concerns about poor nursing care. Policy Paper 12. Birmingham: Health Services Management Centre.

Sawbridge, Y. and Hewison, A. (2012) Taking action on poor practice. *Nursing Standard*, **26** (30), 62–3.

Sawbridge, Y. and Hewison, A. (2013) Thinking about the emotional labour of nursing – supporting nurses to care. *Journal of Health Organization and Management*, **27**, 127–33.

Sawbridge Y and Hewison A. (2014) Making compassionate care the norm starts with our staff. *Health Service Journal* 25 July.

CHAPTER 5

Person-centredness in nursing strategy and policy

Annette Solman & Val Wilson
University of Technology Sydney, Australia

Current context of health care

There has been significant work in better managing health-care services as costs in service delivery escalate due to advances in science and technology, an ageing population, and new and emerging diseases requiring increased access to health care. This has occurred without the expected reciprocal increase in quality and safety of care. In addition it has been recognised that the traditional approaches to health-care planning and delivery do not necessarily meet the needs of consumers, are often fragmented, result in waste within the health-care system and do not reflect best practice. A risk when seeking to provide affordable, responsive health care is to work primarily through the lens of cost reduction to meet efficiency targets, rather than efficiency targets being the outcome of improved quality and safety. Spurgeon et al. (2011) identified the need for increased medical engagement in supporting changing health-care delivery models, and there is evidence of a more positive impact on the quality of care delivery where there is high-level medical engagement. The importance of inter-professional work in the development and implementation of health-care strategy is well recognised (Carney 2007.) The role and functions of the nurse are essential to both the patients' experience of care and the care outcomes, as is the link between person-centred care provision and staff job satisfaction (Lehuluante et al. 2012). Staff leadership development, to build the capacity of an organisation to respond to challenges and capitalise on opportunities, needs to be linked to the organisation's strategic plan, as change is as much about culture as it is strategic outcomes (Dinwoodie et al. 2014).

There are recent examples in health where the focus of care was not through the lens of person-centeredness resulting in poor outcomes for patients, staff and families. The Independent Inquiry into care provided by Mid-Staffordshire NHS Foundation Trust between January 2005 and March 2009, known as the Francis Report, is such an example (Francis 2013). In his letter to Hon. Jeremy Hunt MP, 5 February 2013, Francis emphasised 'the extent of the

Person-Centred Practice in Nursing and Health Care: Theory and Practice, Second Edition.
Edited by Brendan McCormack and Tanya McCance.
© 2017 John Wiley & Sons, Ltd. Published 2017 by John Wiley & Sons, Ltd.

failure of the system shown in this report suggests that a fundamental culture change is needed' (Francis 2013, p. 5). The Person-centred Nursing Framework (McCormack & McCance 2010) outlines the prerequisites of person-centred care, the focus on the care environment and the care processes that can be used, in conjunction with other management processes. This framework can inform the development, implementation and evaluation of strategy in supporting person-centred practices. Parlour et al. (2014) undertook a study that identified statistically a relationship between care delivery that is person centred and a positive patient experience of care, which we know in our own experience of health care delivery to be true.

Health-care strategy

Strategy is about planning to meet the organisation's vision for the future in health-care delivery. Health-care strategy is influenced by:
- political imperatives;
- social determinants that are currently or predicted to impact on health-care delivery;
- emerging disease processes;
- advances in science and technology;
- the population that it serves; and
- the aspirations of the health entity developing the plan.

With so many factors at play it is important to ensure that the patient is at the centre of decision-making.

The intent of strategic planning in health is to provide high-quality, safe care to patients and to support the workforce to meet service delivery needs. A strategic plan is essentially a high-level road map of where the organisation would like to be in 5–10 years' time from a service provision perspective.

A strategic plan will strive to include strategies to enable the organisation:
- to meet the health-care needs of patients;
- develop the workforce capabilities;
- encourage innovation;
- lead medical science and research translation to practice;
- support technological advancement; and
- build financial sustainability.

Realistic and successful strategic plans are developed to align with current health policy, emerging and current health-care challenges and social imperatives. To be realistic and relevant these plans are developed in consultation with the workforce and other key stakeholders, which include patients and their families. They are enacted through operational plans that are generally focused on one key area of the strategy. This approach of distinct operational plans runs the risk to the organisation of not meeting the goals of the strategic plan, due to fragmentation and the potential of oppositional work occurring unintentionally.

The risk can be minimised by the operational plans being explicitly linked back to the strategy document as well as across to all other operational plans that are in place to support achievement of the strategic plan. A regular review of the progress of the strategic plan implementation and review of the operational plans through the lens of being person centred:

- supports meeting the strategic imperatives; and
- is a gauge to identify the extent to which the people of the organisation and service users are on board and satisfied with the direction and changes that are occurring.

Monitoring of the effectiveness of the strategic plan in meeting the goals is supported when the plan elements are cascaded down into the organisation through to the clinical interface. This approach places the ownership of the strategy at different levels within the organisation and creates meaning and momentum in achieving the best for patients and their families along with a capable and responsive workforce. It supports feedback in a timely way of what is not working and what is working well within the practice domain for patients, their families and the staff.

Building leadership capabilities within the health workforce

Complexity in health-care planning and delivery has increased over the years and requires a changing and evolutionary set of leadership skills to meet and respond to these complexities. Kegan and Lahey Laskow (2009) write about the impact of our personal values and beliefs, coupled with organisational culture, in creating immunity to change. They propose that this immunity to change can be overcome through an investment in adaptive leadership development with staff.

Leadership capability development is essential within the workforce as leadership occurs at all levels within health organisations. A cascade approach to leadership development assists in further developing and creating the necessary skills, energy and impetus to continue to grow and develop the self and others to meet the 'wicked problems' we face within the provision of modern health care. An example of a wicked problem in health would be trying to change a large population mindset and behaviour (Conklin 2006), therefore the culture or attitude. An example we are currently working through in our organisation is how to:

- meet the current and increasing demand for access to health care;
- minimise unnecessary wait times for patients;
- best utilise our inpatient beds to meet service demand;
- explore new models of care including hospital in the home and ambulatory care; and
- ensure evidence-based care practices with the elimination of unnecessary clinical variation.

To meet these challenges requires the staff to think and behave differently in the way they engage with their work, each other and the patient; this would mark a cultural shift from the present situation.

What we need now and into the future are approaches and solutions to respond and plan for the future, not merely to deal with current complexities. Investment in human capital is critical to organisations meeting person-centred sustainable health care.

Building a safe, competent professional workforce: leadership development capabilities – 'Our Journey'

To enhance the leadership development capabilities of staff in the health-care organisation required a multi-pronged approach. To focus on the most pressing 'wicked problems' of the organisation we are engaged in a multi-professional programme that focuses on adaptive leadership development capability. Much has been written about the transformational leader in inspiring a shared vision and working with staff to achieve the organisation's key objectives, through leading the way and using charismatic approaches to staff engagement within a framework of transformation of processes, systems, culture and work practices (Kouzes & Posner 2002). The transformational leader requires the additional skills of adaptive leadership to be truly effective within the context of a changing health-care environment and to meet consumer expectations.

Adaptive leadership within the transformational leadership capabilities is not well documented in the literature. We believe that the transformational leader must have the capabilities of adaptive leadership to truly transform the health-care system's ways of working and thinking about health care (Box 5.1).

Box 5.1 Adaptive leadership supports staff (Heifetz et al. 2009, p. 8).

- Not race to a solution, rather it encourages a deep understanding of the issue.
- Diagnose the issue with the generation of multiple hypotheses.
- Include stakeholder's perceptions of the issue.
- Encourage the same use of language to enhance communication about the issue.
- Identify a number of possible actions based on observations and interpretations to test out for impact.

The adaptive leadership programme currently in place within our organisation is supported by facilitators external to the organisation who have expertise in the theory of adaptive leadership. The internal programme is then supported with internal facilitators working with groups of staff on one of five key strategic priority areas that are challenging to move forwards as these are adaptive challenges that need to be understood and met.

Our organisation has for many years and continues to offer International Practice Development Foundation Schools to support staff development in person-centredness and to enhance the culture of patient- and staff-centred care within day-to-day work practices. The impact of this investment is seen with the majority of ward areas, led by the ward Nursing Unit Manager (Wilson et al. 2013), actively engaged in quality improvement programmes of work to enhance the experience of care for patients, their families and for staff. These programmes of work are mostly within the umbrella of the Teamwork Leadership and Change/Essentials of Care framework, which focuses on meaningful engagement with the patients, family and staff in the delivery of high quality health care.

A range of other leadership programmes are offered that focus on individual leadership development capability through the staff learning about quality improvement or service clinical redesign methodologies. These programmes assist with monitoring clinical practice and variation, supporting processes of change to enhanced clinical practice and in their individual leadership capability development to meaningfully engage and work with others. The range of leadership programmes within our organisation support the delivery of safe, coordinated, responsive and high-quality care for both patients and staff.

Engaging stakeholders

As with all strategic plans there are many pieces of work progressing simultaneously; this is of itself a challenge to effective stakeholder engagement and communication. Stakeholder engagement within the context of change is essential to understanding the views, opinions, opportunities and risks of a proposed strategy.

A range of approaches have been used, including Claims, Concerns and Issues (CCI) (Guba & Lincoln 1989), survey and open forums; at times these have been met with staff indicating that their feedback was not acknowledged or valued as the decision made was not in line with their views. This highlights a bigger issue of focusing on and understanding the culture for these major pieces of work, which, on reflection, would have lent themselves to adaptive leadership practices. See Box 5.2 for an approach and reflection of this approach to change.

Box 5.2 The 'Claims, Concerns and Issues' (CCI) approach.

A method we often use is the 'Claims, Concerns and Issues' (CCI) approach, where we work to obtain stakeholder engagement (a key component of the Person-centred Nursing Framework), and the approach is generally positively received. The challenge is and continues to be major organisational change work in gaining meaningful stakeholder engagement on the issue without the issue being blurred by individual agendas and emotions and becoming clouded by history. Honouring the history and the staff contribution is an important recognition of the work that has gone before. We acknowledge that this is something we need to emphasise more in the change work than we have done previously; it would be enhanced through adaptive leadership capabilities.

Wilkins (1989) writes of the need to build on existing strengths within the new direction. The Person-centred Nursing Framework has been used to inform the approach to consultation.

Person-centred care example from practice

The case of an organisational restructure highlights stakeholder engagement. The restructure was focused on bringing a number of entities together to form one organisation across two main campuses. Both entities involved had a history steeped in tradition, were closely associated and were premier services in their own right. The decision was made at a government level to create a specialty health children's network within Sydney, after a major Special Commission of Inquiry Acute Care Services in NSW Public Hospitals by Peter Garling (2008). A sound governance structure was established with clear processes and systems. Davidson et al. (2015) write of the importance of sound governance in achieving quality and safety in health-care delivery (p. 131). A strategic plan was developed with stakeholder engagement through open forums, small group sessions and other mechanisms. As a component of creating this new entity nursing was to be restructured to form a networked approach to nursing services. Box 5.3 highlights the process.

Box 5.3 Creating a different nursing structure.

A position was proposed, nursing staff were consulted and a mechanism for feedback was established. The nursing staff of both hospitals and other staff actively contributed to designing a different nursing structure from the initial proposal.

The proposed revised structure was functional; it was thought to address the needs for professional nursing leadership at both hospitals, ensured there was a senior nurse position within the Executive and provided a nursing structure for advancement within leadership and management for nursing staff.

The restructure of nursing was an important and an emotive issue. Engagement of the nursing staff was significant as they wanted to ensure that the right decision was being made for the right reasons. This nursing structure was informed by the broader consultation with the nursing staff. This resulted in a change to include a key professional, an issue that was not addressed in the proposed initial restructure; this change is now in place.

The approach reflects the Person-centred Nursing Framework in the need for meaningful engagement with stakeholders; in supporting shared decision-making; and considering the care environment to support the best outcomes.

To gauge staff engagement in the operationalising of corporate strategy and to assess the sense of staff satisfaction over time with the strategy implementation, it is important to be person centred. There are a number of ways that this can be undertaken. In health there are government multi-dimensional staff satisfaction surveys that have been in place for some time, with annual reports made available to each health organisation. A whole of health report is also made available in some jurisdictions, where you can see how your organisation compares with another and track progress on key points over time.

The Person-Centred Nursing Index (PCNI) is used as part of a longitudinal study in one of the hospitals where we work. White and Wilson (2015) report that this survey provides information about how the nurses feel regarding working in the hospital as well as the care they provide (p. 13). A high-level de-identified organisational report is generated that supports senior nursing management and the Executive in understanding the trends and seeking opportunities to enhance areas that are of concern.

Box 5.4 outlines the intent of the work and approach used. It highlights understanding the place of prerequisites of knowing the self, professional competence, commitment to the job, clarity of values and beliefs, and importance of a therapeutic care environment within the Person-centred Nursing Framework.

Box 5.4 The Person-Centred Nursing Index (PCNI).

The PCNI measures a number of indicators that includes nursing and work stress, job satisfaction and organisational characteristics. This survey has enabled a deeper understanding of what is important to nursing. The survey enables us to track trends for each element of the tool and to provide feedback to each of the wards on their results. One annual result alerted us to the ongoing sense of instability for the nursing staff through the restructure of the organisation. Nursing managers were encouraged to speak with staff about the results, and there was greater emphasis from management on the progress of the desired change in an attempt to lessen the nurses' feelings of instability. Each year after the results are communicated to the nursing staff of the ward, they are encouraged to engage in discussion about the results and to explore trends, then make decisions about areas to focus on improving or maintaining at the desired level.

Critical incidents occur due to human error and failure within the health system. When reviewing critical incidents it is important to do so through the lens of being person centred. The review of critical incidents Root Cause Analysis (RCA) membership in this health-care organisation resulted in the most senior nurse within the organisation being on the review panel for all RCAs, not just those that involved nursing, which had previously been the norm. This change highlights the importance the organisation places on an interdisciplinary approach to RCA review and on risk mitigation of supporting decisions that may have a consequential impact within the patient care environment; this practice is reflective of the prerequisites of the Person-centred Nursing Framework.

To support review findings and recommendations it is important to have a multi-professional approach to ensure the recommendations are practical and followed up for their impact. Examples of change that supports person-centred care practices within a multi-professional setting are described in Boxes 5.5 and 5.6.

Box 5.5

An example of person-centred practice (relating to prerequisites and the care environment aspects of the person-centred framework) was the identification that the organisation could improve risk mitigation for patients and staff, particularly outside the 8 am–5 pm timeframe, through an early alert system. An early identification and reporting process was identified as a possible solution and implemented as a trial at one of the hospitals. A draft framework and reporting tool was developed and circulated to key stakeholders for their feedback. The feedback was discussed with a key stakeholder group and the Executive. The draft framework was revised a few times after trialling and receiving further feedback. The tool has been communicated and is now being used after hours in this hospital to support pre-emptive measures and to notify progress of patient, staff or environment critical events.

This change supports improving the care processes and person-centred outcomes for patients, family and staff of the hospital and is now included as a risk mitigation strategy.

Box 5.6 Dealing with haemolytic virus Ebola

The recent outbreak of Ebola virus infection in west Africa resulted in a hospital being designated to prepare for a potential presentation of patients suspected of having this virus. A multi-professional team (clinical and non-clinical) formed a committee to review our existing policy, processes and procedures for the care of the patient/family and the safety of staff and the general public in the provision of care. The committee had the patient, family and staff at the centre of its discussion, planning and decision-making, regarding updating the policy and ensuring staff were competent to enact the policy in a safe and effective way. The policy was reviewed against the best available evidence and updated. It was identified that the safe working practices and safe operating procedures would need to be changed, requiring education and training of staff in a different way of working for the care and management of patients and staff regarding this particular virus.

This multi-professional risk mitigation work is a good example of being person centred in the approach to review of the policy and engagement where policy required a review and then simulation was used to test the revised processes for their effectiveness and against the updated policy. A comprehensive staff training package was implemented led by nursing, infection control services and the broader multi-professional team.

Conclusion

Staff involvement in the development, operationalising, impact monitoring and evaluation of organisational strategy, including policy development, is critical to the success of the work and in minimising risk. Engagement across a range of disciplines, professions and levels of management, having person centredness at the forefront of discussion and decision-making, supports quality and safety of patient care and of staff. The person-centred framework, although not used purposely in developing the organisation's strategy, was, however, used for the nursing operational plan; it is heartening to know that the elements of the framework are inherent within the strategic plan. There are many enablers to support person-centred work; these include staff engagement, data that informs us about our quality and safety trends, seeking out the patient and staff experience of receiving and providing care, ongoing capability development of the workforce and continuing the focus on using the person-centred lens on the work that we do every day.

References

Carney, M. (2007) How commitment and involvement influence the development of strategic consensus in health care organizations: the multidisciplinary approach. *Journal of Nursing Management* **15**, 649–58.

Conklin, J. (2006) *Dialogue Mapping: Building Shared Understanding of Wicked Problems*. Chichester, UK: John Wiley & Sons, Ltd.

Davidson, P., Dennison-Himmelfarb, C., Alsadaan, N. (2015) Governance of nursing practice; steps for the quality and safety of healthcare In: Daly J, Speedy S, Jackson D. (eds), *Leadership & Nursing Contemporary Perspectives*, 2nd edn. Churchill Livingstone Elsevier, pp. 130–7.

Dinwoodie, D., Quinn, L., McGuie, J. (2014) Bridging the Strategy/Performance Gap – How Leadership Strategy Drives Business Results. White paper. Greensboro, NC: Centre for Creative Leadership.

Francis, R. (2013) *Report of the Mid-Staffordshire NHS Foundation Trust Public Inquiry*. London: The Stationery Office.

Garling, P. (2008) *Final Report of the Special Commission of Inquiry – Acute Care Services in NSW Public Hospitals*. State of NSW through the Special Commission of Inquiry: Acute Care Services in NSW Public Hospitals.

Guba, E.G. and Lincoln, Y.S. (1989) *Fourth Generation Evaluation*. Thousand Oaks, CA: Sage.

Heifetz, R., Grashow, A., Linsky, M. (2009) *The Practice of Adaptive Leadership: Tools and Tactics for Changing Your Organisation and the World*. Cambridge Leadership Associates. Harvard Business Review Press.

Kegan, R. and Lahey Laskow, L. (2009) *Immunity to Change*. Harvard Business School Publishing Corporation.

Kouzes, J. and Posner, B. (2002) *The Leadership Challenge*. San Francisco CA: Jossey-Bass.

Lehuluante, A., Nilsson, A., Edvardsson, D. (2012) The influence of a person-centred psychosocial unit climate on satisfaction with care and work. *Journal of Nursing Management* **20**, 319–25.

McCormack, B. and McCance, T. (2010) *Person-centred Nursing: Theory and Practice*, 1st edn. Oxford: Wiley-Blackwell.

Parlour, R., Slater, P., McCormack, B., Gallen, A., Kavanagh, P. (2014) The relationship between positive patient experience in acute hospitals and person centred care. *International Journal of Research in Nursing* **5**(10), 25–34.

Spurgeon, P., Mazelan, P.M., Brawell, F. (2011) Medical engagement: a crucial underpinning to organizational performance. *Health Services Management Research* **24**, 114–20.

White, C. and Wilson, V. (2015) A longitudinal study of aspects of a hospital's family-centred nursing: changing practice through data translation. *Journal of Advanced Nursing* **71**, 100–14.

Wilkins, A. (1989) *Developing Corporate Character: How to Successfully Change an Organization Without Destroying It*. San Francisco, CA: Jossey-Bass.

Wilson, V., Patterson, S., Korman, K. (2013) Leadership development: an essential ingredient in supporting nursing unit managers. *Journal of Healthcare Leadership* **5**, 53–62.

CHAPTER 6

Person-centred nursing leadership

Shaun Cardiff

Fontys University of Applied Sciences, Eindhoven, The Netherlands

Person-centredness is often talked about in terms of the practitioner-service user relationship, although the enactment of person-centredness has also been identified as a key attribute to effective workplace cultures (Manley et al. 2011). Once practitioners start to collectively engage with and reflect on the meaning of person-centred cultures, awareness grows of the relevance person-centredness has for their own relationships too (McCance et al. 2013) and the placement of effective staff relationships within the context domain of the Person-centred Nursing Framework.

Leadership is known to have a large impact on workplace/organisational cultures. Kouzes and Posner's (2007) model of transformational leadership seems to be the preferred choice in practice development and person-centred work and literature. However, whilst showing positive outcomes, it can be argued that this model does not fully reflect the core values of person-centredness (Cardiff, 2014). This then raises the question: What would leadership look like if approached with the same values and beliefs underlying person-centred care? This chapter aims to answer this question using a conceptual framework (see Figure 6.2) developed during a 3-year participatory action research study aimed at exploring and developing person-centred leadership.

The leadership dance

Leadership relationships, like all human relationships, evolve constantly and are formed by two or more people interacting. In healthy relationships people feel safe, energised and connected. As we[1] explored person-centredness within leadership relationships, we began to visualise it metaphorically as an Argentine tango between leaders and associates.[2] In the Argentine tango partners respond

---

[1] Use of the term 'we' in this chapter refers to the author (action researcher) and participants/co-researchers (Marie-Louise van Hest, Elleke van der Furth, and Meriam de Boer) as they actively participated in field data analyses and member checked the thesis chapters.
[2] We use the term 'associates' to denote those being led as this portrays the value of equity better than the more commonly used term 'followers'.

Person-Centred Practice in Nursing and Health Care: Theory and Practice, Second Edition.
Edited by Brendan McCormack and Tanya McCance.
© 2017 John Wiley & Sons, Ltd. Published 2017 by John Wiley & Sons, Ltd.

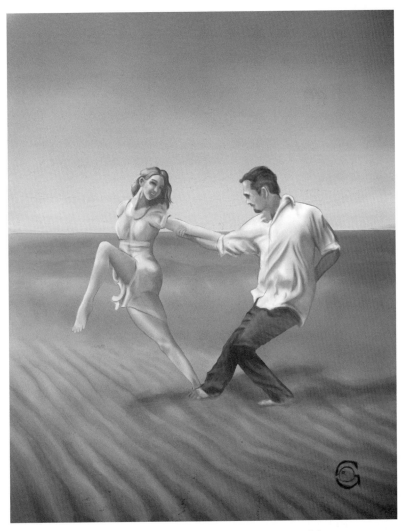

Figure 6.1 A metaphor for person-centred leadership. Artist: George Vink.

to self, other, the music and context in a continuous movement between 'open' and 'closed' embraces (Jensen 2006). Although certain steps characterise the tango, they are not repeated in a set pattern. In a closed embrace the dancers seem to move as one, whilst individuality is clearly visible in an open embrace. Glance quickly at Figure 6.1.

Your gaze may initially be drawn to the female dancer. Her pose is unique, elegant, and she looks competent, exhilarated and free. Look again and see how her partner enables her to safely lean outwards, neither pushing nor pulling her into position. This stance would not have been possible if they were not connected. They are dancing on a sandy beach with a moving shoreline and potentially changeable weather conditions. This requires a different kind of wisdom than dancing inside a studio. Even using the same steps and movement, the imagery

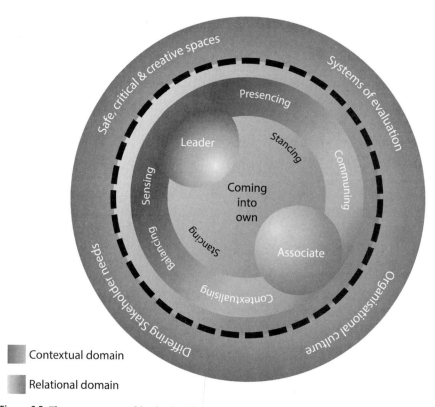

Contextual domain

Relational domain

Figure 6.2 The person-centred leadership framework.

would be different in a studio. Similarly, a change of partners would create a new image too as each couple attends and responds to self, other and context differently.

Like the Argentine tango, we view person-centred leadership as a unique and constantly evolving relationship between people. In line with relational leadership theory (Uhl-Bien 2006), we found that person-centred leaders use a set of attributes and processes for being in relation and relational connectedness. The primary aim of the leader is to enable associate self-actualisation, empowerment and well-being (*coming into own*) within the possibilities and constraints of the context (Figure 6.2).

The relational domain

Embedded in the relational domain of person-centred leadership are six attributes that enable leader *being in relation*, and five processes for *relational connectedness*. Being in relation and relational connectedness help leader *stancing* (positioning self in relation to the other) and enablement of associate *coming into own*.

Leader attributes for being in relation

Contemporary professionals want to be led, not managed (Shelton & Darling 2001) and there is increasing evidence that good health-care practices are built on strong and healthy relationships in cultures that balance 'counting with caring' (Higgs et al. 2014). From an existential humanistic paradigm, leaders lead in relationship with others, and those being led are valued for who they are rather than as a means to an end. Person-centred leaders are authentically other-centred and caring. Being patient, optimistic and open helps them respond appropriately to each associate at each moment in time within each given context, and so helps create conditions for self-actualisation, empowerment and well-being (*coming into own*).

Some leaders may be concerned that these traits (see Box 6.1) prevent professional distancing or foster over-involvement. However, we found that by using intra- and interpersonal intelligences, person-centred leaders are able to move through different levels of engagement with associates, appropriately taking ownership of problems, or leaving problems where they belong. They do not seek followership but mutuality and reciprocity. They use enquiry and emotional intelligence to hear, read and understand the associate's and own state of being, and are willing to show their own vulnerability. But being person-centred does not occur spontaneously. It requires reflexivity, asking: 'What does this person need in order to come into their own? (How) Can I offer them what they need? What are possible consequences of my/our actions? Is this then the right thing to do, and for who?'

Box 6.1 Person-centred leader attributes.

- Authentically other-centred and caring
- Intrapersonal intelligence (knowing self)
- Interpersonal intelligence (knowing other)
- Patience, optimism and openness
- Showing vulnerability
- Reflexivity

Processes for relational connectedness

Many leadership models work from an entity perspective, looking at leader attributes and behaviour rather than social/relational processes (Uhl-Bien 2006). Belonging and feeling recognised and safe are fundamental human needs (Maslow 1943) and nurses want to feel connected to their leaders (Anonson et al. 2013). Seeking inclusion (feeling welcomed, connected and part of a greater whole) without loss of distinctness (directing own agency) fosters survival and thriving (Kegan 1982). When personal and collective goals merge, the individual functions as part of the whole team without losing his or her

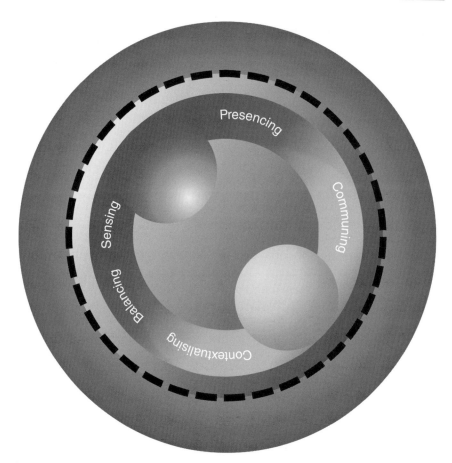

Figure 6.3 Processes for relational connectedness.

individuality (Plas 1996). We identified five processes that enable relational connectedness and related individualism (Figure 6.3).

Sensing is the seeing, hearing, feeling and verifying an associate's state of being. That nurses use their senses to assess service user well-being is well described in acute (Bundgaard et al. 2012) and long-term care (Martin et al. 2012; Sellevold et al. 2013), but not in leadership literature. Hersey et al. (2001) talk of diagnosing associate readiness/development, but their reductionist assessment only focuses on task performance. Person-centred leaders are more holistic. They appreciate how all aspects of human being can influence task performance and how knowledge of a person's being need not be restricted to the personal narrative. Gathering data from different sources such as previous experience, colleague narratives or personnel records, the leader blends and interprets information before undertaking action, and will often seek verification from the associate.

In a person-centred approach to relationships the other is not reduced to one social role, or the here and now. There is recognition of how a person's current being is influenced by the many contexts they inhabit as well as their past, present and future. This viewing and assessing of a person as an embodied and embedded being is named *contextualisation*. Whilst health-care literature continually emphasises the importance of an holistic approach, leadership literature seldom if ever discusses the importance of considering how all aspects of an associate's life may be influencing/influenced by their work. However, we found that such consideration aids leader reflexivity for better/more appropriate associate support within the workplace.

To only consider the needs of one individual at any one time would be advocating individualism rather than related individualism. Being person-centred is about *balancing* the needs of the person before us with those we may (not currently) be engaged with. Decision-making becomes complex in a post-modern world full of diversity, and moral leaders cannot rely on any one set of rigidly applied principles (Thompson 2004). Consequently, leaders often find themselves dialoguing with associates and/or colleagues before deciding on action.

Whilst dialogue strives primarily for mutual understanding, *communing* is action-oriented. Leaders communicate at an intimate level, showing support, seeking understanding, finding a common ground, creating a shared vision and/or making shared decisions. Leader communication competency is widely researched and shown to positively influence patient safety, job satisfaction, nurse retention and healthy work environments, but is often portrayed as unidirectional/leader led, and nurses often do not dare to speak up for themselves (Garon 2012). Groysberg and Slind (2012) state that in person-to-person conversations, leaders intentionally talk 'with' rather than 'to' associates, listening and acknowledging their views so as to develop relational trust, shared ownership and connectedness as well as to prevent divergence and rambling. We also found that communing creatively enhanced a sense of safety, expanded fields of vision and prevented stagnation in semantic discussions.

Presencing is a term found in leadership and organisational change theory; it describes authentic attentiveness and responsiveness, in the moment, to context (Senge et al. 2004; Scouller 2011) rather than between leader and associate. Presencing as 'being and thinking with the other' is described in nursing literature (Baart & Grypdonck 2008; McCormack & McCance 2010). It begins with unconditional openness and beneficent attentiveness (attentiveness for the sake of attentiveness and not as a means to an end). Here a leader tries to understand the associate narrative and build relational connectedness before collaboratively deciding if and how the leader can help. Empathy is described in many leadership models, and has been shown to significantly correlate with job satisfaction, extra effort and effectiveness (Skinner & Spurgeon 2005). However, like McCormack and McCance (2010), we prefer the term (sympathetic) presence as a leader can only use sympathetic imagination (Kontos & Naglie 2007) to try to understand another's unique experience 'as if' it were their own.

Stancing to enable coming into own

Sensing associate (well)being, communing, seeing them in context, balancing needs and showing sympathetic presence enable relational connectedness. A leader can then decide how best to position self in relation to the associate (Figure 6.4). As in the Argentine tango, *stancing* is a constant enactment of attentiveness and responsiveness. It can be seen as beautiful leadership (Ladkin 2008), which requires mastery (understanding self, context and domain with attentiveness to possibilities within the here-and-now), congruency between what is (non)verbally said and done, and ethical purpose.

In contrast to many leadership models, the primary focus of person-centred leaders is associate well-being and empowerment, rather than performance and commitment. We identified four basic stances: leading from the front, sideline, alongside and behind.

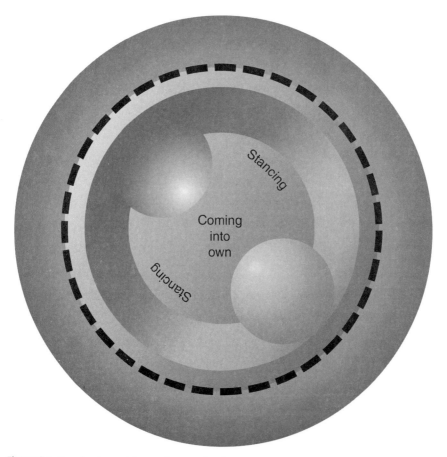

Figure 6.4 Stancing to enable associate coming into own.

In leading from the front a leader offers directive support through role modelling or demonstration. 'Offering' support rather than 'telling' how things should be done respects and fosters associate self-determination. It is the basis for leading from the sideline too. Here a leader communes and/or negotiates support by 'offering' rather than 'selling' instruction (what, when, how and where information).

Sometimes more intense challenge and support is required to help associates move forwards, and a leader may choose to lead from alongside. Actively listening then attentively balancing challenge with support, the leader fosters self-determined action and self-efficacy. At other times leading from behind may be appropriate. The leader takes a step back to create optimum freedom for self-determination. It is not necessarily delegation based on a conviction that the associate can perform independently. The invitation to be self-determinate may have a learning/developmental intent. Either way, the leader considers possible consequences of stepping back (calculated risk-taking) and observing whilst remaining available to intervene if and when necessary. Calculated/considered risk-taking is characteristic of empowering care environments (McCormack & McCance 2010) and innovative leadership (Crenshaw & Yoder-Wise 2013). Benefits include: associate self-awareness, empowerment, self-efficacy, job satisfaction and organisational innovation.

'*Coming into own*' was the phrase clinical leaders frequently used to describe intention and consequences of their leadership. It covered those moments when 'things felt good and right', when people were reaching their potential and/or being their authentic self. Leader fostering of staff well-being and empowerment is supported by NHS NICE guidelines (NICE 2009) and positive leader-associate relationships have been linked to patient outcomes (Wong et al. 2013).

Well-being has two components: the emotional (happiness and satisfaction) and the psychological (reaching one's potential and thriving) (Ménard & Brunet 2011). Empowerment can also be seen as having two components. Structural empowerment comes from the delegation of authority and increased access to organisational information, resources, support and opportunities (MacPhee et al. 2014), whilst psychological empowerment is enhanced by removing conditions fostering powerlessness (Conger & Kanungo 1988). However, descriptions and discussions of empowerment are not always univocal and should be read with an awareness of one's own values and beliefs. For instance, structural empowerment is often described as 'giving power' to associates, whilst post-modern critics argue that associate empowerment can never be truly obtained if leaders control what, when and how associates access information (Spreitzer 2008). We also found that access to information alone was no guarantee for self-directed agency, and so we concluded that empowerment should be both structural and psychological, considering both contextual and personal factors influencing a person's being.

We also encourage leader consideration of individualisation and associate mastery (being the best one can be at something) (Ladkin 2008), as well as performance (which encourages competency comparison and competition).

A person-centred leader considers individual mastery within the context of whole team skill mix and performance. This then creates space for diversity within the team and consequently influences staff recruitment and development strategies. Add to this the principle of participation and leader power ceases to be coercive or 'power-over' associates, but instead becomes coactive or 'power-with' associates (Follett 1940). This focus on individualisation, individual mastery, participation and whole team performance can help leaders create conditions for coming into own.

The contextual domain

Whilst a focus on associate well-being and empowerment is admirable, realism reminds us of the role context plays in leader-associate relationships. Leadership research has often stayed clear of situatedness and contextual influences on day-to-day leader interactions (Ashman & Lawler 2008). We found that contextual factors influence, and are influenced by, the leader-associate relationship. This mutual influencing is denoted in the framework by the perforated line separating the relational and contextual domain (Figure 6.5).

Organisational culture can be simply defined as 'the way things are done around here' (Drennan 1992). Despite the researched benefits of styles such

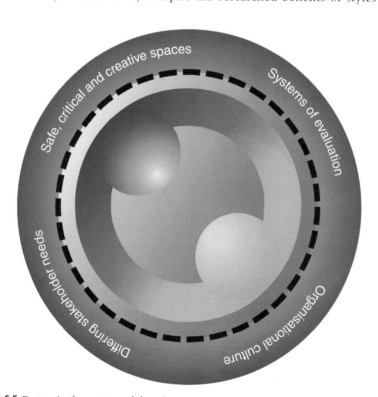

Figure 6.5 Factors in the contextual domain.

as transformational leadership and the knowledge that leadership plays a major role in organisational culture, major incidents such as those described in the Mid-Staffordshire Inquiry (Francis 2013) remind us that autocratic and managerialistic leadership is still predominant in health care. We also faced an organisational culture focused on efficiency and a tradition of nursing and nurses being led by managers and physicians. As the clinical nurse leaders critically and creatively reflected on their own leadership, tensions with the physician team (and physician manager in particular) emerged, but the nursing team and unit idio (micro)culture started to transform.

As the nurse leaders and nursing team became more empowered, physician 'power over' them reduced. Analysing such incidents also revealed the importance of reflexivity as morally reflected action. Leader attentiveness and responsiveness to *differing stakeholder needs* within the context, considering and working with their values and beliefs, can help avoid (interdisciplinary) conflict and the advantaging of some at the expense of others. This entails not only considering the needs of the person at hand, but also those who may not yet be in view.

Enabling associates to come into their own amidst contextual factors such as organisational culture and differing stakeholder needs, often requires facilitated learning and development. Facilitated workplace learning can be professionally and personally empowering (Merriam 1996), and highlighting areas of patient care for critical reflection is a known attribute of effective clinical leadership (Cook & Leathard 2004). Person-centred leaders who feel a responsibility for *creating safe, critical and creative learning spaces* within the clinical workplace can therefore be viewed as facilitators of evidence-based and person-centred care.

Workplace learning may be planned and structured, such as critical and creative reflective enquiries (Cardiff 2012). It may also be unstructured and opportune, such as inviting an associate to decide whether or not to open a closed bed. Regardless, inviting participation and ensuring the absence of negativity starts a process of creating psychological safety for critical learning. Learning can be unsettling as people are asked to suspend disbelief, confront current assumptions and possibly unlearn old ways of being (Mezirow 1981; Schön 1987; Macdonald 2002). We found offering a variety of methods for creative expression fosters psychological safety, raises energy levels, broadens the scope of topics discussed, prevents stagnation in semantic discussions and reveals perspectives that cognitive rationalisation and reasoning may otherwise have kept from the public arena.

The creation and observation of safe, critical and creative spaces can also be used for *systematic evaluation*. How these 'spaces' are created and facilitated will be influenced by the leader-associate relationship, and the content reveals much about what happens in the relationship. Other evaluation data may include patient and staff satisfaction surveys or absenteeism rates, but quantitative data alone would fail to capture the unknown and so not contribute to continued evolution.

Conclusion

Leadership, whether enacted from hierarchical or non-hierarchical positions, is often defined as social influencing: the guiding and supporting of individuals and teams towards predetermined leader/organisational goals. Such definitions imply a unidirectional (leader initiated and led) flow of influence and fail to capture the complexity of people relating in social contexts. There is also the danger that leaders then see their role as exercising 'power over' associates rather than sharing 'power with' them. The person-centred leadership framework presented in this chapter offers a view of leadership based on the same humanistic values as person-centred nursing. Striving for relational connectedness, person-centred leaders primarily aim to enable associate self-actualisation, well-being and empowerment as precursors to individual mastery and team performance.

Leaders' attributes matching person-centred practice prerequisites include being authentically other-centred and caring, intra- and interpersonal intelligence, and reflexivity. Similar processes are also described, such as working with the values and beliefs of the other, viewing them holistically (sensing, balancing and contextualising), sympathetic presence (presencing), shared decision-making (communing) and moving through different levels of engagement (stancing). Person-centred leaders may therefore feel better equipped to develop person-centred cultures.

Focusing on relational connectedness alone is insufficient to enable associate coming into own, as contextual factors such as organisational culture, differing stakeholder needs, safe, critical and creative learning spaces, and evaluation systems will influence how leaders and associates relate. Similarly, how leaders and associates relate will influence how the needs of others are viewed, how learning takes place, how leadership and care are evaluated and the idioculture. At a time when more demands are being placed on fewer people with fewer resources, our interdependency is becoming increasingly obvious. Contemporary leaders, staff and service users may therefore benefit from a leadership style that focuses on developing individuals within a team.

References

Anonson, J., Walker, M., Arries, E., Maposa, S., Telford, P., and Berry, L. (2013) Qualities of exemplary nurse leaders: perspectives of frontline nurses. *Journal of Nursing Management*. doi: 10.1111/jonm.12092

Ashman, I. and Lawler, J. (2008) Existential communication and leadership. *Leadership*, **4** (3), 253–69.

Baart, A. and Grypdonck, M. (2008) *Verpleegkunde en presentie. Een zoektocht in dialoog naar de betekenis van presentie voor verpleegkundige zorg*, The Hague, Lemma.

Bundgaard, K., Nielsen, K., Delmar, C., and Sorensen, E. (2012) What to know and how to get to know? A fieldwork study outlining the understanding of knowing the patient in facilities for short-term stay. *Journal of Advanced Nursing*, **68**, 2280–8.

Cardiff, S. (2012) Critical and creative reflective inquiry: surfacing narratives to enable learning and inform action. *Educational Action Research*, **20**, 605–22.

Cardiff S. (2014) Person-centred leadership: A critical participatory action research study exploring and developing a new style of (clinical) nurse leadership. PhD thesis, University of Ulster, Belfast.

Conger, J. and Kanungo, R. (1988) The empowerment process: integrating theory and practice. *The Academy of Management Review*, **13**, 471–82.

Cook, M. and Leathard, H. (2004) Learning for clinical leadership. *Journal of Nursing Management*, **12**, 436–44.

Crenshaw, J. and Yoder-Wise, P. (2013) Creating an environment for innovation: The risk-taking leadership competency. *Nurse Leader*, **11**, 24–7.

Drennan, D. (1992) *Transforming Company Culture*, McGraw-Hill, London.

Follett, M. (1940) *Dynamic Administration. The Collected Papers of Mary Parker Follett*, Harper & Brothers, New York.

Francis, R. (2013) *Report of the Mid-Staffordshire NHS Foundation Trust Public Inquiry*, Stationery Office, London.

Garon, M. (2012) Speaking up, being heard: registered nurses' perceptions of workplace communication. *Journal of Nursing Management*, **20**, 361–71.

Groysberg, B. and Slind, M. (2012) Leadership is a conversation. *Harvard Business Review*, **90** (6), 76–84.

Hersey, P., Blanchard, K., and Johnson, D. (2001) *Management of Organizational Behavior: Leading Human Resources*, 8th edn, Prentice Hall, New Jersey.

Higgs, J., Croker, A., Tasker, D., Hummel, J., and Patton, N. (eds) (2014) *Health Practice Relationships*, Sense Publishers, Rotterdam.

Jensen M. (2006) *Sensuous and gendered embraces: an investigation into tango dance practices*. MA thesis, Roehampton University. Retrieved from: http://www.i-m-pulse.eclipse.co.uk/MA %20Thesis%20(2).htm

Kegan, R. (1982) *The Evolving Self: Problem and Process in Human Development*, Harvard University Press, Cambridge.

Kontos, P. and Naglie, G. (2007) Bridging theory and practice: Imagination, the body, and person-centred dementia care. *Dementia*, **6**, 549–69.

Kouzes, J. and Posner, B. (2007) *The Leadership Challenge*, 4th edn, Jossey-Bass, San Francisco.

Ladkin, D. (2008) Leading beautifully: How mastery, congruence and purpose create the aesthetic of embodied leadership practice. *The Leadership Quarterly*, **19**, 31–41.

Macdonald, G. (2002) Transformative unlearning: safety, discernment and communities of learning. *Nursing Inquiry*, **9** (3), 170–8.

MacPhee, M., Dahinten, V., Hejazi, J. *et al.* (2014) Testing the effects of an empowerment-based leadership development programme: part 1 – leader outcomes. *Journal of Nursing Management*, **22**, 4–15.

Manley K, Sanders K, Cardiff S, Webster J. (2011) Effective workplace culture: the attributes, enabling factors and consequences of a new concept. *International Practice Development Journal* **1**(2): art. 1. Available at: http://www.fons.org/library/journal/volume1-issue2/article1

Martin A, O' Connor-Fenelon M, Lyons R. (2012) Non-verbal communication between Registered Nurses Intellectual Disability and people with an intellectual disability: An exploratory study of the nurse's experiences. Part 1. *Journal of Intellectual Disabilities* **16**:61–75.

Maslow, A. (1943) A theory of human motivation. *Psychological Review*, **50** (4), 370–96.

McCance T, Gribben B, McCormack B, Laird E. (2013) Promoting person-centred practice within acute care: the impact of culture and context on a facilitated practice development programme. *International Practice Development Journal* **3**(1). Retrieved from: http://www.fons.org/ Resources/Documents/Journal/Vol3No1/IDPJ_0301_02.pdf (accessed 1 February 2016).

McCormack, B. and McCance, T. (2010) *Person-Centred Nursing: Theory and Practice*, Wiley-Blackwell, Oxford.

Ménard, J. and Brunet, L. (2011) Authenticity and well-being in the workplace: a mediation model. *Journal of Managerial Psychology*, **26**, 331–46.

Merriam, S. (1996) Updating our knowledge of adult learning. *The Journal of Continuing Education in the Health Professions*, **16**, 136–43.

Mezirow, J. (1981) A critical theory of adult learning and education. *Adult Education Quarterly*, **32**, 3–24.

NICE (2009) *Promoting mental wellbeing at work*, NHS National Institute for Health and Clinical Excellence, London.

Plas, J. (1996) *Person-Centred Leadership*, Sage Publications, Thousand Oaks, CA.

Schön, D. (1987) *Educating the Reflective Practitioner: Toward a new design for teaching and learning in the professions*, Jossey-Bass, San Francisco.

Scouller J. (2011) *The Three Levels of Leadership: How to develop your leadership presence, knowhow and skill*. Cirencester, UK: Management Books 2000.

Sellevold, G., Egede-Nissen, V., Jakobsen, R., and Sørlie, V. (2013) Quality care for persons experiencing dementia: The significance of relational ethics. *Nursing Ethics*, **20**, 263–72.

Senge, P., Scharmer, C.O., Jaworski, J., and Flowers, B. (2004) *Presence: Human Purpose and the Field of the Future*, SOL, Cambridge.

Shelton, C. and Darling, J. (2001) The quantum skills model in management: a new paradigm to enhance effective leadership. *Leadership & Organization Development Journal*, **22** (6), 264–73.

Skinner, C. and Spurgeon, P. (2005) Valuing empathy and emotional intelligence in health leadership: a study of empathy, leadership behaviour and outcome effectiveness. *Health Services Management Research*, **18**, 1–12.

Spreitzer, G. (2008) Taking stock: A review of more than twenty years of research on empowerment at work, in *The Handbook of Organizational Behavior* (eds C. Cooper and J. Barling), Sage Publications, London, pp. 54–72.

Thompson, L. (2004) Moral leadership in a postmodern world. *Journal of Leadership and Organisational Studies*, **11**, 27–37.

Uhl-Bien, M. (2006) Relational leadership theory: Exploring the social processes of leadership and organizing. *The Leadership Quarterly*, **17** (6), 654–76.

Wong, C., Cummings, G., and Ducharme, L. (2013) The relationship between nursing leadership and patient outcomes: a systematic review update. *Journal of Nursing Management*, **21**, 709–24.

CHAPTER 7

Person-centred nursing education

Deirdre O'Donnell, Neal Cook & Pauline Black
Ulster University, Northern Ireland, UK

While the promotion of person-centred practice among registered nurses has been widely embraced in health-care literature, less attention has been paid to how students are introduced to the principles of person-centredness in undergraduate education programmes. This chapter provides an overview of a developing body of work within one School of Nursing in constructing, implementing and sustaining a person-centred nursing curriculum.

How is person-centredness manifest in nursing curricula?

In order to identify and build on any existing knowledge, the process of constructing a person-centred nursing curriculum began with an exploration of the literature. The initial focus was to become familiar with the extent of published studies pertaining to person-centredness in nursing curricula and to identify and explore any existing pedagogical approaches to the development and promotion of person-centred practice.

A one-year research project was undertaken to conduct a meta-synthesis of person-centredness in nursing curricula. Meta-synthesis involves the integrative secondary analysis and synthesis of findings from a range of existing qualitative studies, which normally share a common theme. The aim of meta-synthesis is to enable the application of qualitative findings to inform the development of practice and the generation of new knowledge that authentically represents the findings of any original studies. The Noblit and Hare methodological approach to meta-synthesis was employed (Noblit & Hare 1988).

A literature search was carried out using key terms derived from a definition of person-centred practice (McCormack 2004). Searches were restricted to those published in English language during the last 10 years. A total of 76 papers were identified from this process and the full sample was reviewed by a group of three academics with expertise in person-centred practice, qualitative methods and/or curriculum development. Following the initial review, 30 papers were considered

Person-Centred Practice in Nursing and Health Care: Theory and Practice, Second Edition.
Edited by Brendan McCormack and Tanya McCance.
© 2017 John Wiley & Sons, Ltd. Published 2017 by John Wiley & Sons, Ltd.

eligible for inclusion. These papers were subsequently considered by an expert panel comprising six independent reviewers. Following completion of the individual review process, all members of the expert panel met to identify areas of consensus and to challenge refutational perspectives.

It was found that, while person-centredness was widely espoused in the literature, there was limited evidence of how this was made operational in curriculum development or how theoretical models or frameworks informed curriculum design or delivery. Four dominant discourses emerged from the meta-synthesis as follows:

Theme 1: Moving beyond mediocrity

Theme 2: Me, myself and I

Theme 3: The curricular suitcase

Theme 4: Learning elevators

The first theme relates to an expressed sense of discontent among nursing academics with the existing models and approaches to curriculum development. There was also a desire to engage in different approaches that bear witness to the ontological basis of nursing that would transcend theory and practice-based learning (Theme 1: Moving beyond mediocrity).

The theme of self-knowledge and the need for teachers and students to have multiple perspectives of self was commonly expressed within the literature. There was a view that there was great merit to be gained from valuing personhood by knowing and caring for all the dimensions of self and developing an empathetic connection with others as if oneself (Theme 2: Me, myself and I).

Significant attention was also paid to the multitude of competing factors that influence and define the content of curricula. There was a predominant theme that nursing curricula are overly influenced by bio-scientific knowledge. Achieving the optimal blend between the art and science of nursing was explored in terms of the value of some traditional core content and the need to shift the focus to embedding core skills that are important to people receiving care, such as communication skills. Dissatisfaction was expressed with the levels of cohesion and integration within and across different subject areas and disciplines in terms of how curricula are constructed (Theme 3: The curricular suitcase).

'Theme 4: Learning elevators' emerged as an expression of the need to prioritise learning experiences that illuminated and crystallised students' understanding of person-centredness. It was suggested that person-centred learning was more likely to occur in safe yet highly challenging learning environments. Where person-centred approaches were reported to occur, these were achieved through service user involvement and through the use of specific teaching and learning methodologies at module level, such as problem-based learning, simulation, role-play and reflection.

The findings from the meta-synthesis provided valuable insights into factors to consider in the development of nursing curricula. The issues arising from the four dominant themes support the view that some nurse teachers are conscious of seeking evidence of the effectiveness and relevance of their teaching and learning strategies. Those who have taken action to address this have emphasised that curriculum change is slow, time consuming and demanding. It was concluded that there is a need for further research to explore how students, educators and clinicians perceive and seek to promote person-centred practice through the experience of nursing education. Furthermore, it was emphasised that there is a need to develop evidence-informed pedagogies so that nurse educators have some confidence and direction in determining effective ways to change their teaching practices to promote learning about person-centred practice.

Educational philosophy

In engaging in curriculum development, the team considered the educational philosophy underpinning the programme in order that the conditions of learning were created to match our vision of how students learn effectively. In engaging with the Person-centred Nursing Framework of McCormack and McCance (2010), the team was cognisant of the need for students to have skills in being able to mould and shape a culture of person-centredness, necessitating them to develop their critical thinking and reflective skills in order to be effective agents of change in practice.

At both practice and educational levels, achieving development in both students and practice necessitates a process that awakens a student to the possibilities and potential by which they are surrounded. This is necessary to enable them to emancipate themselves in order to optimise practice. These concepts are aligned with a critical pedagogical approach to education, emanating from the pioneering work of Paulo Freire (1974).

Freirean principles of education contend that effective education must be transformative. Freire contends that this is achieved through the development of a radical consciousness whereby the student is awakened to having a critical awareness of their relationship with society, history and influential powers (Freire 1972). Being aware is central to developing an understanding of how oneself and others are conditioned by such factors; without awareness one cannot self-actualise and hold the innovative and entrepreneurial skills of contemporary graduates. Within the context of the Person-centred Nursing Framework, these principles filter through many layers, influencing students' abilities to engage with macro-influences, to truly know themselves and to be aware of their beliefs and values, and to have the skills to engage with the complexity of the care environment.

Freire (1972) believed that students come to education blinded by their conditioning, of which they may not be aware. To achieve social awakening, a 'banking' approach to education must be averted, where students are seen as recipients of narrations from teachers. Rather, they must be enlightened through a student-centred approach where educators and students engage in a dialogic process in which they are collaborative explorers of knowledge. This critical engagement shares power, whereby the educator is a mediator of knowledge, harnessing the skills of critical reflection that are core to transformation. This critical awareness and awakening are considered to lead to authentic knowledge, which leads to action that is morally laden.

The role of learning facilitators (including teachers and mentors) is therefore to create the conditions for such critical dialogue through creative, challenging and multi-directional communicative spaces in both the university and practice learning setting. This flourishing approach to education has a strong synergy with the Person-centred Nursing Framework of McCormack and McCance (2010), aligning the curricular structure with the principles of education.

Furthermore, a Freirean approach aligns with Theme 1 of the meta-synthesis, enabling both educators and students to understand the factors that lead to dis-content and empower them to be moral agents of change. It further aligns with Theme 2 in that it embraces a culture of learning that focuses on personhood and knowing self, not in a singular sense, but in a relational, worldly sense. Theme 4 comes alive in a Freirean approach as students are facilitated through critical learning processes that are learning elevators, in illuminating their understand-ing of personhood.

Constructing and sequencing the Person-centred Nursing curriculum

For a curriculum to be developed effectively, consideration needs to be given to the definition and philosophy behind the type of nurse it is hoped will emerge on successful completion of the programme. The processes through which educators support students to learn in a way that prepares them to act autonomously with integrity and keen decision-making skills must be clearly planned and articu-lated. It is often at this stage that discontent with the status quo can be identified and innovative ideas for achieving excellence in education can be shared and explored – this can be seen as an opportunity to move beyond mediocrity and the required minimum standard for registration or certification, principles aligned with critical pedagogy.

The concept of a curriculum does not exist in a standalone state. The historic-ity and socio-political context within which we exist shapes and is shaped by our worldly relationships. The development, planning, delivery and evaluation of education are largely influenced by the beliefs and values of teachers and stu-dents and the culture in which the curriculum exists. It is important for those involved in curriculum planning to develop self-knowledge and insight into the motivation that drives their roles, prior to developing a strategy to create an aligned cultural and curricular reality.

Implicit in the philosophical basis of a person-centred, critical pedagogy is the belief that people who have experience of receiving care are best placed to deter-mine the extent to which care is effective, meaningful and thus person-centred.

In order to develop a person-centred curriculum it was considered imperative that the views of service users should be given due prominence and consideration through authentic dialogic engagement. A research study was conducted to explore service users' and carers' views about programmes that lead to registration as a nurse, and also to evaluate how this feedback impacted on curriculum development. The objectives of the study were to identify views about the design and delivery of programmes that lead to becoming a registered nurse and to map how this feedback influenced curriculum development (Table 7.1). Involvement in this study led to the development of a service users' and carers' forum to further inform education processes and practice.

Once consensus was reached about the overall philosophy of the programme, the values and beliefs of the educators and the values and beliefs both inherent and to be moulded in students were identified. In general, these values and beliefs address the key concepts of person, health, environment and nursing, professionals and education. While the use of single models of nursing to underpin education programmes is considered outdated due to limits in their applicability to all care settings (Boore & Deeny 2012), the Person-centred Nursing

Table 7.1 The impact of service user feedback on curriculum development.

Service user feedback	Actions taken by curriculum development team
'Importance of the person being valued'	Person-centred Curriculum Framework
'We want to feel safe in the classroom'	Code of Practice for Public Engagement in Nursing Education implemented across all programmes
'Visit me at home to understand who I am'	Opportunity for first practice learning experience to take place in the community
'We know what makes a good nurse – being authentic, someone who really listens, who doesn't have to be reminded, who makes time to explain and reassure, who picks up on my feelings, who identifies with me'	Primacy of communication approaches in all learning activities
'Care for yourself as well as your patients'	Theme of self-knowledge developed across curricula
'We would like to give feedback to students about the care they have provided'	All students will receive formative feedback from service users about the care provided
'Don't lose what is special about being students'	Service user involvement with students to explore why students are 'special' to patients and how they can carry this with them during their career
'Get involved with us through volunteering'	Volunteering Charter

Framework of McCormack and McCance (2010) is different in that it focuses on the two key collaborators in care – the nurse and the person – regardless of the setting and it is thus almost universally applicable.

Careful consideration was given to the Quality Assurance Agency (2001) subject benchmarks for nursing and the NMC (Nursing and Midwifery Council 2010) standards for pre-registration nursing education. These outlined domains and outcomes for nursing education focused on public confidence that all nurses in the profession will deliver quality care that meets the needs of all those with whom they come into contact in their roles. Barnett and Coate (2005) suggest a framework for curricula based on three domains of knowing, acting and being to determine the content and structure of curricula. Education programmes are ultimately concerned with knowing, and nursing as a profession is primarily about doing; it is the being aspect that can be ultimately informed by the principles of the Person-centred Nursing Framework and a Freirean approach. In addition, both facilitate not only the key skills of reasoning and decision-making, but also the sensitivity and sense of moral responsibility essential to enable self-determination (McCormack and McCance 2010).

After consideration by the staff of the School of Nursing, the curriculum development steering group explored how the Person-centred Nursing Framework might be used to guide the design of a programme to develop graduate nurses who have the knowledge, skills, values and beliefs to deliver professional, competent, safe and effective care that is person-centred in design, delivery and outcomes. It was envisaged that graduates would have the appropriate value system, ability and commitment to lifelong learning and developing professional practice in tandem with emerging evidence and changes in care delivery systems. Use of the framework was helpful in guiding the team to choose the elements that were essential – the key items to pack into the curricular suitcase. It supported the achievement of integration and cohesion and complements a critical pedagogical approach.

The Person-centred Nursing Framework addresses the prerequisites for person-centred practice, the nature of the environment in which care is provided, the process required to provide the care, and the means to measure the outcomes of the care. The aim of the programme is to produce new graduate nurses who are equipped with the prerequisites and are able to use their knowledge and skills to progressively enhance person-centred nursing by influencing care environments and care processes to produce positive outcomes for people, their carers and families – in other words, agents of transformation.

Utilising the Person-centred Nursing Framework to inform practice development means that nurses bring with them their experiences of practice and the knowledge gained from experience. When integrating Person-centred Nursing Framework into curriculum design, educators must be aware that students may come representing a diversity of experiences of life and previous caring, whilst others may not have that past to reflect upon. Indeed, Freire (1972) views our historicity as central to our authentic knowing of self. There was a need to develop a shared starting point for all students commencing the programme. The framework guided the structuring of learning priorities and the design of learning elevators – the activities and experiences, commensurate with the stage of the programme, that engage students in understanding their practice.

The programme starts by focusing on the attributes of the nurses and how students can develop knowledge of how their beliefs and values can impact on the care that they provide. Students are encouraged to become more self-aware – to help them understand they need to have an insight into who they are before they can help others. They examine the nature of commitment to provide the nursing care that is best for the people for whom they are providing care. The development and practice of effective interpersonal skills to enable them to communicate at a variety of levels is a fundamental outcome in many modules. The development of knowledge and skills to make decisions and prioritise care is also crucial, and students are guided in this process throughout the programme. These key prerequisite qualities are revisited and reflected on in increasing depth throughout the stages of the course.

Once students experience practice learning and progress through the first year, other aspects of the Person-centred Nursing Framework are introduced. The nature of the care environment is highlighted in terms of the composition of the health-care team and the sharing of decision-making and power in effective relationships between staff and the people they provide care for. In the second year, students gain an understanding of the nature and influence of organisational culture and environment that is crucial if they are to make a difference to people by the way they provide care. An appreciation of organisational systems that support innovation and creativity in care-giving is key to the development of entrepreneurial nursing practice during the final year of the programme.

Person-centred care processes are highlighted throughout the course, beginning with a focus on engagement with people requiring care and support and working with their beliefs and values to gain an insight into what it is that is valued by the individual and their family. The need for a holistic perspective in nursing care underpins all activities undertaken by students. Students will develop an awareness of the importance of a sympathetic presence and shared decision-making and will gain the skills necessary to incorporate this into their practice. The need for graduates who are skilled and competent in these aspects of care has been highlighted by feedback from the service user and carer forum, whose input provided a key insight into what nurse characteristics are valued by service users.

The final year brings the ideas of prerequisites, environment and processes together in considering the outcomes of care. The evaluation of outcomes of person-centred care involves knowledge and skills to which students are introduced cumulatively during the programme. From assessing the satisfaction and well-being that people, their carers and families experience when involved with care, to the creation and maintenance of a therapeutic culture based on transformative leadership, the focus is on the creation of graduate nurses who can provide effective person-centred care.

Designing the learning and teaching culture and experience

A crucial aspect was the preparation and support of staff to think differently and to encourage innovative and creative approaches to learning and assessment. The challenge for all staff was to role-model person-centredness as embedded in the role of the educator. This required deeper consideration of our roles in the context of adult education, developing technologies and fiscal pressures. We needed to reflect on how we wanted to interact with students to demonstrate the types of behaviours we wanted students to emulate with those in their care and their working teams. Staff engaged in a series of workshops and creative thinking zones to unpack the concepts of the Person-centred Nursing Framework and identify the beliefs and values held as a team of teachers and educators. Attributes considered essential for effective facilitators included genuineness, and empathy or empathic understanding, as described by Rogers and Freiberg (1994). They also underpin dialogic engagement at the heart of critical pedagogy. This process of reframing traditional approaches resulted in a changing culture within the School driven by the motivation to make the curriculum real (McCormack et al. 2014). As a result a School-wide culture change project was established following the completion of the curriculum, guided by a coordinating group in partnership with an external facilitator. This project aimed to promote a sense of belonging and integration between colleagues, where staff felt autonomous, motivated and responsible for personal and professional development and true participants in decision-making in the School. As a consequence, staff teams work closely to focus on how colleagues can support and challenge each other to live the espoused vision, purpose and values (Box 7.1).

Box 7.1 Culture Change Project.

Vision

The School of Nursing will have a positive influence on the lives of students, staff and all those we engage with and will be recognised nationally and internationally as progressive.

Purpose

Our purpose is to develop a flourishing person-centred culture that:
- positively influences:
  - students' experience and learning
  - staff's experience, learning, development and inquiry
  - people's health-care experience
- establishes and maintains a positive legacy for the university and society.

Values and behaviours framework

	Shared purpose		
	Flourishing students and staff	*Flourishing person-centred culture*	*Positive impact on university and society*
Our values:	Inclusiveness	Integrity	Professionalism
Our commitments to each other	People will feel valued, respected and involved as individuals	People will feel trusted to work in committed and integrated teams to learn from and with each other	People will feel confident and committed to make a difference to society based on their complementary talents and expertise
Standards	• Respect people and their dignity • Be person-centred, positive and caring • Appreciate and celebrate each other • Listen and clearly communicate • Consistently work to nurture and develop the potential of each other	• Consistently work together towards the common purpose • Consistently support each other to reflect, learn and develop • Courage to give and receive feedback • Work with personal and professional commitment and passion • Work as a team with individual and team role clarity • Take responsibility and are accountable for own actions and decisions • Walk the walk	• Deliver the best outcomes for students, the school, university and society within resources available • Draw on the different gifts and talents of all • Always improving • Always using and developing evidence to underpin actions, decisions and professional practice • Maintain equity in work-life balance for self and others

The goal was to actively embed the principles of person-centredness and awareness of Person-centred Nursing Framework into the module designs, teaching plans and the application of concepts to what is being learned. The course teams encouraged approaches to teaching learning and assessment that fostered dialogic student engagement with methodologies selected being determined by the nature of the specified learning outcomes. A number of modules are taught primarily through practical workshops, group work and simulation using a problem-based learning approach coupled with reflection on individual potential and personal flourishing.

It was envisaged that students would progress through stages of learning in both small and large groups, stages that involve students' observation, practice, reflection on their experiences, consolidation and active involvement in the development of confidence and competence in person-centred care throughout the programme from their first year to graduation. Creative approaches to learning were integrated, including reflection, drama, service user assessment and feedback during skills teaching, and service user involvement in classroom teaching. A range of assessment strategies were developed to include assignments based on reflective practice and encouraging innovation to improve person-centred practices. Students were also guided in their engagement with learning outcomes to formulate a range of examination questions that they feel would help them give of their best in a module examination. A selection of these are chosen and supplemented by module coordinators to develop examination papers and rubrics that are student-centred where students can see clear links between learning outcomes and assessment strategies (Biggs and Tang 2011).

The learning and assessment experience is designed to encourage students to become active and motivated learners, who can seek information, question and analyse its validity, and draw appropriate and logical conclusions. Students are encouraged to make connections between theoretical content and practice experiences, thus facilitating an ability to move from understanding practice and applying skills taught to questioning and critiquing practice and proposing possible research or innovation that would contribute to developments or enhancements in practice. This serves to help students understand the symbiotic link between theory and practice in a relational, worldly context. The ethics of professional standards in study, professional practice and research form a theme that crosses the entirety of the course to encompass not just learning in the university setting, but in practice as well.

Service user and carer engagement has been a fundamental component of the development of person-centred learning cultures within the School. The service users' and carers' forum makes a unique and important contribution to the work of the School, and a range of other members of the public contribute to activities across the School, including interviewing and selection of students, clinical skills teaching, involvement in assessment processes, and sharing their experiences with students through seminars and workshops.

Practice learning in the curriculum

The advent of 'Fitness for Practice' approaches in nursing curricula in the last 20 years has led to a competency-based approach to practice learning underpinned by minimum standards with core skills at the heart of assessment (Carr 2008). Minimum standards can feed a culture of mediocrity, and often lie within a banking approach to education. It could be argued that this has deflected from a person-centred approach and influenced, to a degree, an outcome-based approach not centred on the care of people but the achievement of a competency. While it could be further argued that such competency should be grounded in person-centredness, no curricular structure or set of professional standards to date has been centrally constructed around person-centred nursing, albeit influenced by it. Compounding this is the evolving nature of the nurse's role, influenced in part by the expanding role of the health-care assistant, a role that has adopted many traditional aspects of the nurse's role. In this shifting landscape, traditional expectations and preconceptions of nursing can challenge student perceptions as to where the person-centredness lies in practice. Additionally, it is widely reported that students are often attracted to nursing as a result of being motivated by compassion, but that their positive ideals can be lost as they journey through their educational experience as a result of oppressive forces (Adam & Taylor 2014). Adam and Taylor (2014) report that this can be the result of cure being valued above care, a biomedical discourse, and as a result of occupational socialisation, whereby students change their practice to fit and be accepted within the culture that they are learning. This is contrary to truly knowing self and being a transformative change agent. What students do in practice is central to how they develop as a nurse (Carr 2008). As a result, the philosophy of the practice environment must have a synergy with that of the theoretical and curricular structures and philosophies of the course, necessitating a Freirean approach to student learning.

Developing and sustaining the curriculum

Collaborative partnership is vital in developing a curriculum in order to distinguish what each party can bring to it and to bridge variations in perspectives by coming to a collective consciousness. This approach is more likely to achieve stability and sustainability of the course in its co-delivery (MacPhee et al. 2009), while also attending to internal cohesion of the curriculum (Theme 3 of the meta-analysis). Dobalian et al. (2014) identify five elements of effective academic-practice partnerships. Firstly, there must be inter-organisational collaboration, weaving the construction of relationships and processes of both together. At Ulster, this was achieved through developing a steering group for curriculum development that involved practice partners as key stakeholders, and a sub-planning group for the practice element of the programme (Figure 7.1). Secondly, understanding the interface of the blending of the practice and academic cultures is necessary. To achieve this, we sought meaningful involvement of students, service users and mentors to integrate their perspectives into the curriculum planning process. Through ongoing consultation, collaboration, obtaining feedback and seeking agreement, a cohesive structure for the practice learning element of the programme emerged with shared ownership. The third theme identified by Dobalian et al. (2014) is that of identifying practice partners with a key role with educational partners. In Northern Ireland, a Practice

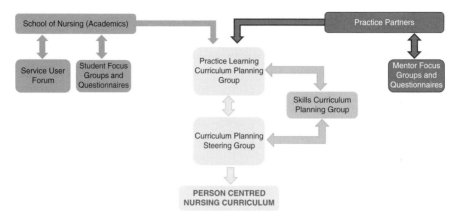

Figure 7.1 Development of Practice Learning Component of Curriculum.

Education Team infrastructure was realised in 2009 and has successfully forged a strong collaborative partnership with the School since then. The fourth theme refers to having a collaborative framework for applying evidence-informed practice in practice. By developing an evidence-informed curriculum and linking this with the framework for learning and assessment in practice, this was achieved. A project team took a participatory action research approach to develop the portfolio for practice learning, which used evidence not only to build it, but also to ensure practice learning and development was grounded in evidence. Finally, Dobalian et al. (2014) identified the need for long-term stability in the relationship. Figure 7.2 identifies the long-term structure set in place to support the delivery of the practice learning element of the programme, which is founded upon ongoing, collaborative and communicative relationships. This relationship is central to the ongoing sustainability of curriculum delivery and creates a communicative space for dialogue not just with educators, but also with students. This is central to critical pedagogy.

Framework for learning in practice

It is essential that the practice-learning element of any curriculum is cohesive and synergistic with the theoretical component (Theme 3 of the meta-synthesis). This required that the Person-centred Nursing Framework underpinned the design of the practice-learning element of the programme in alignment with Freirean principles. However, the NMC Standards for Learning and Assessment in Practice (SLAiP) (Nursing and Midwifery Council 2008) and 2010 pre-registration education standards (Nursing and Midwifery Council 2010) needed to map into any design, alongside those of the Quality Assurance Agency (QAA) and the University (Figure 7.3). This also necessitated reflecting a framework that enveloped all fields of practice across the three years. The tool for achieving the blend of all of

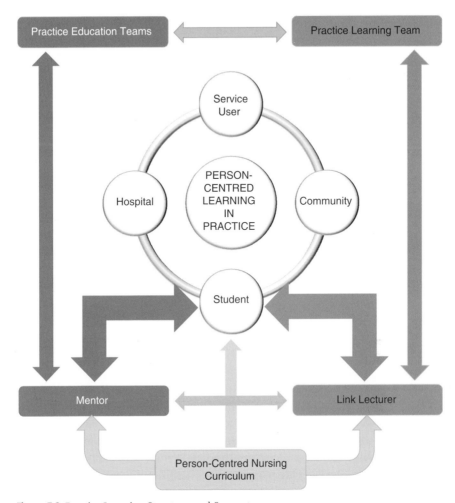

Figure 7.2 Practice Learning Structure and Support.

these factors was a practice-learning portfolio for each year of the programme (Figure 7.4). Through the action research process, it was identified that three core elements would be used to focus student learning within a person-centred, Freirean context:

1 Reflections mapped to learning outcomes.
2 Worksheets mapped to learning outcomes.
3 Service user/carer feedback linked to learning outcomes.

Reflections and worksheets

Adam and Taylor (2014) identified in their research that the use of reflecting on practice learning experiences is central to identifying skills and knowledge underpinning compassionate care; this is supported by the work of Adamson

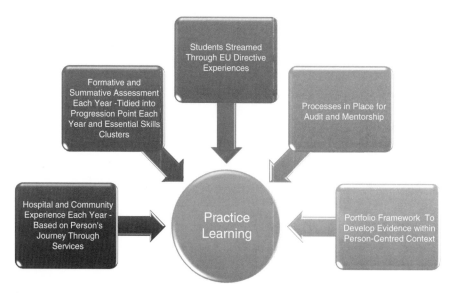

Figure 7.3 Key Components of Practice Learning Structure.

and Dewer (2014). Indeed, this aligned with Theme 2 of the meta-synthesis. In particular, interpersonal skills that are core to compassionate human interactions are developed alongside coping strategies to respond compassionately to the challenging realities of practice, a pursuit with which critical pedagogy must engage. This can negate disengagement from the person and their situation, which can occur due to being overwhelmed, but rather encourages embracing the human reality with compassion (Youngson 2011). Deeper understanding can then be achieved as opposed to trauma or disconnection. Youngson (2011) relays how compassion is a renewable source of energy – facilitating students to develop their skills in being compassionate will therefore offset compassion fatigue. Furthermore, reflective learning engages students in contemplating new knowledge arising from experiences. This can lead to insight into the needs

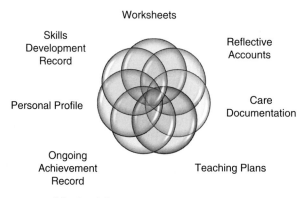

Figure 7.4 Components of the Portfolio.

of the people the students care for, alongside an awareness of the values and influences that govern the nature of that care (Adamson and Dewer 2014), a truly Freirean endeavour. Students then enter a process of cognitively reframing stressful experiences into constructive learning that informs their future compassionate care (Adam and Taylor 2014) and underpins transformative practices. Integrating reflections into practice by valuing them as evidence towards identified practice learning outcomes therefore provided the basis for engaging students with the process of learning to be compassionate, while also valuing that contribution to their learning and development as part of their assessment. Valuing students as people in this regard is central for a wholly engaged approach to critical pedagogy (Freire 1972). It is through this approach that the competency-based approach to practice can remain embedded within a person-centred, compassionate framework without reducing it to a transactional banking educational approach. This was extended into the use of worksheets that are reflective in nature but span core curricular areas on a developmental basis each year. For example, an adult student develops a reflective worksheet in relation to the care of a person with a learning disability in year 1. The complexity and depth of this is built upon in a similar worksheet in year 2 and again in year 3. This enables the bridging of reflection with learning outcomes across core curricular areas and fields of practice in a cumulatively developmental manner across the three years of the programme.

Service user feedback

The experience of being cared for provides invaluable information to the developing student nurse. Adam and Taylor (2014) highlight the necessity to value the integrity and authenticity of human interactions, noting that educational approaches in practice must create mechanisms whereby students are engaged with processes that illuminate such value. Indeed, this is synergistic with Freirean principles. While the NMC (Nursing and Midwifery Council 2010) requires service user involvement in assessment processes in practice, it is not prescriptive about how this is achieved. Through engagement with the Service User Forum in the School, a consultation took place on how this could best be achieved with meaning. This resulted in the development of a Service User/Carer Feedback tool that was integrated as an essential component of evidence for the verification of particular practice learning outcomes. In doing so, an appreciative enquiry philosophy is adopted, in that engaging with feedback from people being cared for informs development and embeds compassion into the assessment processes (Trueland 2009; Adam & Taylor 2014). It is through such an approach that the person remains central to the care being provided, rather than facilitating a competency-task-driven process for achievement that does not consider the human element central to compassionate, person-centred care – Theme 2 of the meta-synthesis.

Mentorship and partnership

Effective mentorship within a supportive practice-learning environment has been evidenced to positively influence student empowerment (Bradbury-Jones et al. 2011). That sense of empowerment underpins how valued a student feels in that learning relationship, as a person, team member and learner (Freire 1972; Bradbury-Jones et al. 2011). Adamson and Dewar (2014) identify that developing skills in delivering compassionate care is predicated upon feeling valued, necessitating an empowered student. This is also central to a Freirean approach. As a result, effective mentorship is central to achieving the development of person-centredness in practice. While the School has a robust and innovative process of ensuring each and every student is allocated to a mentor meeting the NMC (Nursing and Midwifery Council 2008) SLAiP requirements, the change to a curriculum built around the Person-centred Nursing Framework required a strategy to ensure a refocus on the principles of the new approach (Figure 7.5). A cohesive preparation strategy was essential to offset any variation in preparation and support often experienced by mentors (Gurling 2011). However, such a shift in the structure and philosophy of the programme meant that practice partners need a period of time for adjustment not only to a new programme, but also to a new culture of learning. Ongoing support and liaising with practice partners through the Practice Education Teams infrastructure engendered a partnership approach that existed in designing the programme to permeate into support for its delivery in practice, central to cohesion – Theme 3. To complement this approach, a comprehensive handbook was collaboratively developed, within which clear roles of the student, mentor and link lecturer emerged. These were developed with each relevant stakeholder and complemented the NMC (2008) SLAiP. This role clarity was essential to stabilise the support network for both students and those supporting them (Gurling 2011). To further promote stability, link lecturers were identified for each practice setting to ensure continuity of relationships and promote support for curriculum delivery, including monitoring the quality of the learning experience through partnership, feedback and educational audit.

Conclusion

The development of person-centred nursing education remains a work in progress as the living curriculum unfolds and matures in response to the perceptions and experiences of students and learning facilitators. It has been our experience that the roots of person-centredness can be firmly and explicitly established through nursing education. The alignment of educational and practice philosophies enabled us to craft an undergraduate nursing curriculum with the capacity to create the conditions for learning where person-centred practice could be recognised, valued, expected and delivered.

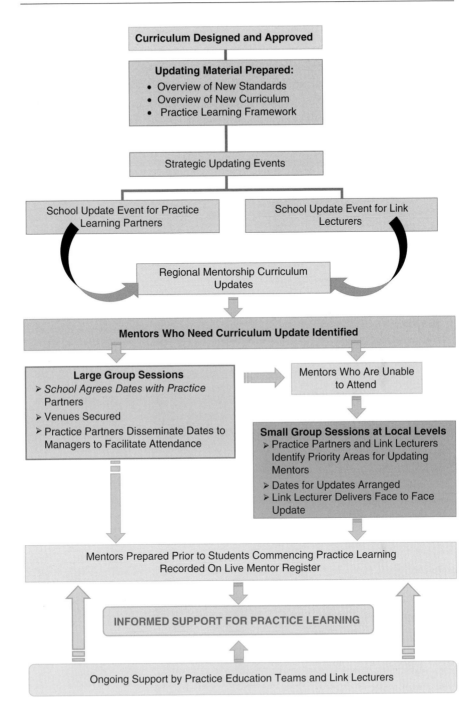

Figure 7.5 Mentor Curriculum Update Strategy.

Undertaking a meta-synthesis led to critical consciousness raising and the identification of factors considered to be influential in the realisation of person-centredness in the curriculum. This enabled a cohesive, value-laden approach to engaging in sculpting a curriculum through dialogue, alignment of values, and integration of professional requirements and standards.

A body of ongoing research is associated with the development of person-centred undergraduate nursing. The findings of these studies will seek to inform our understanding of how students conceptualise person-centredness and provide evidence of teaching and learning approaches that are effective in this regard.

References

Adam, D. and Taylor, R. (2014) Compassionate care: Empowering students through nurse education. *Nurse Education Today*, **34**, 1242–5.

Adamson, E. and Dewar, B. (2014) Compassionate care: Student nurses' learning through reflection and the use of story. *Nurse Education in Practice*, **15**, 155–61. doi: 10.1016/j.nepr.2014.08.002

Barnett, R. and Coate, K. (2005) *Engaging the Curriculum in Higher Education*, Open University Press, Maidenhead, UK.

Biggs, J. and Tang, C. (2011) *Teaching for Quality Learning at University*, 4th edn, Open University Press, Maidenhead, UK.

Boore, J. and Deeny, P. (2012) *Nursing Education: Planning and Delivering the Curriculum*, Sage, London.

Bradbury-Jones, C., Sambrook, S., and Irvine, F. (2011) Empowerment and being valued: A phenomenological study of nursing students' experiences of clinical practice. *Nurse Education Today*, **31**, 368–72.

Carr, G. (2008) Changes in nurse education: Delivering the curriculum. *Nurse Education Today*, **28**, 120–7.

Dobalian, A., Bowman, C., Wyte-Lake, T., Pearson, M., Dougherty, M., and Needleman, J. (2014) The critical elements of effective academic-practice partnerships: a framework derived from the Department of Veterans Affairs Nursing Academy. *BMC Nursing*, **13**, 1–31.

Freire, P. (1972) *Pedagogy of the Oppressed*, Herder and Herder, New York.

Freire P. (1974) *Education for Critical Consciousness*. London: Bloomsbury Academic (2013 reprint).

Gurling, J. (2011) Link mentorship: improving support for pre-registration students and mentors. *British Journal of Community Nursing*, **16**, 435–40.

MacPhee M, Wejr P, Davis M, Semeniuk P, Scarborough K. (2009) Practice and academic nurse educators: finding common ground. *International Journal of Nursing Education Scholarship* **6**: art. 32. doi: 10.2202/1548-923X.1882.

McCormack, B. (2004) Person-centredness in gerontological nursing: an overview of the literature. *International Journal of Older People Nursing*, **13** (3), 31–8.

McCormack, B. and McCance, T. (2010) *Person-Centred Nursing: Theory and Practice*, Wiley-Blackwell, Oxford.

McCormack B, McGowan B, McGonigle M, Goode D, Black P, Sinclair M. (2014) Exploring 'self' as a person-centred academic, through critical creativity. *International Practice Development Journal* **4**(2): art. 3. Available at: http://www.fons.org/library/journal/volume4-issue2/article3 (accessed 2 February 2016).

Noblit, G. and Hare, R. (1988) *Meta-Ethnography: Synthesising Qualitative Studies*, Sage, Newbury Park.

Nursing and Midwifery Council (2008) *Standards to support learning and assessment in practice*. London: NMC.

Nursing and Midwifery Council (2010) *Standards for pre-registration nursing education*. Nursing and Midwifery Council: London. Available at: http://standards.nmc-uk.org/PublishedDocuments/Standards%20for%20pre-registration%20nursing%20education%2016082010.pdf (accessed 2 February 2016).

Quality Assurance Agency (QAA) (2001) *Benchmark statement: Health care programmes – nursing*. Gloucester, UK: Quality Assurance Agency for Higher Education. Available at: http://www.qaa.ac.uk/en/Publications/Documents/Subject-benchmark-statement-Health-care-programmes---Nursing.pdf (accessed 2 February 2016).

Rogers, C. and Freiberg, H.J. (1994) *Freedom to Learn*, 3rd edn, Prentice Hall, Upper Saddle River, NJ.

Trueland, J. (2009) Compassion through human connection. *Nursing Standard*, **23** (48), 19.

Youngson, R. (2011) Compassion in healthcare – the missing dimension of healthcare reform? in *Caregiver Stress and Staff Support in Illness, Dying and Bereavement* (ed I. Renzenbrink), Oxford University Press, Oxford, pp. 37–49.

CHAPTER 8

Person-centred research

Belinda Dewar[1], Aisling McBride[2] & Cathy Sharp[3]

[1] University of the West of Scotland, UK
[2] University of the West of Scotland, Hamilton, Scotland
[3] Research for Real Edinburgh, Scotland, UK

Research that explores person-centredness has adopted a range of methodologies. This chapter presents one methodology – that of appreciative action research. I begin by sketching out the principles of appreciative action research and then present an argument for the use of this methodology for research into person-centredness. This is illustrated through case examples about how these principles are promoted in practice. I include an introduction to the caring conversations framework that supports animation of the appreciative dialogue in practice as well as promoting person-centred caring cultures. In conclusion, the chapter suggests that affirmation, provocation, inquiry and collaboration are core elements that enhance a more hopeful and improvisational approach to innovation in health and social care.

Introduction

The health and social care landscape is characterised by paradox, ambiguity and complexity, and now more than ever before there is a need for an approach to inquiry that can accommodate the challenges of the dynamic world of practice, the variety of people with whom practitioners work, and the dominant discourse of helplessness, negativity and control.

A range of participative research methodologies have been used to explore person centredness (Glasson 2006; McCormack et al. 2011; Manley et al. 2014). Participative methodologies, such as action research, are appropriate as they align with principles of person-centredness in that they aim to be inclusive, democratic and collaborative. In addition they support people to learn from experience and support the blending of research and practice, which fits well with the discipline of nursing (Cowling 2001).

What is appreciative action research?

Action research 'seeks to bring together action and reflection, theory and practice, in participation with others, in the pursuit of practical solutions to issues of pressing concern to people' (Reason & Bradbury 2001, p. 1). In this sense it is a problem-solving approach that aims to create practical knowledge through inquiry. Appreciative inquiry shares the social constructivist foundations of action research and aspires to the same goals, that is, to work towards emancipatory transformation (Reason & Bradbury 2001; Grant & Humphries 2006; Reed 2007). Yet, appreciative inquiry has a distinctive positive and generative philosophical stance that claims to:

> unleash a positive revolution of conversation and changes in organisations by unseating existing reified patterns of discourse, creating space for new voices and new discoveries, and expanding circles of dialogue to provide a community of support for innovative action.
>
> *Ludema et al. (2001, p. 189)*

Appreciative inquiry has been used in an array of differing organisational contexts to transform practice by developing theory of what 'gives life' to an organisation, and what it is that works well (Carter 2006; Dewar & Mackay 2010; Bellinger & Elliot 2011; Rubin et al. 2011; Doggett & Lewis 2013). From this premise, theory embedded in the direct experiences of stakeholders can be developed to allow the focus of any 'action' taken forward to be based on 'the most positive core – their values, visions, achievements, and best practices' (Watkins & Mohr 2001, p. xxxi).

The principles of appreciative inquiry are:

- that inquiry begins with appreciation of what works well and what is valued;
- that it is applicable to the system in which the inquiry takes place and is validated in action;
- that the inquiry should be provocative, encourage reflection in and on action and create new knowledge compelling to the organisation members;
- that it is collaborative, in the sense that participants must be part of the design and execution of the inquiry (Bushe & Kassam 2005).

Here I argue that action research that uses an explicit appreciative focus of inquiry, and so of how problems are framed in the first place, enables practitioners to make ongoing judgements about what will be 'life giving'. This deliberate stance away from a deficit-focus enables practitioners to respect the complexities of situations they face and keep conversations person-centred and generative whilst exploring vulnerabilities, fears, distress and criticism as well as 'moments of excellence' (Fry 2014, p. 48).

In this way, appreciative inquiry shares the core of all person-centred approaches in shifting from focusing on the negative (the problems and deficiencies) in people to recognising and so releasing people's potential (strengths and abilities).

Appreciative action research (AAR) has been described by Egan and Lancaster (2005) and tested out by Dewar (2010) as an approach that combines the principles of emancipatory action research with those of appreciative inquiry (AI). The framework for appreciative action research shown in Figure 8.1, developed and tested by Dewar (2010), combines these key principles into one

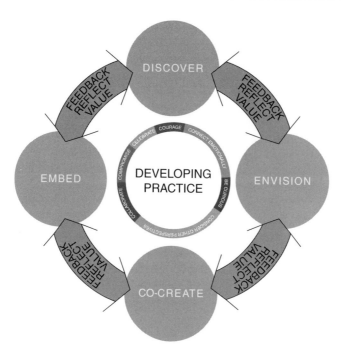

Figure 8.1 Appreciative action research. Source: Dewar and MacBride (2014). Reproduced with permission from Rory Dewar.

framework. This ensures that the positive perspective of appreciative inquiry is combined with a systematic approach to experimentation in practice, the taking of action, reflection on action, and evaluation of processes and outcomes. Evaluation is built into the day-to-day process of the inquiry and is a process of continuous reflection, valuing and feedback.

The approach of appreciative action research goes through a number of phases, which it is helpful to make explicit. It starts with the *discovery* of what is working well – what excites us in our work; what makes a difference to staff, people that use services and their families; what are we proud of; why do things work well; what helps it to happen; how do we make sense of what is believed and said about the system at its best? It also looks at and explores what matters and what is valued.

We then feed back learning from the discovery phase to work with people to *envision* the desired future. This is followed by *co-creating* with all those involved ways of achieving the ideal and developing strategies to articulate learning and achievements. And finally the phase of *embed*, which is about embedding new developments in routine practice, and considering what people need to continue learning and flourishing.

Throughout all of this there is a need to create opportunities for processes of feedback reflection and valuing. In these processes, conversations and language matter in how we make sense of what is going on and consider possibilities. We do this through *appreciative dialogue*, which is:

> dialogue in the sense of enabling us to talk to each other about what we aspire to do, and appreciative in the sense of supporting people to engage in meaningful conversations that help them analyse and articulate what works well and when. This raises these positive practices to consciousness and motivates practitioners to make this way of behaving happen more often.
>
> *Dewar and Sharp (2013, p. 2)*

Appreciative action research as a relational practice

The relationships existing between people in an organisation or system *are* the organisation, and form the basis of its strength or weakness. We know that the quality of relationships determines outcomes for staff experience and well-being as well as patient and family well-being and care experience (Nolan et al. 2006).

Appreciative action research celebrates both individual and mutual successes to create a positive relational language of inquiry and dialogue. An appreciative stance to inquiry is inevitably a form of relational practice as it has to be done 'with' rather than 'to' people. Strengths attributed to the appreciative approach include engagement, inclusivity and collaboration encouraging the acknowledgement of experiences and also individual skills (Trajkovski et al. 2012).

The various diverse formal roles within health care, such as nurse, clinician, patient, health-care assistant or relative, can act as a barrier to authentic relationships if a dialogue of mutual understanding is not encouraged. An appreciative stance enables a more humanistic, authentic and relational approach to research and practice development that helps people to step out from their formal ascribed or assumed roles and be more fully present with each other; what John Rowan (2001) calls 'research as if people were human' (Rowan 2001, p. 121)

What is important for person-centred practice or relational practice is that the philosophical values of exploring the uniqueness, wholeness and essence of human life *in the context of one another* are central to the research design. A framework of caring conversations has been developed to support appreciative dialogue and explore possibilities in relationship. It is this appreciative dialogue that helps us to engage in all the phases of AAR and may additionally support practitioners to evoke the Person-centred Nursing framework (McCormack & McCance 2010). The caring conversations framework arose through analysis of more than 240 hours of observation of practice, and eliciting stories about the experience of caring in an acute ward for older people (Dewar 2011; Dewar & Nolan 2013). The study was conducted as AAR (Dewar & Mackay 2010).

Table 8.1 Caring conversations to promote appreciative dialogue.

Be courageous	What would happen if I did something or did nothing? What would it take to give it a go?
Connect emotionally	How do you feel about what I have said?
Be curious	Help me to understand what happened? What do you care about or hope for? What do you notice? What are you wondering about?
Collaborate	Is there anyone else who could help us with this? How can we work together?
Consider other perspectives	What would others say?
Compromise	What is the ideal and what would you settle for? How can we achieve this together?
Celebrate	What has worked well and why? What do we value?

The framework asks that we consider seven key attributes in our interactions aimed at supporting learning and action (the seven Cs). These are illustrated in Table 8.1.

The caring conversations are the 'how' of AAR. The framework guides people to have different kinds of conversations that are appreciative, provocative, more open and inquiring. Some evidence suggests that Caring Conversations help to achieve relationship-centred practice where the senses of security, belonging, continuity, purpose, achievement and significance (the Senses Framework) are fulfilled (Dewar & Nolan 2013).

Related practice inquiry tools developed by practitioners and researchers to help care staff have Caring Conversations, including the Positive Inquiry tool, emotional touchpoints and the use of photo elicitation (Dewar et al. 2010; Dewar 2012). These practice inquiry tools have been used effectively in a range of settings, including care homes and with community-based health-care staff, to explore patient and family experience and to learn from a range of staff involved in caring across health and social care boundaries (Sharp et al. 2013; Dewar & MacBride 2014).

Core principles of appreciative action research

Through using the framework of caring conversations and associated practice tools we are able to highlight three important elements to AAR that enhance the relational and person-centred elements of this approach to inquiry. These are:
- Affirmation as provocation and innovation
- Collaborative inquiry as intervention
- Improvisation.

The next sections will explore these specific principles and use examples to illustrate their use in practice alongside suggestions for supporting the utilisation of the Person-centred Nursing framework (McCormack & McCance 2010).

Affirmation as provocation and innovation

The term provocation is perhaps best understood when aligned with positivity. Provocation here means that which is intended to excite, intrigue, dare, arrest thought or interrupt flow. It helps us to look at things from a different vantage point aimed at challenging assumptions, and say out loud that which is often not said, with the ultimate purpose of creating possibilities for thinking (and acting) in a different way. In this respect, it is a form of disruptive innovation, in the sense of novelty, but one that does not invoke defensiveness.

It has been suggested that an incremental approach to innovation that adopts and recombines things that already exist in new ways is more likely to be effective in health and social care (Mulgan 2013; Pennacchia 2013). I have found that asking appreciative and provocative questions and encouraging dialogue about hopes, passions, values and emotions are valuable ways to drive 'incremental or additive innovation' by building on the best of what already exists, and so in this way be transformational.

To be positive and provocative in unison in the context of health care and practice development means to question assumptions of how things are; is there another way to do something that may be more supportive to all within that practice setting? Is that possible? Could it be explored further? It worked well on an occasion, why was that? Barrett and Cooperrider (1990, p. 232) claim that a good metaphor 'provokes new thought, excites us with novel perspectives and enables us to see the world with fresh perspectives'. A generative metaphor is both a positive and provocative statement intended to enable an alternative perspective on practice to bring about transformational change by harnessing the potential that already exists within an organisation. The development of each 'generative metaphor' stems from the direct experiences of the people who work within that organisation or system. This stimulates the exploration of the possibility of positive change stretching beyond any current problematic situation (Richer et al. 2010).

Generative metaphors that emerged from the direct experiences and conversations within an older people acute care setting had a significant impact on future action (Dewar 2011).

As facilitators, noticing and being playful with language 'from a posture of empathy rather than attack' (Ludema et al. 2001, p. 197) is one of the most significant ways in which we have supported practitioners to explore taken-for-granted assumptions, develop a language of possibility and create generative metaphors.

I noticed, for example, that one support worker referred to a lady she was caring for as 'the lady who likes to be on the move a lot of the time'. The positivity of this statement struck me. I shared what we had noticed with the support worker, who reflected on this and shared other insights. This prompted others to say they often referred to those residents as 'wanderers', but that this way of saying things was better as it did not label the person, but explicitly identified what she liked doing, even if at times this behaviour was difficult for staff to manage.

Such dialogue is *generative*; this one curious encounter with language prompted staff to engage in a whole process of inquiry about the language they used. They developed a language poster to start noting and sharing language they valued, was person-centred and could be developed (Dewar & MacBride 2014).

The prerequisites stated in McCormack and McCance's (2010) Person-centred Nursing framework highlight what is required of the practitioner to enable person-centred care. Qualities such as 'knowing self', 'developed interpersonal skills', and clarity on 'beliefs and values' may require to be nurtured. To move away from 'task' orientation to care, to that of a therapeutic relational interaction – these qualities are essential (McCormack et al. 2010b). Opening up dialogue that is positive in its provocation of questioning why certain language and patterns of care are followed could aid the enhancement of these prerequisites to person-centred practice.

A skilled facilitator of AAR needs to be able to nurture this kind of appreciative dialogue and inquiry. They have to develop language 'antennae' to notice and help others notice beautiful utterances. In addition they need to notice language that does not feel person-centred or relational and be courageous in tactfully interrupting dominant negative discourses and supporting others to reframe this in a sensitive and inspiring manner.

Collaborative inquiry as intervention

The moment we ask a question we begin to create a change. Inquiry is explicit, and asking the right questions is perceived as a first-step intervention that provides a meaningful platform for further development and discovery (Cooperrider et al. 2008, p. 9). One of the most impactful things an appreciative inquirer does is to articulate questions as an invitation to inquire together. The questions we ask set the stage for what we 'find', and what we 'discover' creates the stories that lead to conversations about how the organisation will construct its future.

The My Home Life leadership support programme aims to promote quality of life for those living, dying, visiting and working in care homes through relationship-centred and evidence-based practice (NCHR&D 2007). The programme has appreciative inquiry, relationship-centred practice and caring conversations as its underpinning philosophy. Appreciative questioning became a different way of working for some practitioners. For example, a care home manager talked about how she found it difficult to work in situations when staff did not appear to 'get on' and were constantly bickering. She would normally bring them into the office and ask what the problem was. Through using appreciative questioning she learnt to reframe the questions she was asking. The manager was able to change her language from one of problem-solving to one of inquiring and learning together. She wondered and was curious about what was happening and what could happen. She started to ask:

How do you feel about what is happening in your relationship?

How would you like to feel?

What could be different?

Suppose you come to work tomorrow and it is all working well what would this look like?

Is there one small step you could take together to move towards the way you would like it to be?

Necessary elements of the Person-centred Nursing framework within the care environment are 'effective staff relations', 'power sharing' and 'potential for innovation and risk taking' (McCormack & McCance 2010). The use of appreciative collaborative inquiring could go some may in supporting these key aspects of the care environment. Being open and finding new ways of working that can have a positive impact for all require both sharing power and taking a risk in using a different approach. Additionally, with conflicting demands often directed towards care staff, having the *courage* to ask appreciative questions alongside a willingness to *compromise*, may encourage an ability to remain 'present' and maintain supportive, authentic relations within interdisciplinary teams for the benefit of a person-centred care environment for all.

Improvisation

In their review of appreciative inquiry as an approach for changing social systems, Bushe and Kassam (2005) suggest that appreciative inquiry can be transformational where it focuses on changing how people *think* instead of what they *do*, and supports self-organising (improvisational) change processes that flow from new ideas.

It is important to note that when we advocate 'action' in AAR this relates to bringing to life insights from conversations through active experimentation in practice, rather than advocating specific actions; the 'new actions' are co-designed in the light of the new thinking.

Bushe and Kassam (2005) warn against implementation – a specific tangible change achieved that had been agreed upon by assumed key decision-makers. They prefer the concept of improvisation, where numerous diverse ideas for development are pursued by a range of actors and where there are many changes that link to a deeper fundamental change in how the organisation is perceived.

An example of a deeper fundamental shift to a new way of thinking was highlighted in one study using AAR. Participants believed the process had changed their approach to what they felt was sometimes characteristic of learned helplessness, where they responded to things negatively and often felt powerless to change things. Instead, the process enabled a way of being more characteristic of 'learned hopefulness', in which they now felt they had a framework in place that helped them to explore possibilities with people even in the face of difficulties (Dewar 2011).

Examples of outcomes pursued by a range of participants in AAR projects have included:

- celebrating more openly what works well;
- engaging at an emotional level to learn and act upon the things that matter to people;
- developing ways in which caring acts can move from the unconscious to the conscious and collective;
- being more aware of defensiveness and working hard to enhance engagement;
- encouraging wider and more collaborative inquiry;
- devolving responsibility for noticing how things are, offering ideas and trying out new ways of doing things;
- challenging organisational thinking about implementation and roll-out to a model of progressive wider adoption through nurture and positive 'contagion'.

These changed the way practitioners worked and provided a meaningful and personalised vision for maintaining compassionate caring activities within the care settings.

Barrett (1998) draws on the metaphor of improvisation in jazz as a prototype for developing organisational cultures where people are enabled to experiment and learn in collaborative action. He makes the case that improvisation is happening all the time in organisations, but that successful improvisation is not a haphazard or accidental process; just as 'musicians prepare themselves to be spontaneous', practitioners can prepare organisations to learn while in the process of acting. This perspective is a hopeful, appreciative one rooted in belief in the human capacity to think afresh, generate novel solutions and create something new and interesting by learning in action. Important elements of improvisation are illustrated in Box 8.1.

Box 8.1 Elements of improvisation.

- Trial-and-error thinking – being open to making 'mistakes'.
- Feedback.
- Planning ahead as play.
- Challenging habits, routines or conventional practices.
- Taking turns to 'lead' (going solo) with accompaniment from supporters.
- Suspension of the tendency to criticise, judge or express disbelief.
- Developing supporting behaviours including good listening.
- Acknowledging achievements including rewarding those who support others and making room for contributions from peers.
- Designing more interdependence into tasks to enhance responsive capacity.
- Willingness to take risk and see errors as a source of learning and new lines of inquiry.
- Embrace the unknown.
- Cultivate serious play as a fruitful, meaningful activity that remains open to cues from the environment.

There are numerous examples of these elements of improvisation in our practice experience of using AAR supported by the caring conversations framework and practice tools. One example is detailed in Box 8.2.

Box 8.2 Case example of improvisation.

When working in one of the ward areas I noticed that a member of staff and a visitor went up to a lady in a four bedded bay and pulled the curtains around the bed – they sat down and the visitor said to the patient that she wanted to let her know that her mum had died that morning – she wanted to tell her because the patient and her mum had struck up a good friendship when they were both in the bay – her mum had been moved to a single room a few days ago, where she died.

   This was beautiful practice – when I celebrated this with the member of staff and asked her what prompted her to do this – she said that she had asked the bereaved family if there was anything else that she could do for them and they said they wanted her to tell Jean, the patient, that their mother had died. The member of staff said she felt nervous to do this – worrying that it might not be appropriate – it was not something she normally did – but it also got her thinking why not. Thinking quickly on her feet she wondered what would help her to do this – she asked the bereaved relative if they could do this together.

   Staff on the ward debated this practice of telling people that a fellow patient had died and made decisions about when to do this – the action became amplified and done by more people more of the time – the fact that it had already been done ensured that it was possible. But in addition we learnt about the process of asking curious questions to hear another perspective, to consider ourselves how we feel about that perspective and what would help us to do this – collaborating with another, in this case the relative, to help to give courage to do this. The process of hearing another perspective and considering it even if it seemed to go against normal practice and using the patient or relative themselves to help to do something differently were key lessons the staff took to look at other situations.

Conclusion

I argue that AAR is an appropriate methodology for exploring and developing person-centred cultures. It offers a significantly different approach to the necessary transformation of health and social care that goes through the 'front door of enthusiasm' (Ludema et al. 2001, p. 191).

   Evidence from practice suggests these tools have been helpful, particularly in relation to enhancing relationships and achieving positive person-centred outcomes for those involved. The caring conversations framework and the practice tools developed go some way in helping to support others in the craftful application of the principles of AAR into practice, and may aid the implementation of the Person-centred Nursing framework (McCormack & McCance 2010).

   Appreciative caring conversations promote appreciation and affirmation, which, in turn, provoke generative inquiry into existing ways of thinking and acting. By noticing the best of what already exists and bringing that to more collective awareness they enable innovation that feels 'doable' and hopeful. They don't impose solutions from elsewhere but help to share responsibility for development and change, strengthening collaboration amongst staff and between staff, patients or residents and their relatives. They provide feedback and actionable new knowledge about what matters to people, whether they are managers, staff, patients or relatives. The practice tools can only be enacted in relationship: their effectiveness rests on the qualities of genuine inquiry, empathy and authenticity that cannot be mandated or 'rolled-out' but that must be nurtured at all levels in health and social care.

Appreciative action research must include methods that are appreciative and provocative: build on what is working well; support people to have the courage to challenge dominant ideologies; and be confident and curious to really explore what matters to those who give and receive care. The glue that enables the above to happen is caring conversations. We suggest that it is through using a framework for caring conversations more deliberately, that innovation can be realised.

We need to use the framework of caring conversations in appreciative action research to enable us to foreground the practices of affirmation, provocation, inquiry and collaboration as core elements that enhance a more hopeful and improvisational approach to innovation in health and social care. This is the 'how' of the necessary cultural transformation of public service reform.

References

Barrett, F.J. (1998) Creativity and improvisation in jazz and organisations: implications for organizational learning. *Organization Science*, **9** (5), 605–22.

Barrett, F. and Cooperrider, D. (1990) Generative Metaphor Intervention: A new approach for working with systems divided by conflict and caught in defensive perception. *Journal of Applied Behavioural Science*, **26**, 219–39.

Bellinger, A. and Elliot, T. (2011) What are you looking at? The potential of appreciative inquiry as a research approach for social work. *British Journal of Social Work*, **41**, 708–25.

Bushe, G.R. and Kassam, A.F. (2005) When is appreciative inquiry transformational? A meta-case analysis. *Journal of Applied Behavioural Science*, **41**, 161–81.

Carter, B. (2006) One expertise among many – working appreciatively to make miracles instead of finding problems: using appreciative inquiry as a way of reframing research. *Journal of Research*, **11**, 48–63.

Cooperrider, D.L., Whitney, D., and Stavros, J. (2008) *Appreciative Inquiry Handbook: For Leaders of Change*, 2nd edn, Berrett-Koehler Publishers, San Francisco, CA.

Cowling, R.W. (2001) Unitary appreciative inquiry. *Advances in Nursing Practice*, **23** (4), 32–48.

Dewar, B. (2010) Editorial: Appreciative Inquiry. *International Journal of Older People Nursing*, **5**, 290–1.

Dewar, B. and Mackay, R. (2010) Appreciating compassionate care in acute care settings for older people. *International Journal of Older People Nursing*, **5**, 299–308.

Dewar B. (2011) Caring about caring; an appreciative inquiry about compassionate relationship centred care. PhD thesis, Edinburgh Napier University. Retrieved from: http://researchrepository.napier.ac.uk/id/eprint/4845 (accessed 3 February 2016).

Dewar, B. (2012) Using creative methods in practice development to understand and develop compassionate care. *International Practice Development Journal*, **2**, 1–11.

Dewar B and MacBride T. (2014) *Enhancing dignity through caring conversations*. Final Report for Queen's Nursing Institute Scotland. University of the West of Scotland. Available from:

http://myhomelife.uws.ac.uk/scotland/wp-content/uploads/2014/06/Final-report_QNIS_25.08.14.pdf (accessed 3 February 2016).

Dewar, B. and Nolan, M. (2013) Caring about caring: Developing a model to implement compassionate relationship centred care in an older people care setting. *International Journal of Nursing Studies*, **50**, 1247–58.

Dewar, B. and Sharp, C. (2013) Appreciative dialogue for co-facilitation in action research and practice development. *International Practice Development Journal*, **3** (12), 1–7.

Dewar, B., Mackay, R., Smith, S., Pullin, S., and Tocher, R. (2010) Use of emotional touchpoints as a method of tapping into the experience of receiving compassionate care in a hospital setting. *Journal of Research in Nursing*, **15**, 29–41.

Doggett, C. and Lewis, A. (2013) Using appreciative inquiry to facilitate organisational change and develop professional practice within an educational psychology service. *Education and Child Psychology*, **30** (4), 124–43.

Egan, T.M. and Lancaster, C.M. (2005) Comparing appreciative inquiry to action research: OD practitioner perspectives. *Organisational Development Journal*, **23** (2), 29–49.

Fry R. (2014) Appreciative inquiry. In: Coghlan D and Brydon-Miller M. (eds), *The Sage Encyclopaedia of Action Research*. Sage, pp. 44–8.

Glasson, J. (2006) Evaluation of a model of nursing care for older patients using participatory action research in an acute medical ward. *Journal of Clinical Nursing*, **15**, 588–98.

Grant, S. and Humphries, M. (2006) Critical evaluation of appreciative inquiry. *Action Research*, **4**, 401–18.

Ludema JD, Cooperrider DL, Barrett FJ. (2001) Appreciative inquiry: the power of the unconditional positive question. In: Reason P and Bradbury H. (eds), *Handbook of Action Research*. Sage, pp. 155–65.

Manley, K., O'Keefe, H., Jackson, C., Pearce, J., and Smith, S. (2014) A shared purpose framework to deliver person-centred, safe and effective care: Organizational transformation using practice development methodology. *International Practice Development Journal*, **4**, 1–3.

McCormack, B. and McCance, T. (2010) *Person-Centred Nursing: Theory and Practice*, Wiley-Blackwell, Oxford.

McCormack, B., Karlsson, B., Dewing, J., and Lerdel, A. (2010a) Exploring person-centredness: A qualitative meta-synthesis of four studies. *Scandinavian Journal of Caring Sciences*, **24**, 620–34.

McCormack, B., Dewing, B.L. *et al.* (2010b) Developing person-centred practice: Nursing outcomes arising from changes to the care environment in residential settings for older people. *International Journal of Older People*, **5**, 93–107.

McCormack, B., Dewing, J., and McCance, T. (2011) Developing person-centred care: Addressing contextual challenges through practice development. *Journal of Issues in Nursing*, **16** (2), 3.

Mulgan G. (2013) Achieving more for less – the innovators catalyst. Speech to the Advancing Health Care Conference, 19 June, London. Available at: http://www.kingsfund.org.uk/audio-video/geoff-mulgan-achieving-more-less-innovators-catalyst (accessed 3 February 2016).

NCHR&D (National Care Home Research and Development Forum) (2007) *My Home Life: Promoting quality of life in care homes – literature review.* , London: Help the Aged. Available at: www.myhomelife.org.uk (accessed 22 February 2016).

Nolan MK, Brown J, Davies D, Nolan J, Keady J. (2006) The Senses framework: Improving care for older people through a relationship-centred approach. Getting Research Into Practice (GRIP) Report No. 2. Project report. University of Sheffield.

Pennacchia, J. (2013) Exploring the relationships between evidence and innovation in the context of Scotland's social services. *Institute for Research and Innovation in Social Services (IRISS)*.

Reason, P. and Bradbury, H. (eds) (2001) *Handbook of Action Research: Participative Inquiry and Practice*, Sage, London.

Reed, J. (2007) *Appreciative Inquiry: Research for Change*, Sage Publications, London.

Richer, M.C., Ritchie, J., and Marchionni, C. (2010) Appreciative inquiry in health care. *British Journal of Healthcare Management*, **16** (4), 164–72.

Rowan, J. (2001) The humanistic approach, in *Handbook of Action Research* (eds P. Reason and H. Bradbury), Sage, London.

Rubin, R., Kerrell, R., and Roberts, G. (2011) Appreciative inquiry in occupational therapy education. *British Journal of Occupational Therapy*, **74**, 233–40.

Sharp C, Kennedy J, McKenzie I, Dewar B. (2013) *Caring to Ask: how to embed caring conversations into practice across north east Glasgow*. Available at: http://library.nhsggc.org.uk/mediaAssets/CHP%20Glasgow/Caring%20to%20Ask%20-%20%20ISP%20FINAL%20report%20Dec%202013.pdf (accessed 22 February 2016).

Trajkovski, S., Schmied, V., Vickers, M., and Jackson, D. (2012) Implementing the 4D cycle of appreciative inquiry in healthcare: a methodological review. *Journal of Advanced Nursing*, **69**, 1224–34.

Watkins, J.M. and Mohr, B.J. (2001) *Appreciative Inquiry: Change at the speed of imagination*, Jossey-Bass/Pfeiffer, San Francisco, CA.

Developing person-centred cultures: a practice development approach

CHAPTER 9

An overview of practice development

Kim Manley
Canterbury Christ Church University, UK

Introduction

Person-centred care is a philosophy that values individuals' own unique values, personality, personal history and the right of each person to respect, dignity and to participate fully in their life choices. This philosophy in health and social care embraces therapeutic and compassionate relationships between providers and patients/clients (Patterson et al. 2011; Dewar & Nolan 2013) and also between staff (Maben 2008; Kirkley et al. 2011; Maben et al. 2012).

Practice development has a long association with the development and provision of person-centred care, cultures and ways of working. Contemporary practice development is systematic, can contribute to the body of knowledge, focuses on using the workplace as the main resource for learning and development, and seeks to improve health and social care through developing and sustaining person-centred cultures. These cultures enable patients, clients and staff to flourish but also embrace knowledge translation in that the effective generation and use of evidence in practice is dependent on blending different knowledges, including people's own expertise about themselves and their health.

Theoretical research into practice development (Garbett & McCormack 2002; McSherry & Warr 2008; Unsworth 2008) led to it becoming a search term in the British Nursing Index. Today, the purpose of practice development – person-centred care – is language increasingly embedded in policy and practice, research and quality strategies across organisations and systems (Health Foundation 2015; National Voices 2015).

This chapter provides an overview of practice development as a methodology in the context of developing person-centred cultures. It will provide a contemporary analysis of the current evidence base and will conclude with direction for professionals with a range of experience from individual to systems level.

Person-Centred Practice in Nursing and Health Care: Theory and Practice, Second Edition.
Edited by Brendan McCormack and Tanya McCance.
© 2017 John Wiley & Sons, Ltd. Published 2017 by John Wiley & Sons, Ltd.

Practice development: a methodology for developing person centred cultures

Methodology provides a set of principles that guide systematic activity in a particular discipline. For practice development, methodology became explicit in the late 1990s, when it was aligned to critical social science and the enlightenment, empowerment and emancipation of practitioners (Manley 1997; McCormack et al. 1999; Manley & McCormack 2003). Culture, facilitation and outcome evaluation became the focus of emancipatory practice development, affiliated with emancipatory action research and the development of transformational cultures (Manley 1997; Manley & McCormack 2003).

Concept clarification undertaken in parallel (Garbett & McCormack 2002; McSherry & Warr 2008; Unsworth 2008) led to describing the purposes, attributes and outcomes of practice development more specifically as developing person-centred care through working with cultures and contexts, enabling values and beliefs through systematic approaches that focus on learning in and from practice.

Realistic synthesis of the impact of practice development resulted in the identification of key methods (McCormack et al. 2006), summarised in Box 9.1. Major theoretical critique through the International Practice Development Collaborative led to further exploration of fundamental concepts: critical creativity linked to transformational practice development (McCormack & Titchen 2006); person-centredness (McCormack 2004); facilitation (Shaw et al. 2008); active learning (Dewing 2008) and work-based learning (Manley et al. 2009) as well as effective workplace culture (Manley et al. 2011a). In parallel, practice development has also been closely aligned with knowledge translation in that effective evidence translation is dependent on blending different types of evidence about the person, patient views, the local context, clinical experience and research (Rycroft-Malone et al. 2004; Lomas et al. 2005). Similarly, knowledge translation is reliant on skilled holistic facilitation and building enabling contexts and cultures (Rycroft-Malone et al. 2004; Rycroft-Malone 2013). Practice development methodology is summarised through nine principles (Manley et al. 2008) (Box 9.2).

Latterly, practice development as a broad approach to health and social care practice that overlaps improvement methodologies has also begun to be understood as a complex intervention, driven by the need to describe it as a research intervention, It is an approach that specifically uses collaborative, inclusive and participatory approaches to support the transformation of individuals, teams, practice and cultures to enhance the effectiveness of practices enabling all to flourish (Manley et al. 2011b). The concept of flourishing encompasses a person-centred approach (Titchen & McCormack 2010). Table 9.1 uses the five Medical Research Council (MRC, 2008) questions to guide

Box 9.1 Methods for practice development.

Becoming person-centred, ethical, knowing self and others

- Agreeing ethical processes
- Being person-centred
- Knowing 'self' and participants
- Analysing stakeholder roles and ways of engaging stakeholders

Clarifying focus, values, culture

- Clarifying the development focus
- Clarifying values
- Clarifying workplace culture

Developing common direction through collaboration, inclusion and participation

- Collaborative working relationships
- Developing a shared vision
- Developing critical intent
- Developing participatory engagement

Facilitating reflection, ideas, transitions and incentives

- Continuous reflective learning
- Giving space for ideas to flourish
- Developing a reward system
- Facilitating transitions

Using effective strategies for communication, sharing and dissemination

- Good communication strategies
- High challenge and high support
- Implementing processes for sharing and disseminating

Evaluation

- Evaluation

Adapted from McCormack and Titchen (2006). Reproduced with permission of Taylor & Francis.

the expression of practice development as a complex intervention. Whist the epistemological approach informing the MRC differs from that underpinning practice development it is nonetheless useful in reducing ambiguity about what can be expected when used as a programme intervention.

From a realist perspective, practice development would be considered a *social* complex intervention, recognising the influence and impact of context when used.

> **Box 9.2** Nine principles of practice development.
>
> Practice development:
> - Aims to achieve person-centred and evidence-based care that is manifested through human flourishing and a workplace culture of effectiveness in all health-care settings and situations (**Principle 1**).
> - Directs its attention at the micro-systems level – the level at which most health care is experienced and provided – but requires coherent support from interrelated mezzo and macro-systems levels (**Principle 2**).
> - Integrates:
>   - work-based learning with its focus on active learning and formal systems for enabling learning in the workplace to transform care (**Principle 3**);
>   - the development of evidence from practice and the use of evidence in practice (**Principle 4**);
>   - creativity with cognition in order to blend mind, heart and soul energies, enabling practitioners to free their thinking and allow opportunities for human flourishing to emerge (**Principle 5**);
>   - evaluation approaches that are always inclusive, participative and collaborative (**Principle 9**).
> - Is a complex methodology that can be used across health-care teams and interfaces to involve all internal and external stakeholders (**Principle 6**).
> - Uses key methods according to the methodological principles being operationalised and the contextual characteristics of the programme of work (**Principle 7**).
> - Is associated with a set of processes including skilled facilitation that can be translated into a specific skill-set required as near to the interface of care as possible (**Principle 8**).
>
> Adapted from Manley et al. (2008).

Realist evaluation begins with the researcher positing the potential processes through which a programme may work as a prelude to testing them. [p. 6] … Realism utilises contextual thinking to address the issues of 'for whom' and 'in what circumstances' a programme will work. [p. 7]

Pawson and Tilley (2004)

Developing person-centred cultures

Effective workplace cultures espouse and live person-centred values (Manley et al. 2011a),combining these with values about:

1 Working with others – open communication, high support and high challenge, involvement, participation and collaboration with stakeholders, teamwork and leadership development.
2 Effective care – evidence use and development, lifelong learning, positive attitude to change, holistic safety.

Other attributes of effective workplace cultures explain how values such as person-centredness are sustained:

- The values are realised and experienced in practice, there is a shared vision and mission with individual and collective responsibility.
- Adaptability, innovation and creativity maintain workplace effectiveness.

Table 9.1 Practice development as a complex intervention from the perspective of the Medical Research Council (2008) criteria.

MRC question	Practice development
What are you trying to do; what outcome you are aiming for?	• Person-centred care • Contexts and cultures of effectiveness • Human flourishing
How will you bring about change?	Using the Collaboration, Inclusion and Participation (CIP) principles to facilitate: • identification and implementation of shared values and beliefs with stakeholders • learning in and from practice about a specific/generic issue using reflective practice, creative imagination and expression, and active learning to generate self-awareness that then motivates implementation of shared values • systematic change using multiple evidence sources
Does your intervention have a coherent theoretical basis?	• Underpinned by critical social science and critical creativity • Realistic synthesis identifies the methods and CIP principles • Participative and critical action research approaches and stakeholder evaluation provide research approaches that demonstrate principles in action
Have you used this theory systematically to develop the intervention?	Yes, from initial concept analysis of the intervention through to realistic synthesis and concept analysis of related concepts

Can you describe the intervention fully so that it can be implemented properly for the purposes of your evaluation, and replicated by others?	Specific criteria can be used to identify the presence of the intervention; these would include:
	• Developing a shared purpose and values about:
	  ◦ person-centredness
	  ◦ effective ways of working
	• Collaborative, Inclusive and Participative working with stakeholders including patients/clients
	• Focus on systematic use of a range of mixed methods to guide action spirals
	• Includes reflection, learning in and from practice, and the use of creativity

Adapted from Manley et al. (2013).

- Appropriate change is driven by the needs of patients/communities.
- Formal systems exist to continuously enable and evaluate learning; performance and shared governance embed the values in practice.

The stages in a culture change journey demonstrate how these attributes become embedded over time (Figure 9.1). Embedding values such as person-centredness in the workplace is associated with a number of transitions against which progress can be judged. Based on a readiness to want to engage, the journey commences with agreeing values and beliefs; then passes through

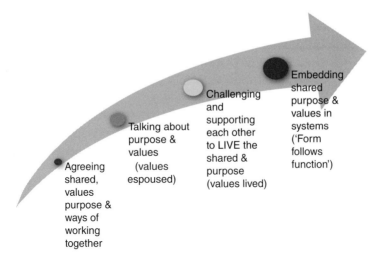

Embedding
shared
purpose &
values in
systems
('Form
follows
function')

Challenging
and
supporting
each other
to LIVE the
shared &
purpose
(values lived)

Talking about
purpose &
values
(values
espoused)

Agreeing
shared,
values
purpose &
ways of
working
together

Figure 9.1 Understanding the culture change journey.

transitions reflected by talking about what these values mean (values espoused); building mutual support and challenge across teams and organisations through feedback to enable values to be lived and inform decision-making; and finally, the introduction of systems (structures and processes) that will continue to embed and sustain values over time, as 'form follows function'. In relation to person-centredness there is a continuum through which individuals and teams progress as they become more person-centred: starting with person-centred moments – ad hoc experiences of person-centredness – through to person-centred care as the underpinning culture of teams and organisations (McCormack et al. 2013).

Hence, the aim of practice development is to develop effective workplace cultures that have embedded within them person-centred processes, systems and ways of working, enabling all to experience person-centredness.

Current evidence base underpinning practice development

When considering the evidence base underpinning practice development in developing person-centred cultures, there are a number of relevant questions to ask:

- How would a person-centred culture be recognised?
- What is the impact of practice development on the development of person-centred cultures?
- What are the specific cultural change strategies that work?
- What difference does a person-centred culture make to health-care outcomes?

When determining how practice development as an approach achieves its impact on culture and establishing the significant aspects of the intervention, there are different philosophical approaches to consider. Culture is a complex social phenomenon and a nebulous social concept, where cause-and-effect relationships are difficult to establish, especially when there are so many multifactorial aspects to consider.

Insights from various research methodologies can contribute different aspects to understanding the culture change journey towards person-centredness, and this premise has guided the examples used rather than narrowly considering whether practice development has made a difference to culture. These insights will inform the future research landscape around the development of person-centred cultures. The diverse examples of different research approaches that follow illustrate this point.

How would a person-centred culture be recognised?

Person-centred cultures would be expected to consistently demonstrate as a social norm, person-centred values in action, based on a deep understanding by staff of what person-centredness means. Methods for identifying cultural attributes include the use of participant and non-participant observation or care and relationships, such as 'Observations of Care' (Royal College of Nursing 2006); Workplace Culture Critical Analysis Tool (WCCAT; McCormack et al. 2009) and other ethnographic approaches such as critical ethnography; and exploring experiences of patients, service users and staff to identify if there is a gap between what is espoused and spoken about and the lived experience of patients, service users and staff. Tools that can be used for this purpose include: emotional touchpoints (Scottish Health Council, 2014); patient stories (Royal College of Nursing 2006); questionnaires, such as the person-centred nursing index (Slater et al. 2009); and documentary analysis.

Kirkley et al. (2011) from a social care perspective, identified that views of person-centred care can often be diverse, and understanding person-centred care was one of five themes that influenced whether organisations were in a position to develop cultures to deliver on it.

Barriers to implementing person-centred care identified by Kirkley et al. (2011) included resource constraints, knowledge, attitudes and personal qualities of staff. Enablers were leadership style, and how managers support and value staff.

What is the impact of practice development on the development of person-centred cultures?

At the national level in Ireland, McCormack and colleagues (2010) implemented a programme in older people services using practice development and the Person-Centred Nursing Framework of McCormack and McCance (2006), using cooperative inquiry. They were able to identify the impact the programme had on staff (nursing and care staff), who achieved many of the prerequisites of the person-centred framework and changed significantly their perceptions of caring towards a non-technical conception. Residents and families also experienced qualitative changes in the care cultures around hope and hopelessness, choice, belonging and connectedness, and meaningful relationships, suggesting that the social norms were changing towards those that are more person-centred. The researchers highlighted the need to constantly support teams in this ongoing endeavour if person-centred cultures were to continue to develop and be sustained.

One comprehensive doctoral study (Osbourne 2009) using longitudinal design sought to evaluate the impact of emancipatory practice development across a large acute teaching hospital in Australia, although the focus was more on developing a context and culture that emphasised inquiry and evidence-based practice rather than person-centredness, which was an aspect of the study. This study was able to show through using an extensive number of validated tools, the effectiveness of practice development methodology in changing the culture and context of care through the attributes of autonomy and control, workplace empowerment and constructive team dynamics, which were connected to engagement with research and evidence inquiry.

The focus on the team culture and engagement approaches that enable workplace empowerment through an organisation-wide programme endorses the view that evaluating workplace culture is a powerful indicator of whether organisational values such as person-centredness are lived out in practice.

Beckett et al. (2013) demonstrated the impact of using practice development in an action research project in inpatient mental health with nursing and multidisciplinary team members, and showed the importance of transformational principles at all levels of the organisation; a solution-based approach resulted in a development plan encompassing person-centred care amongst other themes.

McCance et al. (2013) were also able to affirm the value of using practice development to promote person-centredness through key findings showing: (1) that shared processes enabled engagement; (2) the impact of context on person-centred practice; and (3) the living of person-centred values. Preparedness and willingness to engage were identified as essential precursors. The key processes accounting for these changes included:
- focused on understanding person centeredness;
- developing a shared vision;
- determining the quality of the user experience;
- systematically developing practice;
- celebrating success.

What are the specific cultural change strategies that work?

In addition to those strategies above identified by McCance et al., a review of 82 practice-related projects, funded over ten years and supported by the Foundation of Nursing Studies (FoNS), was undertaken with the aim of identifying insights into creating caring cultures (Manley 2013). The projects were based on practice development, research implementation, practice-based research or a combination of these approaches. An impact framework informed by the attributes of effective cultures was used to evaluate these projects (Manley et al. 2013a). The review aimed to identify the espoused values, beliefs and attitudes, including person-centredness, that influenced the focus of each project, and to ascertain whether these values were more evidenced at the end of the project through documentary analysis. The project also aimed to draw out the processes influential in changing the culture.

The 82 projects were classified into five groups: (1) pure research, (2) implementing evidence, (3) practitioner-led service improvement projects, (4) practitioner-led using practice development principles, and (5) action research with/without practice development principles. Many of the projects involved working with service users in a person-centred way. Practice development typologies (group 4) and also action research (group 5) intentionally addressed workplace culture through working with person-centred values and the patient experience and the other attributes of effective workplace cultures. Group 4 and group 5 projects deliberately used tools and processes to implement values and drew on eclectic approaches to engage and work with stakeholders, working together using practice development principles. These approaches associated with groups 4 and 5 were more successful in making changes and sustaining caring, person-centred and effective workplace cultures, to the extent that this could be concluded for documentary analysis alone. However, none of the projects identified the importance of embedding person-centred values through implementing systems that embed these.

In a collaborative inquiry across three different projects, all drawing on practice development principles to take forward some aspect of person-centred care, 'action hypothesis' was used to identify the strategies that consistently appear to demonstrate similar outcomes (Manley et al. 2013b). Two common trigger points were identified across the three projects, related to developing effective workplace cultures (defined as being person-centred), specifically:

- Lack of common shared purpose/vision in relation to the project focus (Trigger 1).
- Unreceptive/underdeveloped workplace cultures characterised by such factors as lack of feedback processes/systems/evaluation/professional networks, support and challenge (Trigger 2).

The strategies used across the three projects were similar and found to be influential in all three projects to achieve similar outcomes. Figure 9.2 illustrates the action hypothesis resulting for Trigger 2 to demonstrate this synthesis of understanding.

Action hypothesis has much in common with realist evaluation where there is potential for identifying the mechanisms, contexts and outcomes that describe how person-centred cultures are developed. Within a project funded by Health Education England, realistic evaluation has been used to generate four transformation theories that account for how individuals' professional practice and team cultures amongst other aspects can achieve person-centred care through

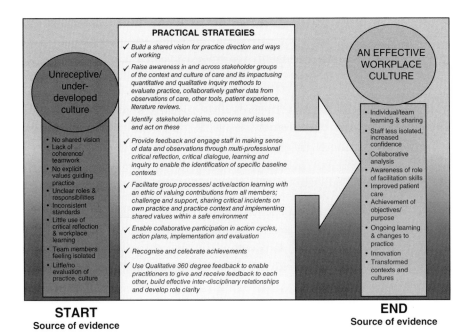

START
Source of evidence

END
Source of evidence

Figure 9.2 Developing a culture of effectiveness. From Manley et al. (2013b).

describing and explaining the relationships between context, mechanisms and outcomes based on extensive reconnaissance through literature analysis and stakeholder engagement. These transformation theories for continuous professional development are linked to indicators at the individual, team, service and organisational levels, including person-centred practice (Jackson et al. 2015).

What difference does a person-centred culture make to health-care outcomes?

There is a growing relationship between person-centred workplace cultures and impact in a number of areas: for example, whether care is experienced as person-centred, whether learning is embedded, research is implemented, and the achievement of staff well-being, quality care and patient safety. The potential for practice development as a complex social intervention to contribute to the broader health-care agenda is proposed through using the attributes of effective workplace cultures as process indicators that signpost the potential for achieving the broader health outcomes (Manley et al. 2011b). This is an area that requires more substantial investigation.

Direction for practitioners with a range of experiences

The purpose of this section is to help practitioners consider how they may either contribute to or facilitate the development of person-centred cultures using practice development through perspectives at four different levels:

- building effective relationships;
- building effective teams and workplaces;
- embedding organisational values in systems;
- building whole systems approaches through clinical systems leadership.

Building effective relationships

Building person-centred relationships is one of the ways that culture can be changed, so practitioners in health and social care settings can begin to influence this by reflecting on their own relationships. Through systematic inquiry at the individual level we need to continue to develop our self-awareness, to know our own values and beliefs, and what these mean in the context of daily work as a practitioner, team member, preceptor, mentor and critical companion. Self-awareness is a prerequisite for enlightenment, becoming empowered and freeing oneself from the things we take for granted in everyday life. Whilst there is much that can be done on one's own in terms of rigorous reflection, it is important to obtain support through clinical supervision, critical companionships or peer support and challenge. This will help us to obtain different perspectives, to push our insights further, to become aware of the consequences of our actions on ourselves and others, and prevent us from deluding ourselves or accepting assumptions uncritically in our relationships or the influence of social norms in the workplace.

Box 9.3 makes five suggestions about building effective relationships that will help you become more person-centred: self-assessment against emotional competence (the prerequisite for effective relationships); developing a rigorous

---

Box 9.3 Developing relationships.

1 **Assess yourself against the emotional competence framework** and areas around emotional intelligence to understand your strengths in relationship building and the areas you need to develop (http://www.eiconsortium.org/pdf/emotional_competence_ framework.pdf).
2 **Develop your approach to rigorous reflection** by testing out a range of different models that support you in this activity.
3 **Obtain feedback from your colleagues about how supportive and how challenging you are** based on the premise that high support and high challenge are required for effective working and that people's perceptions are different. The only way to become more person-centred and getting to know the people we work with is to ask for feedback.
4 **Engagement in appreciative caring conversations** with patients, their families but also colleagues and students too, as identified by Dewar and Nolan (2013):
   - Know who I am and what matters to me?
   - Understand how I feel about my experience?
   - Work with me to shape the things that are done?
5 **Use emotional touchpoints** to find out what matters to patients, relatives, staff and students (Scottish Health Council, 2014).

approach to reflection; obtaining feedback from colleagues about support and challenge; engage in caring conversations (Dewar & Nolan 2013); and using emotional touchpoints (Scottish Health Council 2014).

Building effective teams and workplaces

From the evidence provided above the importance of focusing on the workplace level and the team is emphasised in developing person-centred cultures. If you are in a team leader role in any context then practical suggestions that you may wish to consider include developing role clarity and developing your leadership potential in collaboration with your teams. Both are enablers to effective person-centred workplace cultures at the individual level (Manley et al. 2011a). Developing skills and the behaviours associated with transformational leadership and starting at the team/unit level will be an important focus together with asking yourself and your team the following questions. Does your team have:

- A shared purpose as a team?
- A shared understanding about what person-centred means?
- Agreed ways of working as a team about how you support and challenge each other, use learning and inquiry?
- Regular opportunities to celebrate achievements?

Shared purpose and agreed ways of working, prioritised and sharing learning, and celebrations are all aspects of effective person-centred workplaces for staff as well as patients and service users.

Developing role clarity in yourself and others is a useful way of making explicit what is expected of yourself and others, and through using approaches that are open and direct you can begin to model ways of working that embrace the giving and receiving of feedback, transparent and person-centred approaches. Not all 360-degree feedback approaches focus on these qualities as many are anonymous and electronic; however, qualitative 360-degree feedback is one approach that will help you (Garbett et al. 2007).

Embedding organisational values in systems

To achieve shared person-centred values and purposes across large health and social care organisations requires leadership, resilience and persistent use of practice development principles. The biggest challenge at both organisational and unit level is using these values to guide decision-making and implementing of systems that embed the values across the organisation. Manley et al. (2014a) describe the approach used to achieve such an outcome. A number of ideas (listed below) are identified to embed person-centred values in organisational systems.

- Establishing work-based programmes that focus on self-assessment around person-centred indicators and growing a critical community with the skills needed for culture change.
- Schwartz rounds (King's Fund 2011) focus on providing emotional support to staff in a person-centred way.

- Establishing interdisciplinary quality review teams, including service users, that focus on using cultural tools that focus on person-centredness and provide immediate feedback.
- Establishing link worker systems around organisational purposes so that person-centred care can be embedded in all teams through shared governance.
- Developing accredited wards/departments around shared purposes including person-centredness.
- Ensuring strategies for learning and development and research and development are integrated with shared purposes such as providing person-centred care.

The role of organisational leaders is to constantly model and challenge others to use values and shared purpose to guide decision-making at every level.

Building whole systems approaches through clinical systems leadership

Whole systems ways of working across local health economies is a priority agenda for today's health care, enabling the integration of health and social care in a way that provides better continuity in person-centred approaches. This provides an opportunity for clinical systems leaders with person-centred values to be influential in this agenda.

Practice development principles have been used to identify how local services can be transformed to provide whole systems person-centred approaches around the urgent and emergency care agenda in South East England (Manley et al. 2014b). A key finding was the need for clinical systems leaders with the skills required:

- to enable boundaries and silos to be dismantled and staff enabled to work towards a shared purpose and values across health economies;
- to enable people to be cared for in their own homes or as near as possible;
- for staff to feel valued in a person-centred way and retained in the workplace.

Clinical systems leadership draws on clinical expertise and credibility from different disciplines, but also enables different systems partners to work together towards a shared purpose through being jointly appointed across different contexts in primary and secondary care and drawing on expertise in:

- Leadership to achieve culture change through working with shared purposes achieving integrated ways of working and effective teamwork across primary and secondary care and partner organisations.
- Developing, improving and evaluating person-centred, safe and effective care and services.
- Consultancy functions from client-centred through to organisational and systems level (Caplan & Caplan 1993) and process consultancy approaches (Schein 1999) to enable expertise to be widely accessible.

- Creating learning cultures that use the workplace as the main resource for learning, to maximise opportunities for learning and development, competence development and innovation.

This direction provides opportunities for consultant-level practitioners to influence whole systems from a person-centred perspective.

Conclusion

The chapter has set out to show how an understanding of practice development can enable, develop and sustain person-centred cultures. Practice development has been associated with these purposes since its inception as a methodology with a set of principles that address this. Evidence drawn from various research approaches illustrates both the impact and potential that practice development has for enabling person-centred cultures. The need to make explicit the relationships between the mechanisms, contexts and outcomes through which culture change takes place is cognisant of culture and culture change as social phenomena. Practical strategies and potential directions are presented as ideas for practitioners at different levels in relation to starting or building on their own role as cultural change agents. These strategies focus on establishing and sustaining person-centred cultures from individual professional relationships through to team, organisational and systems leaders.

References

Beckett P, Field J, Molloy L, Yu N, Holmes D, Pile E. (2013) Practice what you preach: developing person-centred culture in inpatient mental health through strengths based, transformational leadership. *Issues in Mental Health Nursing* **34**:595–601.

Caplan, G. and Caplan, R.B. (1993) *Mental Health Consultation and Collaboration*, Jossey-Bass, San Francisco.

Dewar, B. (2002) Evaluation of workbased learning in a community nursing health degree programme: the students' perspective on the impact on practice. *New Capability*, **5**, 10–15.

Dewar, B. and Nolan, M. (2013) Caring about caring: Developing a model to implement compassionate relationship centred care in an older people care setting. *International Journal of Nursing Studies*, **50** (19), 1247–58.

Dewing J. (2008) Becoming and being active learners and creating active learning workplaces: the value of active learning in practice development. In *Manley K, McCormack B*, Wilson V. (eds), *International Practice Development in Nursing and Healthcare*. Oxford: Blackwell Publishing, chapter 14.

Garbett, R. and McCormack, B. (2002) Focus. A concept analysis of practice development. *NT Research*, **7** (2), 87–100.

Garbett, R., Hardy, S., Manley, K., Titchen, A., and McCormack, B. (2007) Developing a qualitative approach to 360 degree feedback to aid understanding and development of clinical expertise. *Nursing Management*, **15**, 342–7.

Health Foundation (2015) *Person-centred care resource centre*. Available at: http://personcentred care.health.org.uk/ (accessed 3 February 2016).

Jackson C, Manley K, Wright T, Martin A. (2015) *Continuing Professional Development (CPD) for quality care: context, mechanisms, outcomes and impact*. Final Report. England Centre for Practice Development.

King's Fund (2011) *Schwartz rounds evaluation*. Available at: http://www.kingsfund.org.uk/publications/schwartz-center-rounds-pilot-evaluation (accessed 3 February 2016).

Kirkley, C., Bamford, C., Poole, M., Arksey, H., Hughes, J., and Bond, J. (2011) The impact of organisational culture on the delivery of person-centred care in services providing respite care and short breaks for people with dementia. *Health and Social Care in the Community*, **19** (4), 438–48.

Lomas, J., Culyer, T., and McCutcheon, C. (2005) *McAuley L, Law S*, Conceptualizing and combining evidence for health system guidance, Canadian Health Services Research Foundation (CHSRF).

Maben, J. (2008) The art of caring: invisible and subordinated? A response to Juliet Corbin: 'Is caring a lost art in nursing?'. *International Journal of Nursing Studies*, **45**, 335–8.

Maben J, Peccei R, Adams M, Robert G, Richardson A, Murrells T. (2012) *Patients' experiences of care and the influence of staff motivation, affect and wellbeing*. Final report. NIHR Service Delivery and Organisation programme.

Manley, K. (1997) A conceptual framework for advanced practice: an action research project operationalising an advanced practitioner/consultant nurse role. *Journal of Clinical Nursing*, **6** (3), 179–90.

Manley, K. (2013) Insights into developing caring cultures: a review of the experience of the Foundation of Nursing Studies (FoNS), , FoNS, London.

Manley, K. and McCormack, B. (2003) Practice development: purpose, methodology, facilitation and evaluation. *Nursing in Critical Care*, **8**, 22–9.

Manley, K., McCormack, B., and Wilson, V. (2008) Introduction, in *International Practice Development in Nursing and Healthcare* (eds K. Manley, B. McCormack, and V. Wilson), Blackwell Publishing, Oxford, pp. 1–16.

Manley, K., Titchen, A., and Hardy, S. (2009) Work based learning in the context of contemporary healthcare education and practice: a concept analysis. *Practice Development in Health Care*, **8** (2), 87–127.

Manley K, Sanders K, Cardiff S, Webster J. (2011a) Effective workplace culture: the attributes, enabling factors and consequences of a new concept. *International Practice Development Journal* **1**(2), art. 1.

Manley K, Crisp J, Moss C. (2011b) Advancing the practice development outcomes agenda within multiple contexts. *International Practice Development Journal* **1**(1), art. 4.

Manley K, Hardy S, Shaw T, Sanders K. (2013a) Outcomes and impact of practice development: a draft framework. In: Manley K. *Insights into developing caring cultures: a review of the experience of the Foundation of Nursing Studies (FoNS)*. London: FoNS, Appendix 2.

Manley, K., Parlour, R., and Yalden, J. (2013b) The use of action hypotheses to demonstrate practice development strategies in action, in *Practice Development in Nursing and Health Care*, 2nd edn (eds B. McCormack, K. Manley, and A. Titchen), Wiley-Blackwell, Oxford, pp. 1–17.

Manley K, O'Keefe H, Jackson C, Pearce J, Smith S. (2014a) A shared purpose framework to deliver person-centred, safe and effective care: organisational transformation using practice development methodology. *International Practice Development Journal* **41**(1), art. 2.

Manley K, Jackson C, Martin A, Apps J, Setchfield I, Oliver G. (2014b) *Transforming urgent & emergency care together phase 1: Final Report*. England Centre for Practice Development.

McCance T, Gribben B, McCormack B, Laird E. (2013) Promoting person-centred practice within acute care: the impact of culture and context on a facilitated practice development programme. *International Practice Development Journal* **3**(1) [2]. Available at: http://www.fons.org/Resources/Documents/Journal/Vol3No1/IDPJ_0301_02.pdf (accessed 3 February 2016).

McCormack, B. (2004) Person-centredness in gerontological nursing: an overview of the literature. *Journal of Clinical Nursing*, **13** (3a), 31–8.

McCormack, B. and McCance, T. (2006) Development of a framework for person-centred nursing. *Journal of Advanced Nursing*, **56**, 472–9.

McCormack, B. and Titchen, A. (2006) Critical creativity: melding, exploding, blending. *Educational Action Research*, **14**, 239–66.

McCormack, B., Manley, K., Kitson, A., Titchen, A., and Harvey, G. (1999) Towards practice development – a vision in reality or reality without vision. *Journal of Nursing Management*, **7** (5), 255–64.

McCormack, B., Dewar, B., Wright, J., Garbett, R., Harvey, G., and Ballantine, K. (2006) *A Realist Synthesis of Evidence Relating to Practice Development: Executive Summary*, NHS Quality Improvement Scotland and NHS Education for Scotland, Edinburgh.

McCormack, B., Henderson, E., Wilson, V., and Wright, J. (2009) Making practice visible: The Workplace Culture Critical Analysis Tool (WCCAT). *Practice Development in Healthcare*, **8**, 28–43.

McCormack, B., Dewing, J., Breslin, L. *et al.* (2010) Developing person-centred practice: nursing outcomes arising from changes to the care environment in residential settings for older people. *International Journal of Older People Nursing*, **5** (2), 93–107.

McCormack, B., Manley, K., and Titchen, A. (2013) Introduction, in *Practice Development in Nursing and Health Care*, 2nd edn (eds B. McCormack, K. Manley, and A. Titchen), Wiley-Blackwell, Oxford, pp. 1–17.

McSherry R and Warr J. (2008) Introducing practice development to facilitate excellence in care. In: McSherry R and Warr J. (eds), *An Introduction to Excellence in Practice Development in Health and Social Care*. Maidenhead, UK: Open University Press-McGraw-Hill Education, chapter 1.

Medical Research council (MRC) (2008) *Developing and evaluating complex interventions: new guidance*. London: MRC. Available from: www.mrc.ac.uk/complexinterventionsguidance (accessed 3 February 2016).

National Voices (2015) *Prioritising person-centred care – the evidence*. Website: http://www.nationalvoices.org.uk/evidence (accessed 3 February 2016).

Osborne S. (2009) Testing the effectiveness of a practice development intervention on changing the culture of evidence based practice in an acute environment. PhD thesis, Queensland University of Technology School of Nursing Institute of Health and Biomedical Innovation.

Patterson M, Nolan M, Rick J, Brown J, Adams R, Musson G. (2011) *From metrics to meaning: culture change and quality of acute hospital care for older people. National Institute for Health Research Service Delivery and Organisation programme*. Available at: http://www.nets.nihr.ac.uk/__data/assets/pdf_file/0015/81402/ES-08-1501-93.pdf (accessed 3 February 2016).

Pawson R and Tilley N. (2004) *Realist evaluation*. Available at: http://www.communitymatters.com.au/RE_chapter.pdf (accessed 3 February 2016).

Royal College of Nursing (2006) *Workplace Resources for Practice Development*, RCN, London.

Rycroft-Malone J. (2013) How you might use PARIHS to deliver safe and effective care. In: McCormack B, Manley K, Titchen A. (eds), *Practice Development in Nursing and Healthcare*, 2nd edn. Oxford: Wiley-Blackwell, chapter 7.

Rycroft-Malone, J., Seers, K., Titchen, A., Harvey, G., Kitson, A., and McCormack, B. (2004) What counts as evidence in evidence-based practice. *Journal of Advanced Nursing*, **47**, 81–90.

Rycroft-Malone, J., McCormack, B., Hutchinson, A.M. *et al.* (2012) Realist synthesis: illustrating the method for implementation research. *Implementation Science*, **7** (1), 33.

Schein, E.H. (1999) *Process Consultation Revisited: Building the Helping Relationship*, Organizational Development Series, Prentice Hall.

Scottish Health Council (2014) *Emotional touchpoints*. Available at: http://www.scottishhealthcouncil.org/patient__public_participation/participation_toolkit/emotional_touchpoints.aspx (accessed 3 February 2016).

Shaw T, Dewing J, Young R, Devlin M, Boomer C, Legius M. (2008) Enabling practice development: delving into the concept of facilitation from a practitioner perspective. In: Manley K, McCormack B, Wilson V. (eds), *International Practice Development in Nursing and Healthcare.* Oxford: Blackwell Publishing, chapter 8.

Slater, P., McCormack, B., and Bunting, B. (2009) The development and pilot testing of an instrument to measure nurse's working environment: The Nursing Context Index. *Worldviews on Evidence-Based Nursing,* **6** (3), 173–82.

Titchen, A. and McCormack, B. (2010) Dancing with stones: critical creativity as methodology for human flourishing. *Educational Action Research,* **18**, 531–54.

Unsworth, J. (2008) Practice development: a concept analysis. *Journal of Nursing Management,* **8** (6), 317–26.

CHAPTER 10

Creating flourishing workplaces

Jan Dewing & Brendan McCormack
Queen Margaret University, Edinburgh, UK

Introduction

Imagine a workplace or an organisation where person-centred care is the reality
for the majority of people for most of the time, by teams who have established
person-centred patterns of care and ways of working embedded in a workplace
culture that is person-centred; all of which is held within a person-centred corporate culture – an ideal perhaps? We can't recall having ever experienced, in
totality, this type of organisation. However, we have encountered in different
organisations various aspects of person-centredness as we've just set out here.
The ultimate aim of such a person-centred organisation, we will argue, is to
create a place and related conditions where people flourish. So this chapter is
primarily about the outcome of flourishing within person-centred workplaces. It
will also touch on the notion of the person-centred organisation in its totality and
the mysterious idea(l) of sustainability. We make parallel connections between
person-centredness and human flourishing to help us set out the attributes of
a person-centred workplace culture, and introduce a model developed by one
of the authors (J.D.), from research and scholarship, to illustrate our discussion. This model can provide a useful heuristic for describing the movement and
progress of person-centredness in the workplace as organisations move towards
flourishing. Readers are asked to note that person-centredness here, unless otherwise stated, is an inclusive idea that includes employees and those receiving
services and care.

Person-centredness and human flourishing

When we consider what person-centredness is for – the intention – we argue
that person-centredness is ultimately concerned with human flourishing. In
Chapter 2 McCormack and McCance defined person-centredness as:

> an approach to practice established through the formation and fostering of *healthful* rela-
> tionships between *all care providers, service users and others significant to them in their lives.*

Person-Centred Practice in Nursing and Health Care: Theory and Practice, Second Edition.
Edited by Brendan McCormack and Tanya McCance.
© 2017 John Wiley & Sons, Ltd. Published 2017 by John Wiley & Sons, Ltd.

It is underpinned by values of respect for persons, individual right to self-determination, mutual respect and understanding. It is enabled by cultures of empowerment that foster continuous approaches to practice development [emphasis added].

Whilst this definition does not explicitly state an outcome from person-centredness, implicit in the definition is a focus on effective relationships that are healthful, where healthfulness is focused on respecting individual needs, wants and desires that result in a positive experience for all concerned – or, as we would argue, contributing to the condition of human flourishing. Therefore, flourishing is a desirable outcome of person-centredness. Generally speaking, human flourishing is about individuals being in a continued state of well-being and being at their best for prolonged periods of time (Seligman 2012, p. 70), and when they're not, having the resilience to bounce back stronger. Heron and Reason (1997) view human flourishing as a focus on maximising individuals' achievement of their potential for growth and development as they change the circumstances and relations of their lives at individual, group, community and societal levels (Titchen & McCormack 2010). Drawing on ecological and transformative perspectives, McCormack and Titchen (2014, p. 19) suggest that:

Human flourishing occurs when we bound and frame naturally co-existing energies, when we embrace the known and yet to be known, when we embody contrasts and when we achieve stillness and harmony. When we flourish we give and receive loving kindness.

This idea that to flourish is both a giving and receiving of energy is important in healthful relationships that are reciprocal and that have the ultimate goal of all persons flourishing.

However, whilst the ideal of person-centred relationships that are healthful is for everyone to flourish, there are some situations for persons, related to health and health care, where flourishing will not occur. Nevertheless, we still need to be mindful of supporting the enabling factors of flourishing because some aspects of flourishing could occur and because it is the morally right thing to do. Although flourishing will be addressed in other ways in this book (see Chapter 11), we want to add to these contributions with a perspective from the field of positive psychology.

In this field researchers do not talk about person-centredness per se; however, central tenets of the discipline are well-being, thriving and flourishing, in which we can see a direct resonance with person-centredness. Seligman (2011) articulated the importance and significance of well-being. He began his articulation of this with three elements he argues are essential for well-being: (i) experiencing positive emotion; (ii) engagement and being absorbed; and (iii) having meaning in life through belonging to and serving something one believes to be bigger than oneself. As a consequence of learning from subsequent research, he has added to these, to form what he now refers to as PERMA: positive emotion, engagement, relationships, meaning, and accomplishment (Seligman 2011, p. 16). These he suggests are the five essential conditions necessary for flourishing. What is of particular interest to us, as practice developers, is that Seligman argues, based on his research findings, that it is possible to build PERMA within individuals, teams and even whole organisations. Gaffney (2012, p. 6) has adapted Seligman's model and proposes four essential elements necessary for flourishing. These are given in Box 10.1.

Box 10.1 Four essential elements for flourishing (after Gaffney 2012).

1 *Challenge*: Some call or demand for you to do something, to get over an obstacle, to engage with some life task, to make something happen.
2 *Connectivity*: Being attuned to what is happening inside you and outside you. Connectivity orientates you to the challenge and gets you ready to deal with it.
3 *Autonomy*: Feeling free to move and to act in pursuit of the challenge. This gives you the energy to get going and sets the direction of travel.
4 *Using valued competencies*: The experience of using your talents, especially the strengths you most value in yourself, to the full.

Gaffney argues that the best kind of challenge is one that we 'own'. That does not mean that we have to identify or plan the challenge ourselves as sometimes we can find ourselves being challenged, not of our choice but because of a context we are in. In the context of practice development, we have identified these as 'critical moments' when we have a choice to grow, develop and transform or not. However, irrespective of the challenge and where it comes from, Gaffney (2012, p. 8) further argues that flourishing requires 'connectivity' or 'psychological attunement'.

Although others, including Sabi (2013), challenge the view that it is possible to build PERMA, our experience of practice development and working with individuals and teams would suggest that it is possible, but that it is also fragile and context-dependent. Seligman seems to focus primarily on the internal world of persons and seems to suggest that PERMA is the responsibility of individuals. However, we all live and work in communities that are culturally, historically and politically influenced. Critical social theory informs us that these external social and cultural factors bear down on the person and contain and restrain individuals and groups from the freedom to act. It is these forces that need containing or overthrowing for human flourishing to occur. Becoming an emotionally intelligent person will contribute in part to realising PERMA and flourishing in the workplace or to living well with a health-related condition; however, external social structures and perceived power relations are also influencing forces (Schutte & Loi 2014). McCormack et al. (2013) argue that there is ample evidence to suggest that strong connections between team members, between team members and the values and goals of an organisation, and between the organisation and the personal values of employees, create effective workplaces and, indeed, environments that flourish. There is equally strong evidence to illustrate the impact of what are termed 'psychologically unsafe' environments, that is, environments that are disrespectful of persons (Brown & McCormack 2011).

What is a flourishing organisation?

A good place to start is to ask ourselves *what is a person-centred workplace and a person-centred organisation?* How would you know you were in it? What would you see? What would you hear and how would you feel? Person-centred workplaces and organisations, by definition, need to be focused on the people they support and provide services for; but not simply on the work, treatment and 'care' or support needs but on what matters to the person given who they are and where they are in their life and in relation to the person's aspirations and wishes. Trying to do this on a large scale provides huge challenges – but huge opportunities too. Williams and Sanderson (2015), drawing on their experiences within UK health care, propose seven elements they believe are the foundation for person-centred organisations: visionary leadership; shared values and beliefs; outcomes for individuals; community focus; empowered and valued staff; individual and organisational learning, and partnership. We wouldn't argue with any of these, although they are fairly general. There has to be something else, something more specific. Cameron (2010), for example, suggests five strategies that would be seen in flourishing organisations:

- Capitalising on the inherent human inclination towards positive energy.
- Managing financial and economic challenges virtuously.
- Focusing on abundance gaps.
- Creating positive energy in the face of challenges.
- Implementing positive practices even where they don't seem to be valued.

These broad-based strategies capture the essence of PERMA as set out by Seligman (2011, pp. 16–20). They are also useful in helping us appreciate that flourishing can take place in organisations where there are challenges due to tough internal and/or external business forces – a current reality for most, whether in public or private health-care services.

We felt that something more specific and more strategic was needed to position and visualise the development needed within the nursing and health-care context, where there was a blending together, in a dynamic way, of some of the principles underpinning person-centred practice and positive psychology. The rest of this chapter will focus on a model that seeks to describe and illustrate the movement towards flourishing in the workplace.

The Compliance, Service Improvement and Innovation Model (CoSII)

The origins for the model began within a three-year practice development programme between The University of Wollongong and Uniting Care Ageing in New South Wales, Australia. The programme's focus was on developing and evaluating person-centred cultures across one region of a national organisation with a view to transferability and upscaling (Dewing et al. 2010, p. 163; 2014). In one of the workshops we drew out ideas for the coming years' development activities. The mapping of the development activities then led to a discussion where we tried to uncover what essential attributes were driving our journey towards person-centredness. We hypothesised that these were positive forms of energy and the momentum of movement. These two attributes were left in their raw state for a while. Then a systematic method was used to begin to develop a model that drew on the two attributes of energy and movement. Critical discussion, within the International Person-centred Practice Research Community of Practice (ICoP), offered a forum where an early iteration of the model presented here was critiqued. Since then, four assumptions and three, threefold core concepts representing movement towards a flourishing culture have been proposed; note these are still embedded within the notions of energy and movement:

Assumptions:

• Movement towards an inclination for flourishing.
• Movement away from patient-centredness towards person-centredness as central to achieving flourishing for all individuals, teams and workplaces.
• Movement away from external rewards to internal rewards for individuals and teams in being person-centred.
• Movement away from a technical focus on efficiency and effectiveness and its measurement in organisations towards an integrated system of virtuous practices and evaluation.

Threefold concepts:

• Compliance/Person-centred moments/Performing
• Improvement/Person-centred patterns/Thriving
• Innovation/Person-centred cultures/Flourishing

An unpublished review of the literature relating to these concepts and assumptions led to the 'three circles' mode, subsequently called the CoSII model. The model has been further tested within a programme of practice development activity in an NHS Trust in England. The current model, although very much still a work in progress, is depicted in Figure 10.1.

We will now describe the key components of the model, beginning with the horizontal and vertical axes. The model aims to present the forces and key features within workplaces and the organisation that work to enable persons to experience more positive emotion, high levels of engagement, meaningful relationships, acquire meaning, and feel a sense of accomplishment (Seligman 2011, pp. 18, 124).

Absorptive capacity and capability

Absorptive capacity is an organisation's ability to identify, assimilate, transform and apply external knowledge it considers valuable. There is always a limit to the rate or quantity of scientific or technological information that an organisation (or parts of it) can absorb at any one time (Cohen & Levinthal 1990).

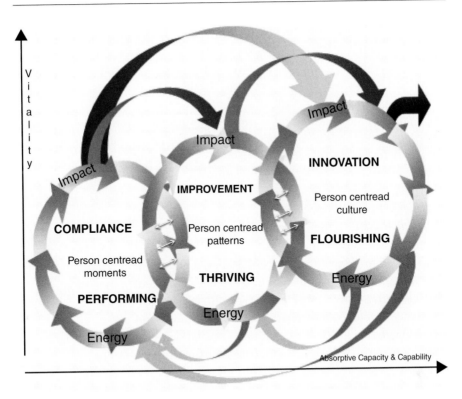

Figure 10.1 The Compliance Service Improvement and Innovation Model (CoSII). Source: Dewing et al. (2015). Reproduced with permission of Foundation of Nursing Studies.

Having the capacity for absorption is considered essential for knowledge mobilisation. The term mobilisation is used here as it indicates a shifting focus from traditional management of knowledge (teaching and training) to the provision of space that enables people to act and apply their sense making, toward greater collective understanding and where people make decisions together to achieve genuine outcomes (Hasan & Crawford 2007). The latter is much more of a positive fit with ideas of person-centredness. Of even more relevance to us is that the focus is on the development of systems to support knowledge creation and innovation at the level of a group or community, rather than with individuals or with a few people at senior management level. In the CoSII model we specifically include the translation of all types of knowledge from knowledge 'about' to knowledge on 'how to'. There are a number of factors that influence knowledge mobilisation. For example, Lane and Rogers (2011) claim organisations consider the value of knowledge according to their mission and the interests of their members to absorb different types of knowledge. The type and quality of relationships between different stakeholder groups in an organisation, such as those between general management and clinicians and practitioners, are strong factors in influencing how knowledge mobilisation does or does not take place and what the movement of knowledge looks like (Greenhalgh et al. 2004). Further, Rycroft-Malone et al. (2013) propose that successful implementation of evidence-based knowledge into practice is a planned facilitated process in which individuals, teams and context are major factors. The resources and strengths within an organisation and within a team represent the capabilities available. These will include: human capital (numbers of people, knowledge levels, skills and experience); physical and material resources; strategy and planning; financial and IT resources. Therefore, we have blended in capability as well as capacity. Kislov et al. (2014) set out four principles that fit well with the blended absorption axis in this model because of their focus on capability and capacity as dynamic entities. They are:

- moving from the notion of 'building' capacity towards 'developing' capacity in a health-care organisation;
- moving from passive involvement in formal education and training towards active continuous participation in knowledge mobilisation practices;
- moving from lower order project-specific capabilities towards higher order generic capabilities allowing flexibility and innovation;
- moving from single-level to multi-level capability development involving transitions between individuals, groups and organisational learning.

Vitality

Vitality has been generally considered as having sufficient physical and mental energy. We like this concept as it can be seen in a number of Western and Eastern traditions. Vitality, or the energy available to a person (chi, ki or bayu), is said to be an indicator of health and motivation (Ryan & Deci 2008). When vitality is present, persons experience a sense of enthusiasm and aliveness. Vitality is associated with feelings of vigour and positive emotions, and can be associated with calmness and being grounded. Subjective vitality, unlike other forms of energy (such as anger, anxiety, or arousal), is a form of energy that a person can harness and coordinate for intentional and purposeful action. Ryan and Deci (2008) point to a number of experimental and field studies suggesting that vitality and energy are enhanced by activities that satisfy core human needs for relatedness, competence and autonomy. We would also add that good physical health is a prerequisite. Therefore, in relation to the prerequisites for vitality as an employee or service user, being in meaningful relationships, the demonstration of competence and having subjective feelings of autonomy are essential – elements that are consistent with the prerequisites of McCormack and McCance's Person-centred Nursing Framework (see Chapter 3). Vitality is necessary for growth and resilience, which in turn are necessary for flourishing. Depending on the focus of activities in the workplace and the way in which they are carried out, energy levels may become depleted or enhanced. A nurse may feel energised as a result of being with a person they are caring for, or from being in an education session. A service user may feel energised or tired after being provided with care. Activities carried out positively will lead to renewal of energy and over time will add to an increased sense of vitality. By activities we mean anything and everything from the apparently simplest of tasks (e.g. talking to another person, reading or writing an email) through to complex multi-factorial tasks either within the team or with persons receiving care (e.g. adapting to a new manager or team leader, a new role, implementing new guidelines, or taking part in a service improvement project).

Within both the domains of absorptive capacity/capability and vitality, the matrix of time is present. There are some developmental processes that simply require more time than others (Jones & Woodhead 2015). Maximising communication in networks and forward-looking leaders who invest in staff and have positive management practices can positively reduce the time needed for knowledge absorption (Tu et al. 2006). However, no matter how much capacity 'building' and energy is put in, individuals and teams will always need time to search out naturally occurring opportunities(Kouzes & Posner 2012) and to absorb new knowledge and to learn how to translate this into everyday practice. As McCormack and Titchen (2014, p. 15) have argued, 'creating different and complementary spaces for different purposes is an important consideration in enabling human flourishing.'

First impressions of CoSII

The heart of the model shows the three circles. There is also the possibility of moving on from innovation/person-centred culture/flourishing to something else. At this point we do not know what that will look like. Something else will evolve in time. There is a sense of the model being complex; although it is simply a series of repeating arrows. This, we hope, illustrates both the complexity and the repeated patterns inherent within workplace cultures and large organisations. It can engender images of a moving snowball, a glowing firework or a whirlwind. All these may be positive or equally they can be negative, depending on your perspective and imagination.

The three cycles in the model have overlapping arrows and indicate the concepts of energy and impact within the workplace or organisation. The arrows here represent the synergistic relationship between the types and levels of energy and impact in the workplace or organisation. Positive energy will contribute significantly to positive impact, whereas negative energy leads to poor impact and possibly even to negative impact. The notion of engagement is also hidden within these arrows. Engagement is both a process of and an outcome from collaboration, inclusion and participation (Dewing & McCormack 2015).

Necessarily, there is an overlap between each cycle. The small linear arrows in the overlap spaces indicate that the space can expand or contract according to how effectively or not the four core principles (Kislov et al. 2014) are being realised. Therefore, workplaces and organisations are never, in entirety, in one cycle only. There are a number of assumptions, values, artefacts and behaviours

(Schein 2010, pp. 23–33) that can generally be found within each cycle, and often these exist despite values, vision and mission statements that might insist otherwise.

The large arrows, external to the circles and moving between each of them, indicate the combined relationship and effects of the positive influencing forces (moving forwards and upwards) or negative influencing forces (moving backwards and downwards).

The effective workplace culture model by Manley et al. (2011) shows the antecedents, attributes and outcomes of the effective workplace culture viewed through a practice development lens, and the Person-centred Nursing Framework (McCormack & McCance 2010, p. 61) indicates the essential attributes of a conducive care environment. The CoSII model adds to these by suggesting that there are complex sets of energies and forces that come into play when working towards achieving an innovative and flourishing workplace and organisational culture where person-centredness is the norm. Getting out of the first cycle for example, or 'outperforming' the compliance/performing cycle requires a huge amount of investment in energy creation and absorptive capacity and capability. It also requires a ceiling to be put on the energy that is used up by compliance activities such as monitoring and routine measurement. Many of the methods and tools that are used in compliance-focused organisations focus on reducing error and minimising the impact of error; although necessary, these are not effective when applied to an agenda that is about innovation. The school of Positive Organisational Scholarship (POS) recommends methodologies with a positive lens; assuming an affirming bias; focusing on positive deviant performance and examination of the best people and their performances (Cameron & McNaughton 2014). Changes in rules and practice should be driven by learning what is and is not working in supporting individuals. Using a small set of value-based skills at all levels of the system will drive change throughout the system. Using these skills in conjunction with selected quality management and organisational development tools will improve quality of life and increase organisational effectiveness and efficiency.

Research in international business indicates that outperforming requires three core activities: organisational structures and functions where innovation is core to all business; workplace cultures that enable innovation to thrive; and processes (and we would say people too) that help others to convert ideas into innovation plans and actions. At the point where the compliance and service improvement cultures overlap, the innovation investment is usually regarded as developmental and 'nice to do' if there is time and money. We argue that in order to move forwards, and certainly to move beyond the service improvement culture, an innovative way of being needs to become fundamental to everyday business in health care. For this to be nurtured, a number of core driving forces need to be put in place or strengthened (see Box 10.2). We have adapted these from a recent report by the IBM Institute for Business Value (IBM 2015).

Box 10.2 Core driving forces for innovation.

1 Innovation needs aligning with strategy and aims.
2 Structures in workplace and the whole organisations need to adapt to be open and welcoming of innovation.
3 Invest in people who can lead innovation from within the workplace.
4 Leaders to have a skill set around innovation and work with managers to ensure compliance is achieved but does not dominate.
5 Encourage innovative ideas, dialogue and activities in all workplaces.
6 Sustain innovation momentum during times of adversity.
7 Generate new ideas from a wider range of sources.
8 Invest in learning and education that focuses on everyone's contribution to innovation.
9 Fund innovation.
10 Measure and evaluate innovation outcomes.

Adapted from IBM (2015).

Sustainability

The CoSII model has an inclination towards being positive and optimistic as demanded by the underpinning assumptions. Code (1999) advises caution here, that we should beware the dynamic charm that the notion of flourishing can invoke. Certainly, flourishing for one should not be at a cost of not flourishing for others. Code draws on the work of Cuomo (1998), to argue that flourishing requires more than self-capability (we have replaced the term mastery with capability here), it needs to be combined with social, cultural and political capability to ensure that 'habitats' are developed where people can work well together.

> We are embedded beings who create work in a social context, toiling shared soil in the hopes that our labour bears fruit. It is up to all of us whether this soil is enriched or depleted, whether it nurtures diverse and vital produce or allows predictable crops to take root and run rampant. The notion of sustainable culture forces us … to figure out how to improve them [our workplace cultures].
>
> *Taylor (2014)*

Summary

In a model where movement and energy predominate, sustainability is found in persons and processes rather than in structures. It is an ever increasing reality that no health-care structures are permanent, and in fact they are being reorganised on a more frequent basis than ever before. Those workplaces and organisations that place more importance on energy capacity and capability development ultimately should have outcomes that relate to thriving and flourishing for all, and should recover more quickly from adversity and trying times. It is our contention therefore, that for a workplace or an organisation to claim person-centredness, it must also have a commitment to creating flourishing organisational characteristics, whilst at the same time recognising that this is not achieved through one-off projects, but instead is embedded in the DNA of the organisation.

References

Brown, D. and McCormack, B. (2011) Developing the practice context to enable more effective pain management with older people: An action research approach. *Implementation Science*, **6** (9), 1–14.

Cameron, K. (2010) Five keys to flourishing in trying times. *Executive Forum Winter*, pp., 45–51.

Cameron, K. and McNaughton, J. (2014) Positive organisational change. *Journal of Applied Behavioural Science*, **50** (4), 445–62.

Code, L. (1999) Flourishing. *Ethics and The Environment*, **4**, 63–72.

Cohen, W. and Levinthal, D. (1990) Absorptive capacity: a new perspective on learning and innovation. *Administrative Science Quarterly*, **35** (1), 128–52.

Cuomo, C.J. (1998) *Feminism and Ecological Communities; An Ethic of Flourishing*, Routledge, London.

Dewing J and McCormack B. (2015) Engagement: a critique of the concept and its application to person-centred care. *International Practice Development Journal* **5** (Suppl.):[6]. Available at: http://www.fons.org/Resources/Documents/Journal/Vol5Suppl/IPDJ_05(suppl)_06.pdf (accessed 15 February 2016).

Dewing, J., Dowse, H., Eldridge, P. *et al.* (2010) Person-centred practice at Uniting Care Ageing, New South Wales, in *Person-Centred Nursing: Theory and Practice* (eds B. McCormack and T. McCance), Wiley-Blackwell, Oxford, pp. 163–8.

Dewing, J., Downs, J., and Frei, I.-A. (2013) Strategic practice development work, in *Practice Development in Nursing and Health Care: A Foundation Text*, 2nd edn (eds B. McCormack, K. Manley, and A. Titchen), Wiley-Blackwell, Oxford.

Dewing J, Harmon AM, Nolan J. (2014) The Aspire to Inspire programme in aged care: the final chapter, one year on. *International Practice Development Journal* **4**(1). Available at: http://www.fons.org/library/journal/volume4-issue1/article9 (accessed 4 February 2016).

Gaffney, M. (2012) *Flourishing: How to Achieve a Deeper Sense of Well-being, Meaning and Purpose - Even when Facing Adversity*, Penguin, London.

Greenhalgh, T., Robert, G., McFarlane, F., Bate, P., and Kyriakidou, O. (2004) Diffusion of innovations in service organisations: systematic review and recommendations. *The Millbank Quarterly*, **82** (4), 581–629.

Hasan H and Crawford K. (2007) Knowledge mobilisation in communities through socio-technical system. *Knowledge Management Research and Practice* **5**/4:237–48.

Heron, J. and Reason, P. (1997) A participatory inquiry paradigm. *Qualitative Inquiry*, **3** (3), 274–94.

IBM (2015) *More than magic: How the most successful organizations innovate. IBM Institute for Business Value*. Available at: http://www.slideshare.net/FiweSystems/more-than-magic-bengt-eliasson-smarter-commerce-day-2015 (accessed 15 February 2016).

Jones, B. and Woodhead, T. (2015) *Building the Foundations for Improvement: Learning Report*, The Health Foundation, London.

Kislov R, Waterman H, Harvey G, Boaden R. (2014) Rethinking capacity building for knowledge mobilisation: developing multilevel capabilities in healthcare organisations. *Implementation Science* **9**:166. Available at: http://www.implementationscience.com/content/9/1/166 (accessed 4 February 2016).

Kouzes, J. and Posner, B. (2012) *The Leadership Challenge*, 5th edn, Jossey-Bass, London.

Lane JP and Rogers JD. (2011) Engaging national organisations for knowledge translation: comparative case studies in knowledge value mapping. *Implementation Science* **6**:106. Available at: http://www.implementationscience.com/content/6/1/106 (accessed 4 February 2016).

Manley K, Sanders K, Cardiff S, Webster J. (2011) Effective workplace culture: the attributes, enabling factors and consequences of a new concept. *International Practice Development Journal* **1**(2). Available at: http://www.fons.org/Resources/Documents/Journal/Vol1No2/IPDJ_0102_01.pdf (accessed 4 February 2016).

McCormack, B. and McCance, T. (2010) *Person-Centred Nursing: Theory and Practice*, Wiley-Blackwell, Oxford.

McCormack B and Titchen A. (2014) No beginning, no end: an ecology of human flourishing. *International Practice Development Journal* **4**(2), art. 2. Available at: http://www.fons.org/library/journal/volume4-issue2/article2 (accessed 4 February 2016).

McCormack, B., Titchen, A., and Manley, K. (2013) The contextual web of practice development, in *Practice Development in Nursing*, vol. **2** (eds B. McCormack, K. Manley, and A. Titchen), Wiley-Blackwell Publishing, Oxford, pp. 275–95.

Ryan, R.M. and Deci, E.L. (2008) From ego depletion to vitality: theory and findings concerning the facilitation of energy available to self. *Social and Personality Psychology Compass*, **2** (2), 702–17.

Rycroft-Malone J, Seers K, Chandler J et al. (2013) The role of evidence, context and facilitation in an implementation trial: implications for the development of the PARIHS framework. *Implementation Science* **8**:28. Available at: http://www.implementationscience.com/content/8/1/28 (accessed 4 February 2016).

Sabi, A. (2013) Whose flourishing? Which Aristotelianism? *Society*, **50**, 587–91.

Schein, E.H. (2010) *Organizational Culture and Leadership*, 4th edn, Jossey-Bass, San Francisco.

Schutte, N.S. and Loi, N.M. (2014) Connections between emotional intelligence and workplace flourishing. *Personality and Individual Differences*, **66**, 134–9.

Seligman, M. (2011) *Flourish: A New Understanding of Happiness and Well-being and How to Achieve Them*, Nicholas Brealey, London.

Seligman, M. (2012) *Flourish: A Visionary New Understanding of Happiness and Well-being*, Simon and Schuster, New York.

Taylor (2014) cited by Popova M on the Brain Pickings website: http://www.brainpickings.org/2015/02/05/the-peoples-platform-astra-taylor/?mc_cid=62a64daceb&mc_eid=0fd40c7f5f (accessed 4 February 2016).

Titchen, A. and McCormack, B. (2010) Dancing with stones: critical creativity as methodology for human flourishing. *Educational Action Research*, **18**, 531–54.

Tu Q, Vonderembse M, Ragu-Nathan TS. (2006) Absorptive capacity: Enhancing the assimilation of time-based manufacturing practices. *Journal of Operations Management* **24**(5). Available at: http://scholarworks.rit.edu/article/579 (accessed 4 February 2016).

Wiliams R and Sanderson H. (2015) *What are we learning about person centred organisations?* Available at: http://creativeoptionsregina.ca/wp-content/uploads/2015/03/What-are-We-Learning-About-Person-Centred-Organizations.pdf (accessed 4 February 2016).

CHAPTER 11

Helping health-care practitioners to flourish: critical companionship at work

Angie Titchen[1] & Karen Hammond[2]

[1] Ulster University, Northern Ireland, UK
[2] East Kent Hospitals University Foundation Trust, Kent, UK

Opening space

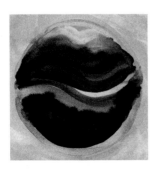

Human flourishing occurs when we bound and frame naturally co-existing energies, when we embrace the known and yet to be known, when we embody contrasts and when we achieve stillness and harmony. When we flourish we give and receive loving kindness

Definition and image from
McCormack and Titchen (2014, p. 19)

Person-centredness is central to helping practitioners to flourish at work. It manifests through relationships between colleagues and between practitioners and service users. These are relationships based on respect for persons, compassion, kindness, self-determination, mutual respect, trust and understanding. Such relationships are brought alive by working intentionally with the Person-centred Nursing Framework (McCormack & McCance 2006). Critical companionship (CC) (Titchen 2001, 2004) is a person-centred relationship that can help practitioners to develop the domains (prerequisites, care environment and care processes) of the Person-centred Nursing Framework. The companion aims to be a visible, living embodiment of person-centredness, helping practitioners to flourish through the relationship and by flowing and spiralling through inner and outer turbulence that occurs through change and transformation. CC is made visible through a metaphor of accompanying an individual or group on a co-learning/inquiry journey within their everyday practice and a conceptual framework.

Person-Centred Practice in Nursing and Health Care: Theory and Practice, Second Edition.
Edited by Brendan McCormack and Tanya McCance.
© 2017 John Wiley & Sons, Ltd. Published 2017 by John Wiley & Sons, Ltd.

We are critical companions helping each other in a critical-creative inquiry in which Karen is exploring her own development of CC in her practice development facilitator role and Angie is deepening her understanding of how she does CC in a critical creativity worldview. When we were invited to write this chapter we decided that we would use a 'faction' genre, which is fiction based on 'fact', derived from our own and others' empirical research and experience. We want to give you a taste of how CC can contribute to developing and sustaining person-centred cultures through helping practitioners to become person-centred by exploring self, reflectively and critically, and using that knowledge and understanding to change their approaches to practice and engagement with service users.

The chapter tells the story of how imaginary critical companionships were set up to embed the Person-centred Nursing Framework in a large NHS Foundation Hospital Trust that integrates hospitals in different towns with rural-based clinics. We show you how two companions use the PCN and CC frameworks to create spaces for practitioners' self-reflection and critique as they learn in and from practice. We draw on two other frameworks concerned with human flourishing (Titchen & McCormack 2010; McCormack & Titchen 2014) to touch lightly on the idea that it is the professional artistry of the critical companion that effectively creates the conditions for human flourishing.

Preparing the ground for critical companionship

Five years ago, a national quality inspection was carried out in the Trust and the report highlighted the need for culture change, beginning at the top. A new Chief Executive, Linda, was then appointed to lead the change. In her previous post as a Director of Nursing and Allied Health Professions, Linda had been a passionate supporter of staff who were using an emancipatory practice development approach (Manley et al. 2004) to create person-centred cultures throughout the organisation. She had seen the impact of such cultures on service users' experiences of their care and had observed that culture change seemed to come about by paying attention to person-centred relationships between staff and service users and colleagues. In her new post, Linda set to work to help the hospital executive team become more person-centred in the way they worked together and with hospital staff, and to experience the challenges of transforming their relationships and ways of working and the need for support for themselves and all staff in creating person-centred cultures.

Simultaneously, Linda developed a proposal for a Trust-wide, inter-professional practice development programme to support transformation. A cornerstone of the programme would be to support experienced practitioners, clinical leaders and managers in developing facilitation skills. They would learn how to help their staff and the people they work with develop and strengthen their capacity to create person-centred care environments in their workplace and acquire care process and practice development skills. Joanna, a physio-therapist with experience in primary and acute care, practice development and research, was appointed to join the executive team as the practice development programme director. Joanna had impressed Linda at her interview by her vision of using the Person-centred Nursing Framework as an energising, dynamic framework to guide change, and the CC framework as a strategy for facilitating the change.

Joanna had explained then, 'Here is a mandala[1] of the CC framework superimposed on the person-centred framework, which I have symbolised by three spirals at the centre (Figure 11.1). Within the spirals (which have no beginning and no end), learning and inquiry spaces flow across the three domains of the Person-centred Nursing Framework. In other words, when companions work in a space in one domain there is an effect in the others too. In reality, these spirals are bigger than CC, but I have designed it this way to fore-ground CC at this point.'

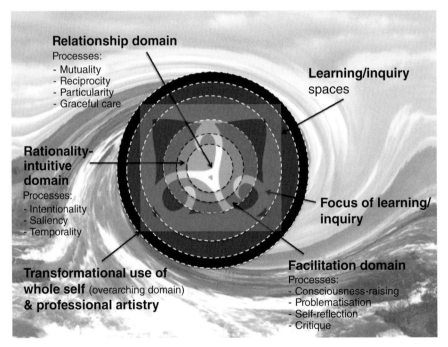

Figure 11.1 Key components of the CC framework (for full framework, see Titchen 2001, 2004).

---

[1] A mandala is an ancient circular or square symbol showing the parts and whole of something and the relationships between the parts and the whole.

She went on, 'There are four CC domains and each one has specific processes and strategies. The dotted lines show the potential for the processes to be brought together in a kind of improvisation according to the uniqueness of each person, context and situation and what is needed.'

Later, after Joanna had taken up her post, Linda wanted to check that she had understood how the two frameworks would work together. 'So let me get this right, Joanna, the idea would be that we could support these experienced people in becoming critical companions whose work would promote the development of the whole of the Person-centred Nursing Framework and, in turn, they could help others, in their workplace to become companions. Over time, the strategy could snowball across the Trust?'

'Exactly', replied Joanna. She takes a deep breath and suggests to Linda that they could become critical companions to help each other work effectively with both frameworks across the organisation. Linda accepted.

Becoming critical companions

Over the next few months, Joanna set up a practice development support group and introduced them to the CC framework. She suggested that they start to reflect on their facilitation practice by identifying which processes they were using. She gave them a handout with the mandala (Figure 11.1) and a brief description of each domain and its processes to put in their metaphorical pockets.

The *Relationship domain* has four processes. *Particularity* is about knowing the other(s) as a whole person in their situation and contexts, so as to devise helping strategies that are likely to work for that person or group. *Reciprocity* is about giving and receiving gifts of care, concern and wisdom. That makes the relationship more equal. *Graceful care* means authentically engaging the other as a whole person with the whole of oneself and being kind/present/emotionally engaged but balanced. *Mutuality* is dependent on all three processes and it is about working with other(s) in a genuine partnership with shared decision-making about everything.

The *Facilitation domain* also has four processes. *Consciousness-raising* is concerned with enabling conscious awareness of taken-for-granted assumptions, embodied wisdom and the carrying of culture in the body, discourse and language. *Problematisation* is about helping others to see problems that they are not aware of, or reframing problems to help others see things from different perspectives. The *self-reflection* means helping people to reflect on themselves and their practices to develop self-knowledge and to be able to evaluate their impact in interaction with others. And finally, *critique* involves engaging in critical-creative dialogue with oneself and others to co-create and contest new knowledge and understanding.

The *Rationality-intuitive domain* drives the use of the other domains. *Intentionality* is being deliberate, purposeful cognitively and intuitively; *saliency* is about knowing what matters/what is significant/what needs to be paid attention to);

and *temporality* is concerned with attending to past, present, future time, timing, timeliness, pacing and anticipating.

The *transformational use of self domain* is overarching and is enabled by *professional artistry* (Titchen 2009). Professional artistry is the means through which the critical companion blends, 'dances' or improvises any combination of the domains, processes and their strategies to meet the particular needs of people being helped in relation to their particular experiences, contexts and situations.

Over the next year, group members use this summary to help them to analyse and develop critical companionship within their current roles.

Linda is very supportive both to the group and individuals, and both she and Joanna become CCs to key individuals in the Trust. With this high profile across the domains of the Person-centred Nursing Framework, as well as celebration of progress all round, the snowballing effect they were hoping for is just beginning to happen.

Bounding and framing the turbulence of practice change

Nine months ago, James, a charge nurse in the cardiac unit, invited Chrissie, a clinical educator in the Surgical Directorate, to be his critical companion whilst undertaking a clinical leadership course. In their first sessions, she helped him to tell her what each part of the Person-centred Nursing Framework meant to him and then encouraged him to explore the prerequisites in relation to himself. Over the next few months, he chose to examine his values and beliefs and knowing himself, in conjunction with the 360° appraisal he was undertaking as part of the leadership programme. Through this process, he discovered he needed to manage his behaviours and understand their impact on himself and others. The story begins after he first made this discovery.

James steps into my office, 'I've had enough!' he says. 'I can't do it any more!' His angry tone, wide eyes and pained expression, alert me to his distress and I know I need to help him right now. But I am mindful of the relentless, rhythmic beat of the cardiac unit pulsing in the background (*temporality*).

'This place is all wrong and unfair. I am really worked up!'

Recognising the window of opportunity and the urgent need for me to open a dialogue space (*saliency* and *temporality*), I say, 'James, do you have 15 mins now?'

'Yes.'

I say, 'OK, please shut the door and sit down.' (*graceful care*) I think, 'How and where should I start?' Critical questions flow across my mind. What strategies am I going to draw on (*intentionality*)? How will I gather the salient issues in this situation where time is so limited? How can I help James to learn from the past, present and the future in this moment (*temporality*)?

In this very moment, I am minded of a metaphor of music . My thoughts tune into the gathering orchestral instruments, which, for me, represent the domains of the PCN and CC frameworks, as well as the elements of human flourishing (Figure 11.2).

I imagine a harp. I embrace it and begin to pluck the strings to improvise a melodic, harmonious tune of human flourishing. Using all the strings of my knowledge and skills, I draw together the sounds of my *professional artistry* (Figure 11.3) to help James in this personal moment. I am aware of grasping the situaton rapidly with my embodied, artistic and spiritual *intelligences* (they are like my antennae!) and *synthesising* my theoretical knowledge with my personal knowledge of James (*particularity*) in my body and my imagination. I feel a surge of energy as I interplay these dimensions of professional artistry, in what seems like milliseconds. I know deep inside myself that my strategy is very likely to work for James and to help him become more reflexive about his impact on others.

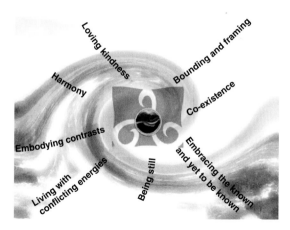

Figure 11.2 The elements of human flourishing (from McCormack & Titchen 2014).

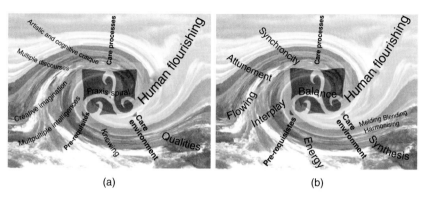

(a)   (b)

Figure 11.3 (a) The dimensions of professional artistry. **(b)** The more invisible processes (from Titchen 2009).

I take paper and pen. I draw a central hub in the centre of the page, telling James this circle represents him. Then I add spokes off this circle to represent his concerns, which we will fill in together. Dipping into my embodied knowing of creativity, I draw this out so we could see and focus on the real issues (*saliency, intentionality, consciousness-raising*). I do this because James feels hopeless about the hugeness of the problem that he sees as a weakness within the hospital *care environment* and beyond his control. I also recognise that I am working with the human flourishing elements of *bounding and framing* and *embracing the known and yet to be known* elements of human flourishing (Figure 11.2).

By putting a frame around a tiny part of the musical score, as it were, I am putting boundaries on the problem to make it feel more manageable for James (*problematisation*). I hope also that the *bounding and framing* element of human flourishing (Figure 11.2) will help James to flourish over time as he begins to understand the bigger musical score of person-centred cultures through understanding himself better. So the hub and spokes are a way of helping James critique what he knows and get a sense or feeling of what he does not yet know and then work with it (*self-reflection*). My aim also is to help him to *live with conflicting energies*.

'So, James, tell me what is happening for you?'

James replies: 'You know that I have been working with Joanne on creating a Trust-wide vision of person-centred, effective cultures within the Trust?' I nod; 'And that you have been helping me to understand the importance in the Person-centred Nursing Framework in relation to the care environment and how important it is to attend to these areas to enable person-centred cultures? Well, something has come up that flies in the face of such a culture in our unit. And I just feel so frustrated.'

'First, a member of staff is going to be disciplined and I am concerned that she will not be able to get another job because she won't be able to get a reference. Second, there was a similar issue two years ago and nothing has been done. It's so unfair !'

His words hit the air thick and fast. He draws very little breath. He just needs to express himself.

I make notes within the spokes, so he can see that I am actively listening and capturing his issues (*particularity, intentionality*). I am also role-modelling a way that we can capture our reflections for further analysis. But now is not the right time to tell him this because it would seem irrelevant and he is too emotional (*multiple intelligences*). I will point it out to him later (*temporality*).

He continues: 'Our line manager is letting the staff down by not completing tasks that she should. This is really difficult for other members of staff, as they can't challenge her. And another thing, on nights, a team member is being really lazy and is not doing his share of work. That makes it difficult for everyone else! And I have just had two weeks off and I was really relaxed. Now I am back, it's hard to settle back in.'

I notice that James's body language changes as he unloads these thoughts and feelings. His face relaxes and is less contorted. I ask, 'Is there anything else, James?' (*particularity*)

'No', he replies.

Then I take another piece of paper and draw Stephen Covey's (2004) circle of influence and circle of concern. I use the example of world hunger to show how it works and he clearly sees the connection with his own situation.

The 'Ah ha' moment!!

I know he has got it because he automatically begins to explore the issues he has raised. He begins to evaluate his situation into what he could influence and change and what he couldn't change.

He continues: 'Actually, I have done all I can to support the woman being disciplined and, maybe, I don't know all the facts! Also, I have offered to do a reference. I know that we are trying to develop an effective, person-centred workplace culture, which includes developing supportive organisational systems, but, professionally, I recognise that this issue still needs to be addressed.'

He ponders. I hold the space in stillness (Figures 11.2 and 11.4). I know that *movement* often occurs *in stillness* and that as a critical companion, I have to create the conditions for it to happen.

James continues: 'I know the line manager is being supported with leadership and management issues and I have met with the lazy person on nights.'

James smiles. 'It's good to be back from my holiday. While I was away I read about the Person-centred Nursing Framework and I feel it has changed me and offered me a different view point. I guess it will take more of our companion sessions to explore my reactions in depth, but I can't believe how much better I

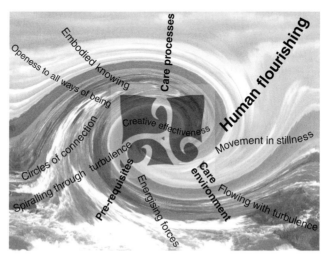

Figure 11.4 Methodological principles for creating the conditions for human flourishing (from Titchen & McCormack 2010).

feel. I know I have a short fuse and that it adversely effects my working relationships with patients and staff. And I know I am ranting about my line manager not living a person-centred culture when I am not doing it myself right now! But at least, I can see that the way you just helped me to turn my negativity into positive energy, and doing it quickly, is something that I could learn to do for myself, so that I can be person-centred with staff and patients and model a person-centred culture, even when I feel angry about something! It's all about learning to flow with turbulence, rather than getting sucked into it. Would you help me learn to do what you did today with me - with the staff in the midst of the working day?'

I am beaming; 'I would love to, James.'

James nods and stands up; 'Thanks, Chrissie, for listening and helping me to clarify things. I'll see you later to fix up a session.'

He went back into the busyness of the unit and reconnected harmoniously to the rhythmic beat.

When James closed the door I was amazed at what I had achieved in 15 minutes. I wondered whether the effective action I had taken was something to do with my deepening professional artistry. I think this might be the transformative 'magic' that others often comment on when they work with me. I am going to formulate a new learning inquiry question about my professional artistry and its relationship with human flourishing as I think the two are possibly connected. I'll ask James if he would help me to learn by giving me feedback on what I do within our companionship. Goodness, I feel really excited!

Postscript

A year later, James pops his head around Chrissie's door. 'Chrissie, I wanted to tell you what the staff have just said in the team meeting. Over the last months, they have experienced a consistent change in me, both working with patients and with them. When there has been an issue and they have been expecting me to bite heads off, they say I have responded in ways that are truly person-centred – respectful, compassionate, tailored to the person and situation. They keep expecting me to be angry and go off into a rant, but I don't! And they say that they are watching me and learning from me how to change their relationships with patients, families and team members. I am a role-model!'

'However, I also know that there is still a lot for me to learn about being and doing person-centred leadership and practice! But it is so exhilarating to see the unit culture beginning, at last, to become more person-centred. Do you know something – four team members have asked me to be their critical companion and help them, as a group, to develop the care processes of the Person-centred Nursing Framework!? Although I feel that I have learned something about CC from observing you and helping you with your inquiry into professional artistry, I would really appreciate your support in becoming a critical companion for them.'

Tears welled up as a golden glow suffused Chrissie to the core of her being. 'I would be delighted', she said.

References

Covey, S. (2004) *The Seven Habits of Highly Effective People*, Bath Press, Bath.

Manley, K., McCormack, B., and Garbett, R. (2004) *Practice Development in Nursing*, Blackwell Publishing, Oxford.

McCormack, B. and McCance, T. (2006) Development of a framework for person-centred nursing. *Journal of Advanced Nursing*, **56** (5), 1–8.

McCormack B and Titchen A. (2014) No beginning, no end: An ecology of human flourishing. *International Practice Development Journal* **4**(2) [2]. Available at: http://www.fons.org/library/journal/volume4-issue2/article2 (accessed 4 February 2016).

Titchen, A. (2001) Critical companionship: a conceptual framework for developing expertise, in *Practice Knowledge and Expertise in the Health Professions* (eds J. Higgs and A. Titchen), Butterworth Heinemann, Oxford, pp. 80–90.

Titchen, A. (2004) Helping relationships for practice development: Critical companionship, in *Practice Development in Nursing* (eds B. McCormack, K. Manley, and R. Garbett), Blackwell Publishing, Oxford, pp. 148–74.

Titchen, A. (2009) Developing expertise through nurturing professional artistry in the workplace, in *Revealing Nursing Expertise through Practitioner Inquiry* (eds S. Hardy, A. Titchen, B. McCormack, and K. Manley), Wiley-Blackwell, Oxford, pp. 219–43.

Titchen, A. and McCormack, B. (2010) Dancing with stones: Critical creativity as methodology for human flourishing. *Educational Action Research: An International Journal*, **18** (4), 531–54.

CHAPTER 12

Navigating organisational change: being a person-centred facilitator

Famke van Lieshout

Fontys University of Applied Sciences, Eindhoven, The Netherlands

Worldwide, health-care practice is facing societal and political changes and challenges. Initiatives for organisational change alternate rapidly to respond to these developments. There is an ever increasing number of initiatives in which the human dimension of caring gains explicit attention; the development of person-centred care is illustrative of this. Facilitation is vital in effective implementation of person-centred care in health-care practice (McCormack & McCance 2010); this could be performed by management, team leaders, advanced nurse practitioners or consultants. Also, by practitioner (action) researchers, who aim to develop practice and to study this development simultaneously (Kemmis et al. 2014).

Each of these professionals can choose from a wide variety of facilitation approaches. Deciding on a certain approach is guided by the value system a person holds, which often also characterises them as facilitators. In my doctoral study, I facilitated the development of an effective workplace culture in clinical practice through participatory action research. In order to achieve congruency between my facilitation, the research topic and methodology, I adopted an holistic and emancipatory/enabling facilitation approach that was supported by humanistic and person-centred values. However, realising this in practice was no mean feat. Four themes, identified in this study, will be presented in this chapter and could help when working with the person-centred framework (McCormack & McCance 2010) in order to be and to become a person-centred facilitator.

Person-centred facilitation

Person-centredness is a normative-value approach to relationships and is characterised by values of respect, mutual respect, understanding and the right to self-determination. These values can, metaphorically speaking, be a rudder for decision-making, consciously or pre-consciously, in the development of

---

Person-Centred Practice in Nursing and Health Care: Theory and Practice, Second Edition.
Edited by Brendan McCormack and Tanya McCance.
© 2017 John Wiley & Sons, Ltd. Published 2017 by John Wiley & Sons, Ltd.

relationships. Person-centredness is often associated with care relationships. However, Rogers (1980) defines it also as any helping relationship aimed at growth: 'person-centredness is a philosophy, an approach to life, a way of being, which fits any situation in which growth – of a person, group or community – is part of the goal' (p. xvii). Facilitation is most simply regarded as 'the helping of others to change their current situation' (Harvey et al. 2002) and as a holistic means of enabling practitioner emancipation, development of self and effective workplace cultures. Combining these concepts of person-centredness and facilitation results in 'person-centred facilitation' as a specific type of relation-ship where person-centred values are lived and (personal) connectedness and reciprocity foster mutual growth (van Lieshout & Cardiff 2015). This mutual growth can both liberate people from restrictive views, traditions and practices that inhibit their flourishing, and enhance commitment for developing and sustaining ethical organisational change. Participation in the change process and in person-centred relationships is essential for such ethical change.

Although humanistic and person-centred values were embodied in my daily actions, these were challenged when I engaged with individuals, teams and contexts in the study. I experienced that my value system and my interrelated philosophical stance and facilitation approach, were continuously subjected to intra-personal, inter-personal and contextual influences and therefore were in a constant state of change. Values supportive of being person-centred were alternated with values that were less supportive of being person-centred. Hence, remaining person-centred in the many relationships I engaged in, as a practice development facilitator, could not be taken for granted and became a main focus for reflection and action.

The person-centred framework of McCormack and McCance (2010), although it has a focus on nursing relationships, is also perceived to be helpful in reflecting on relationships in the facilitation of change. It emphasises those key concepts that are relevant for engaging in person-centred relationships, helps to under-stand person-centredness and guides action. The framework, however, does not prescribe specific actions that could be taken when facing complexity as a person-centred facilitator in practice. For this reason, I will focus on four specific themes in this chapter, which I will argue can help when working with the framework to develop and sustain person-centred relationships, in particular when involved in facilitating organisational change.

Working with the person-centred framework

This idea of linking new themes to the framework is drawn from my doctoral study, in which the central focus was an extensive reflexive analysis of my lived experience as a person-centred facilitator in developing practice through partici-patory action research (van Lieshout 2013). Themes were identified from storied data, which were collected in a 2-year period of facilitating practice development, and considered in relation to existing literature. The themes that were identified in the analysis were central in the development of a mid-range theory on essential conditions for facilitating organisational change. The themes are:

- knowing the context;
- balancing being and doing;
- creating a system of support;
- achieving synchronicity.

These will be described and linked to relevant elements of the person-centred framework.

Theme: knowing the context

It is argued that the ability to use a person-centred approach is heavily influenced by the care environment (McCabe 2004) – that is, the context. Context is complex and dynamic as it concerns the interplay of culture, leadership, behaviours, relationships and evidence. Culture in particular is considered to shape the dynamics and to have an impact on relationships. Culture holds a set of values and beliefs that become noticeable in collaborative working, and impact on the way people do things in their context.

The culture I worked in during my study indicated issues of hierarchy and the valuing of a more traditional stance in research. For instance, when I presented my study proposal to higher management, to gain permission to work with a selected unit, they wanted to know in advance what my actions would be, whilst this could not be answered as the study had an emerging design. Also, in my engagement with the unit leader I experienced a constant struggle in working together with the team to reflect on practice and to identify issues for action. The leader was suspicious of my role as an external facilitator and often withheld initiatives for collaborative action and for exchanging information. In sharing some preliminary findings on workplace culture to management, they felt offended and doubted my competencies. Signs of a blame culture were evident here.

Practitioners were disappointed in the organisation. They felt they were 'marionettes in the game of change' and their individual talents were not seen. Also, the formation of teams was constantly changed by management, which required practitioners to constantly fine-tune with others. All these issues and values that were characteristic for an overall culture in context, made practitioners hold back from engaging in a relationship with me in order to change their practice. These hindered the realisation of person-centred processes – those of shared decision-making and working with the team's values and beliefs. Specific preparatory action in building relationships was required for these processes to be realised.

I also experienced (sub-)cultures where openness and autonomy were valued. In my engagement with advanced practice nurses, perceived as clinical leaders, we regularly shared our observations about practice and were open about our strengths and limitations in bringing about change. This enabled discussion of the meaning of being in relation with the other and achieving full engagement. These cultures were thus more supportive of processes of engagement and thus the realisation of person-centred relationships.

KEY MESSAGE: Spending time to get to know a person's or team's context, in particular understanding its culture and working with this deliberately, enables processes that will contribute to the development of person-centred relationships.

Theme: balancing being and doing

Context, as illustrated in the previous paragraph, consists of multiple cultures. While practising, a facilitator becomes directly exposed to the multiple values and beliefs of these cultures, and needs to understand and to work with these. There is a likelihood that she or he might become overwhelmed and caught up by the cultural dynamics, contextual layeredness and complexity. Hence, it might happen that the relationship building and organisational change are without success, leading to the facilitator losing their balance. In the research study, the concept of balance is defined as congruency between the concepts of 'being' and 'doing', which refers to the constant tension between values of context, personal values and, particularly in organisational change, values underlying an approach to facilitation. It was only 'by doing' in practice that I became aware of my 'being', of those values I was able to bring into practice and those I had not embodied and was not yet able to bring adequately into practice.

For example, on seeing a great potential for development in practice but a unit leader hardly receptive to change, my eagerness to structure, to decide for others on themes and to come into action myself, became ever stronger. I became impatient and concerned about delaying the practice development process. I noticed these were characteristics of context I actually criticised, but now socialised with. This caused feelings of losing ground and brought up emotions of uncertainty and a loss of self-confidence in being person-centred. This impacted on my focus and also on building person-centred relationships. My awareness and confusion with self, made me keep a distance from individuals and practitioner teams. This distance hindered my authentic engagement with others, to have sympathetic presence or compassion with the other (van Lieshout et al. 2015), and to work with their values and beliefs. Therefore, I felt that I failed in role modelling person-centredness, which in turn strengthened my feeling of imbalance. Still, there were times I experienced balance. For instance, when I facilitated a workshop in practice, with university colleagues as co-facilitators, and where valuable data were shared in a creative way. A distinctive feature of these balanced moments was that I stayed close to my own values, worked collaboratively and had reflexive dialogues with colleagues. As a result different values and ways of knowledge were blended. In this way I was more able to provide those 'physical' or more 'holistic' needs of others, which was supportive to the development of person-centred relationships.

KEY MESSAGE: Acknowledging 'where you are at' in terms of being person-centred, and appreciating this, as part of the framework's prerequisite of knowing 'self', enables the development of person-centred relationships too.

Theme: creating a system of support

In the study it is suggested that taking time for reflection and reflexivity is supportive to the development of person-centred relationships, as they help with knowing 'self' and with 'knowing the context'. It is argued in the literature that this can be done best with others as they help to show the self-to-self (Kemmis et al. 2014). A system of critical companions creates reflexive spaces, which enables a facilitator to know context and self, but more importantly to know how these elements interplay. This interplay is made less explicit and visual in the person-centred framework. This could suggest there is some fixed linearity between these elements. However, practice shows differently and stresses the importance of understanding the interplay between elements.

While facilitating during the study, I believed that the complexity I encountered in facilitating action research was just part of the process and something I needed to learn to deal with. I did not want to bother my supervisors, as critical companions, about these trivialities and focused merely on 'doing' in practice, perceiving this as something separate from my 'being'. This resulted in me becoming caught up in practice, repetition of actions, no progress in practice and me becoming imbalanced. Engaging with others in practice while not making efficient use of a support system, and being driven by values of autonomy and proving self, hindered me in the study to take sufficient time to reflect and to be flexible in my strategies for action. This challenged me to adapt to different contexts and to become person-centred in relationships. While engaging in an extensive reflexive analysis with my system of support, through dialogue and creative arts, different ways of knowing were blended, values and beliefs were articulated and person-centredness was role modelled. This helped me in gaining new insights, in defining alternative person-centred actions, to develop expertise and so to achieve balance.

KEY MESSAGE: Creating a system of support in which you are open about self, focus on knowing the interplay between context and self, and work on the development of self, can enable the realisation of person-centred relationships.

Theme: achieving synchronicity

A fourth theme connects the previous themes, which enable or hinder the realisation of person-centred relationships. The dynamic interplay of these themes is necessary for achieving synchronicity in the relationship between the facilitator and others. Synchronicity, in the study, is described as a momentary outcome of the interplay between context, self and system of support. It is described as a forward momentum in which a stance is taken in the relationship that maximises the potential for mutual growth. The relationship then becomes central and no longer the individuals. It is further characterised by connectedness, reciprocal adequacy and synchronised working. In the study, I decided to leave the practice setting after the first orientation phase of the study as I observed no progress in the development of practice and to make sense of data that I had collected. The analysis became the central focus of the study and I did not return to practice. Also the unit did not exist anymore, so synchronicity in these relationships was not achieved. However, I experienced synchronous working in my relationship with my system of support.

KEY MESSAGE: This final theme links to the central 'ring', person-centred outcomes, in the McCormack and McCance framework. For achieving synchronicity and thus for realising person-centred relationships, one should pay attention to themes of context, balance and support that enable or hinder working with elements of the framework.

Moving along with context *and* self

Since its introduction, the Person-centred Nursing Framework of McCormack and McCance has been widely used in nursing practice, and in other relational practices, such as in the facilitation of practice development and thus organisational change. Framework designs usually include key concepts and elements, but often seem static and linear. At first sight the person-centred framework also appears to be flat, simplistic and somewhat idealistic. The different rings of the framework, displaying those prerequisites – organisational attributes that are needed to bring processes into practice and to achieve effective person-centred (nursing) relationships – are actually more diffused than presented. In their study, Cardiff and van Hest (2010) attempted to change this by changing the framework into a windmill, where the metaphor shows how bits and parts are working together. In reality, person-centred concepts and elements are ever dynamic and interplaying as they involve human interactions. Persons, including self, are not static entities; they learn every day in relation with others and constantly change perspectives. Therefore, realising person-centred values in everyday (relational) practice is challenging as it is constantly subject to different cultures and change. I would even argue that this process is complex and messy rather than orderly and structured.

The process is complex, as living these values in practice is a responsive, embedded and embodied process, which is enmeshed within a web of many parts that reciprocally influence each other, and co-emerges with the context (Snoeren 2015). This differs from being complicated, wherein the parts and the way they interact are identifiable and observable and consistently lead to the same result; they do not transcend themselves in the process, as occurs in a complex process (Davis & Sumara 2005). Through this complexity, elements come to life and gain a deeper meaning. Therefore it is essential to appreciate this complexity and to work with it, to respond to changes in context and in self when engaging in and developing person-centred relationships.

The four themes drawn from my doctoral study and described in this chapter demonstrate the vividness of the framework in facilitative practice and how to engage with the complexity of culture in different contexts as a facilitator. Even though attention has not been given to all elements of the framework, the discussion of how the four themes could impact on developing and remaining person-centred in caring or facilitative relationships, in everyday dynamic practice, could in all probability be applicable to the other elements too.

Working with the framework requires a constant dynamic movement between self and context, with regard to making decisions about the extent to which and how person-centred processes can be practised in a specific moment of time, place and with whom. Being person-centred in one situation doesn't mean being person-centred in another situation. In my experience a technical approach and a more emancipatory approach in facilitation (Harvey et al. 2002) can both be person-centred. It all depends on the situation and where you are at yourself in working with person-centred values as a facilitator. The important aspect to remember is that you need to keep moving along with context and self. This navigational process requires a huge amount of flexibility, perseverance and creativity, but also thorough preparatory groundwork.

A key finding in my study (van Lieshout 2013) is the importance of preparatory groundwork by a facilitator and their system of support, to avoid entering a practice setting too soon. This prevents a facilitator from becoming caught up in the complexity of context and becoming imbalanced. This could result in a facilitator becoming caught up in the complexity of context and becoming imbalanced. This has been shown to put a strain upon living person-centred values into facilitative actions and synchronicity to fail. A framework called 'Taking Action For Action' (TAFA), with principles for action, has been developed as part of this study to help diagnose the interplay between oneself, context and the system of support. This is based on the mid-range theory of essential conditions for facilitating organisational change, which include the four key themes presented in this chapter. These principles relate to actions orientated towards understanding the context, those relating to understanding oneself as a (person-centred) facilitator, and most importantly to the interplay between these actions. Further, these principles for action also help to understand what is needed from a facilitator's support system.

These actions are not restricted as preparatory to relational processes, but also are of use during these processes and can become part of recurring spaces for reflection and reflexivity; they build on the notion of Carr and Kemmis (1986) of making 'wise and prudent judgements about what would constitute an appropriate expression of the good, in future facilitative action in particular situations in practice contexts [p. 190]. These actions require sufficient time as rushing them could have a detrimental impact on the development of person-centred relationships in nursing care or in organisational change.'

Summary

Navigating organisational change can be more successful when adopting a person-centred facilitation approach. Besides enabling growth, I suggest it also enables an 'ethic of care' for both practitioners and facilitator in discovering and working with complexity and emotions involved in practice change. Being person-centred while engaging with others in facilitating organisational change, however, is not a straightforward process. It requires deliberate and constant navigational action by all who are engaged in the development of a person-centred relationship. The themes of context, balance, support and synchronicity can help when one works with the person-centred framework in developing and sustaining person-centred relationships in everyday dynamic practice.

References

Cardiff, S. and van Hest, M. (2010) Journeying from 'I have a dream' towards 'Yes, we can': A dialogue about leading the development of person-centred nursing, in *Person-Centred Nursing: Theory and Practice* (eds B. McCormack and T. McCance), Wiley-Blackwell, Oxford, pp. 152–8.

Carr, W. and Kemmis, S. (1986) *Becoming Critical. Education, Knowledge and Action Research*, Deakin University Press, Melbourne.

Davis, B. and Sumara, D.J. (2005) Complexity science and educational action research: Towards a pragmatics of transformation. *Educational Action Research*, **13** (3), 453–64. doi: 10.1080/09650790500200291

Harvey, G., Loftus-Hills, A., Rycroft Malone, J. *et al.* (2002) Getting evidence into practice: the role and function of facilitation. *Journal of Advanced Nursing*, **37** (6), 577–88.

Kemmis, S., McTaggart, R., and Nixon, R. (2014) *The Action Research Planner, Doing Critical Participatory Action Research*. Singapore, Springer Science.

McCabe, C. (2004) Nurse-patient communication: an exploration of patients' experiences. *Journal of Clinical Nursing*, **13**, 41–9.

McCormack, B. and McCance, T. (2006) Development of a framework for person-centred nursing. *Journal of Advanced Nursing*, **56** (5), 472–79.

McCormack, B. and McCance, T. (2010) *Person-Centred Nursing: Theory and Practice*, Wiley-Blackwell, Oxford.

Rogers, C.R. (1980) *A Way of Being*, Houghton Mifflin, Boston.

Snoeren M. (2015) Working = Learning. A complexity approach to workplace learning within residential care for older people. PhD thesis, Vrije Universiteit van Amsterdam, Amsterdam.

van Lieshout F. (2013) Taking Action for Action. A study of the interplay between contextual and facilitator characteristics in developing an effective workplace culture in a Dutch hospital setting, through action research. PhD thesis, University of Ulster, Belfast, UK.

van Lieshout F and Cardiff S. (2015) Reflections on being and becoming a person-centred facilitator. *International Practice Development Journal* **5**(Special issue): art. 4. Available at: http://www.fons.org/library/journal/volume5-person-centredness-suppl/article4 (accessed 4 February 2016).

van Lieshout, F., Titchen, A., McCormack, B., and McCance, T. (2015) Compassion in facilitating the development of person-centred health care practice. *Journal of Compassionate Health Care*, **2**, 5. doi: 10.1186/s40639-015-0014-3

SECTION IV

Adapting the principles of person-centred practice

CHAPTER 13

A narrative approach to person-centredness with older people in residential long-term care

Catherine Buckley
St Luke's Home Education Centre, Cork, Republic of Ireland

Introduction

This chapter outlines the development of a Framework of Narrative Practice to be utilised in the assessment, planning, implementation and evaluation of care in long-term care settings for older people. Although, the framework is new and aims to guide staff who wish to develop care through a narrative approach, it does incorporate aspects of the Person-centred Nursing Framework of McCormack and McCance (2006, 2010). Its primary purpose is to implement a narrative-based approach to help nurses operationalise person-centred care.

Placing the study in context

Increasing regulation internationally and the need to provide services that are driven by a quality agenda has prompted the need for services that are based on best practice evidence, continuously improve quality and are service user driven (Department of Health and Children 2003). In Ireland both the National Standards for Residential Care Settings (Health Information Quality Authority 2007) and the Nursing and Midwifery Regulator's (An Bord Altranais 2009) Professional Guidance for Nurses Working with Older People have been established to promote high quality care. The 2006 version of the Person-centred Nursing Framework (McCormack & McCance 2006) was previously used as the underpinning philosophy for a national collaborative practice development programme in the Republic of Ireland (the National Person-centred Care Practice Development Programme: McCormack et al. 2010). However, during the implementation of this programme, it became evident that the life experiences of residents in residential care were not taken into account when planning or developing their care. The impetus for the study described in this chapter

Person-Centred Practice in Nursing and Health Care: Theory and Practice, Second Edition.
Edited by Brendan McCormack and Tanya McCance.
© 2017 John Wiley & Sons, Ltd. Published 2017 by John Wiley & Sons, Ltd.

stems from both my personal involvement in the National Person-centred Care Practice Development Programme as an internal facilitator, and my background as a practice development facilitator in a residential setting for older people. The lack of understanding among staff regarding the importance of life history and the absence of a suitable framework for nurses to utilise in obtaining this information when planning care, provided a further impetus.

The study described here is based on my doctoral research, which was conducted in the Republic of Ireland in a residential care setting for older people. This was an 18-month collaborative action research practice development programme with Clinical Nurse Managers (CNM) ($n = 4$), registered nurses ($n = 20$), support workers ($n = 14$) and residents ($n = 37$) in two units within this setting.

The relationship between narrative and person-centredness

The study is underpinned by theories of emancipatory practice development (Manley & McCormack 2004), person-centred practice (McCormack & McCance 2006, 2010) and narrative inquiry (Heidegger 1962; Polkinghorne 1988; Ricoeur 1991). Both practice development (PD) and person-centred care (PCC) have been linked in the literature for a number of years, with many writers outlining their interdependent relationships and often hypothesising that one cannot be implemented without the other (Manley et al. 2008; Dewar & MacKay 2010; McCormack & McCance 2010). Indeed, their symbiotic relationship has been well defined in a number of studies that have used these methodologies as theoretical underpinnings or frameworks on which to pin the research approach (Lamont et al. 2009; McCormack et al. 2010; Brown & McCormack 2011). McCormack (2004) in an editorial for the *Journal of Nursing Research* goes so far as to declare the central focus of PD as 'the development of increased effectiveness in person-centred practice'.

So how does a narrative approach to care fit with these two approaches, and is there room for it within these reciprocal concepts? It can be argued that narrative not only connects to sociology, literature and history (Richardson 2000), but also the tenets of narrative connect it to practice and by extension to person-centred care. Narrative has been described as 'the primary schema through which human experience is made meaningful' (Polkinghorne 1988, p. 125) and is a way of maintaining and creating order out of experience. It also links the individual to his or her context. Therefore how people become who they are is because of the way they have engaged with the contexts they have been part of (McCance et al. 2011). These contexts are constantly changing, and this affects the way persons learn. Central to the Person-centred Nursing Framework is 'knowing self' and by extension knowing others. It involves knowing the values of the patient but also being clear about one's own values and beliefs. Narrative approaches promote a culture of caring because they value the voice of not only the storyteller but also that of the listener/re-teller (Bochner 2001). Knowledge, that is, narrative knowledge, can promote a more caring relationship where the narrative can influence the way care is carried out or planned. Narrative deals with meanings, contexts and perspectives, and this is similar to the Person-centred Nursing Framework that enables understanding. It privileges a person-centred approach by making the person and their story central to the event.

Aims and objectives

The aim of the study was to develop and evaluate a methodological framework for a narrative-based approach to practice development and person-centred care in residential aged care settings.

The objectives were:

1 How does narrative help to achieve a depth of understanding of the life-world of older adults in residential care?
2 To what extent does the implementation of a narrative approach to care enable nurses to operationalise person-centred care?
3 How do nurses make sense of narrative experiences in the assessment, planning, delivery and evaluation of care?

Operationalising the study methodology

The study was conducted over two phases. Phase 1 was concerned with the development of a methodological framework that was based in part on the Person-centred Nursing Framework of McCormack and McCance (2010), and Phase 2 was concerned with implementing and evaluating that framework in practice, taking an action research approach.

In Phase 1 a total of four focus groups consisting of 12 nurses were conducted where participants explored the concepts of person-centredness and narrative. The interviews were analysed using an adaptation of the creative hermeneutic data analysis approach (Boomer & McCormack 2010) and questions developed by Hsu and McCormack (2010). Eight residents considered the relevance of narrative and person-centred care to older people and how this would impact on their daily lives in residential care settings. The construction of the framework of narrative practice was based on the conceptual understanding the nurses and residents had of what elements of narrative and person-centredness were important for good quality care and good quality of life for residents in residential care settings. This conceptualisation was based in part on the theoretical underpinnings of the Person-centred Nursing Framework (McCormack & McCance 2010) and secondary data analysis of narratives ($n = 46$) of older adults in residential care. This led to the development of the Framework of Narrative Practice (Figure 13.1). The framework has two key components. The

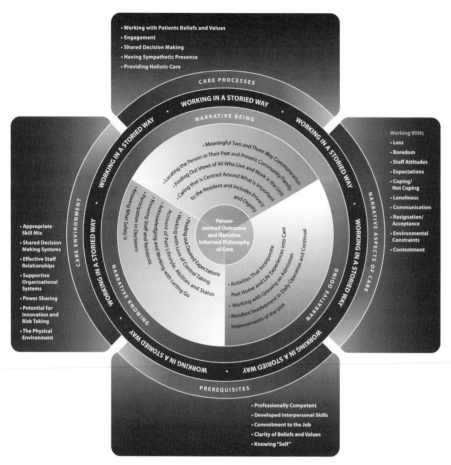

Figure 13.1 Framework of Narrative Practice.

first component comprises the foundational pillars, which consists of three pillars from the Person-centred Nursing Framework – prerequisites, the care environment and care processes – and an additional pillar, 'narrative aspects of care' based on the key themes. The second component comprises the operational elements: narrative knowing, narrative being and narrative doing. The pictorial representation of this framework indicates how the foundational aspects of the framework provide a base for the development of person-centred care and the relationship that needs to occur between the operational elements of the framework in order to enable staff to work in a storied way. The development of this framework is discussed in more detail elsewhere (Buckley et al. 2014).

Implementing the framework in practice

The framework was implemented using an action research approach over eight reflective work-based learning sessions on two residential units for older adults.

A total of 37 residents and 38 staff took part in the sessions and the ongoing work-based learning activities that occurred between the sessions. Identifying the culture and gaining an understanding of the framework of narrative practice was an ongoing exercise throughout the lifetime of the study. However, at the beginning of the study it was important to identify the existing culture and the basic assumptions held by staff and residents about how care was carried out, so that staff could identify what an effective culture was. Using the framework of narrative practice during the programme days enabled the identification of three action cycles. Essentially these were:

- narrative practice and culture identification;
- developing narrative ways of working;
- working in a storied way.

Throughout the process staff utilised the framework of narrative practice to inform their discussions of these three cycles and their understandings of person-centredness. They took account of both the pillars of the framework – prerequisites, care processes, care environment and narrative aspects of care – and the operational elements – narrative being, narrative knowing and narrative doing – in all their learning activities.

Key outcomes

In this study the Framework of Narrative Practice, which is based on the Person-centred Nursing Framework, was used as a tool to help staff identify existing culture and practices and as a guiding framework to develop strategies to improve care. Areas that staff worked with were communication, homely environment, meals and mealtimes, and having more activities with and for the residents. Key outcomes from the implementation of this framework in practice were based on narrative knowing, being and doing, and centred around:

1 How people responded to change.
2 The development of shared understandings.
3 Intentional action.

These outcomes had close adherence to elements of the Person-centred Nursing Framework, and this will be discussed in the following section.

How people responded to change (knowing)

Involvement and engagement in change can range from resistance (both active and passive), through conformity, to engagement and championing (Herscovitch & Meyer 2002). Responding to change is often exhibited by showing support for change and by a combination of emotional normative and continuing commitment to change. In this study, change was embraced in differing ways on both units. Engagement in the Person-centred Nursing Framework occurs in both the environment and care processes. This engagement centres around shared decision-making and knowledge of self, others and professional expertise. Initially in their engagement with the implementation, both units demonstrated enthusiasm and a desire to be engaged and involved in the study. They participated fully in the work-based learning sessions when they occurred, and in both units the staff were very knowledgeable about the structure of the framework and how to operationalise it. However, the staff on Unit 2 exhibited a more inclusive and collaborative person-centred approach with the residents, in the way they engaged them in the gathering of information and in the implementation of the framework in practice. Their engagement was proactive and they exhibited what Hynes et al. (2012) describe as engagement with different voices and acknowledgement of different worldviews. This demonstrated both connectedness with the residents and a willingness to acknowledge the values and beliefs of others by engaging in shared decision-making. On Unit 1 there was a stop/start element to their engagement, and this prevented staff from fully participating in both the work-based learning programme days and the activities that occurred between these days. Their engagement in the project was passive. There was a lack of connection between the practitioners and the residents. While staff identified the values of the residents and had knowledge of the person they did not put this into practice. Engagement is a key element of the Person-centred Nursing framework and is seen in the care processes. According to Fuimano (2004), emotionally intelligent practitioners are more connected and authentic. By reflecting on their practice, nurses are able to assess their authenticity. This in turn enables them to engage in a way that recognises the individuality of the patient and promotes their personhood.

The development of shared understanding (being)

Knowing self and others is an essential component of the framework of narrative practice and of person-centred practice (McCormack & McCance 2010). Staff reflected in and on practice and developed shared understandings of the identified culture. They investigated residents' understandings of the existing culture and obtained their views on improvements through interviews and observations of care. They used this knowledge to varying degrees across the two units to develop action plans that looked at the perceptions and understandings they had of the existing culture.

The culture in which a person exists shapes the self's identity and ultimate being. It is a basic human function to share knowledge within a system where roles are defined. According to Baumeister (2011) this system is called culture, or in other words the process we as humans have for making sense of our lives. This system depends on good communication. In the Person-centred Nursing Framework (McCormack & McCance 2010) communication is described under the prerequisites and in particular in developed interpersonal skills. McCormack and McCance (2010) describe it as 'the ability of the practitioner to communicate at a variety of levels with others'. Using the Framework of Narrative Practice enabled staff to communicate with residents, relatives and other staff in a way that valued what was important for the residents in maintaining a good quality of life within the centre. This demonstrated both effective verbal and non-verbal interactions and a commitment to collaborating to find solutions that were mutually acceptable. It further enabled collaborative understandings about new ways of working that centred on: improving types and methods of communication; maintaining a homely environment; the experience of meals and mealtimes; and having more activities with and for the residents.

Working with communication and interpersonal skills on Unit 1 involved developing a suite of communication tools that staff felt would improve communication between staff, particularly the temporary staff, and help improve the care experience for the residents.

> this is a good method of ensuring the safety of the resident as well as ensuring their likes and dislikes are known by new staff.
>
> *Participant Clinical Nurse Manager*

On Unit 2, staff worked the communication theme in a three-pronged approach. Initially they implemented life story books or memory boards for those who were unable to complete books. Family members of residents who were cognitively unable to complete the story books, were given a copy of life story guidelines and encouraged to engage in the process. This process facilitated shared decision-making and involvement of families and significant others in the care experience. Staff reported that the life story books provided information that helped them develop individualised care and activities for the residents that centred on their past life experiences. In an effort to address and improve intercommunication between staff, the unit commenced a policy of all grades of staff being involved in the handover report. They initiated a schedule of staff nights out to increase social interaction and as a way of team building and increasing team work. In this way they promoted effective staff relationships and an equal sharing of power that values contributions and ideas of all staff members. They further worked on approaches to ensure that everyone had an opportunity to present new ideas at team meetings and to develop ways of trialling and evaluating those ideas. In addressing both the meal and mealtimes and the homely environment themes, staff purchased tablecloths and menu boards for the unit and ensured that the tables were set for meals as they would be in the resident's home. In response to suggestions from residents, several changes were undertaken to make the unit more homely. Relatives and residents were encouraged to bring their own soft furnishings and pictures from home, and these were displayed around the residents' bed spaces. Enabling these changes to occur showed that staff were willing to try new approaches and also to take some risks. It also indicated that staff were aware of the importance of the physical environment.

Intentional action (doing)

Intentional action is based on the beliefs and values of the agent (the person or persons involved in the action), the belief that they can effect change, and that the environment (culture) will be altered by that change (Burks 2001). The Framework of Narrative Practice was conceptualised to provide guidance for staff to take intentional action when working with older people in residential care settings. Similarly the Person-centred Nursing Framework acknowledges the importance of recognising the beliefs and values of both staff and residents in both the prerequisites and the care processes elements of the framework. Our lived experience and our personhood within our social environment is inherently important in maintaining and providing meaning within the context of the intentional actions we take (Popova 2014). According to Popova (2014) intentionality is a process of interaction between agents, and it is through this interaction that we ultimately define who we are. In the Framework of Narrative Practice the operational elements – narrative being, narrative knowing and narrative doing – provide a structure for staff to help with integrating the personal narrative of the resident with the narrative of their existing circumstances and environment. The intent is to enable a more comprehensive understanding of the actions and responses of the resident to change, and in turn enable staff to act intentionally by providing care that is based on this understanding. Intentional action is also concerned with the process of communication (Kihlström & Israel 2002). Knowing the self and others enables communication that identifies the desires and needs of the residents.

Implications from the findings in the context of person-centredness

Narrative goes beyond merely telling a story; it includes the reason for telling that story and the way that story is understood. In narrative communication there is reciprocity between the intent of the story and understanding or making sense of the story (Popova 2014). The Framework of Narrative Practice presented in this chapter, uses narrative being, narrative knowing and narrative doing, along with narrative aspects of care and the pillars of the Person-centred Nursing Framework (McCormack & McCance 2010), with the intention of enabling staff to work in a storied way. It draws on the premise that stories and person-centred practice are interactive processes that enable participatory sense-making between narrators and listeners, leading to meaningful action. It is through this understanding that communicative action takes place. The act of communicative action is what Habermas (1984) refers to as mutually judging and understanding narrative expressions and using these expressions to promote person-centred practice. The framework promotes the use of communicative spaces in order to promote critical reflection and to enable collaborative action, which in turn will lead to person-centred practice.

References

An Bord Altranais (2009) *Professional guidance for nurses working with older people*, An Bord Altranais, Dublin.

Baumeister, R.F. (2011) Self and identity: A brief overview of what they are, what they do, and how they work. *Annals of the New York Academy of Sciences*, **1234**, 48–55.

Bochner, A. (2001) Narrative's virtues. *Qualitative Inquiry*, **7** (2), 131–57.

Boomer, C.A. and McCormack, B. (2010) Creating the conditions for growth: a collaborative practice development programme for clinical nurse leaders. *Journal of Nursing Management*, **18** (6), 633–44.

Brown, D. and McCormack, B.G. (2011) Developing the practice context to enable more effective pain management with older people: an action research approach. *Implementation Science*, **6** (9), 1–14.

Buckley, C., McCormack, B., and Ryan, A. (2014) Valuing narrative in the care of older people: a framework of narrative practice for older adult residential care settings. *Journal of Clinical Nursing*, **23**, 2565–77.

Burks, K.J. (2001) Intentional action. *Journal of Advanced Nursing*, **34**, 668–75.

Department of Health and Children (2003) *The Health Service Reform Programme*, Stationery Office, Dublin.

Dewar, B. and Mackay, R. (2010) Appreciating and developing compassionate care in an acute hospital setting caring for older people. *International Journal of Older People Nursing*, **5** (4), 299–308.

Fuimano, J. (2004) Raise your emotional intelligence. *Nursing Management*, **35** (7), 10–12.

Habermas J. (1984) *The Theory of Communicative Action: Vol. 1. Reason and the Rationalization of Society* (trans. McCarthy T.). Boston: Beacon.

Health Information Quality Authority (HIQA) (2007) *National Standards for Residential Care Settings*, Health Information Quality Authority, Dublin.

Heidegger, M. (1962) *Being and Time*, Blackwell Publishers, Oxford.

Herscovitch, L. and Meyer, J.P. (2002) Commitment to organizational change: extension of a three-component model. *Journal of Applied Psychology*, **87**, 474.

Hsu, M. and McCormack, B. (2010) The experience of applying a narrative research approach with older people. *Journal of Nursing Research*, **18** (4), 249–56.

Hynes, G., Coghlan, D., and McCarron, M. (2012) Participation as a multi-voiced process: Action research in the acute hospital environment. *Action Research*, **10** (3), 293–312.

Kihlström, A. and Israel, J. (2002) Communicative or strategic action – an examination of fundamental issues in the theory of communicative action. *International Journal of Social Welfare*, **11** (3), 210–18.

Lamont, S., Walker, P., and Brunero, S. (2009) 'Teaching an old dog new tricks': A practice development approach to organizational change in mental health. *Practice Development in Health Care*, **8** (2), 65–76.

Manley, K. and McCormack, B. (2004) Practice development: Purpose, methodology, facilitation and evaluation, in *Practice Development in Nursing* (eds B. McCormack, K. Manley, and R. Garbett), Blackwell Publishing, Oxford, pp. 33–50.

Manley, K., McCormack, B., and Wilson, V. (2008) Introduction, in *Practice Development in Nursing: International perspectives* (eds K. Manley, B. McCormack, and V. Wilson), Blackwell, Oxford, pp. 1–16.

McCance, T., McCormack, B., and Dewing, J. (2011) An exploration of person-centredness in practice. *OJIN: The Online Journal of Issues in Nursing*, **16** (2).

McCormack, B. (2004) Person-centredness in gerontological nursing: An overview of the literature. *International Journal of Older People Nursing*, **13** (3a), 31–8.

McCormack, B. and McCance, T. (2006) Developing a framework for person-centred nursing. *Journal of Advanced Nursing*, **56** (5), 1–8.

McCormack, B. and McCance, T. (2010) *Person-Centred Nursing: Theory and Practice*, Wiley-Blackwell, Oxford.

McCormack, B., Dewing, J., Breslin, L. *et al.* (2010) *The Implementation of a Model of Person Centred Practice in Older Persons Settings, Final Report*. Dublin, Health Services Executive.

Polkinghorne, D.E. (1988) *Narrative Knowing and the Human Sciences*, Suny Press.

Popova, Y.B. (2014) Narrativity and enaction: the social nature of literary narrative understanding. *Frontiers in Psychology* **5**, 895. doi: 10.3389/fpsyg.2014.00895 (accessed 5 February 2016).

Richardson, B. (2000) Recent concepts of narrative and the narratives of narrative theory. *Style*, **34** (2), 168–75.

Ricoeur, P. (1991) Life in quest of narrative, in *On Paul Ricoeur: Narrative and Interpretation* (ed D. Woods), Routledge, London.

CHAPTER 14

Person-centred health services for children

Val Wilson[1,2] & Annette Solman[2]

[1] *Sydney Children's Hospitals Network, Sydney, Australia*
[2] *University of Technology Sydney, Australia*

Introduction

The concept of person-centred practice provides nurses with a framework for undertsanding the complexity of the health-care setting. It is applicable across differing care contexts (from acute care to rehabilitation to care within the home), and flexible enough to take into account the needs of patients of all ages. At its heart is the need for those who work in such contexts to focus on delivery of care that achieves outcomes that benefit the patient, their family and themselves. Providing such care not only nurtures the patient and supports the family, but also ensures staff invest in creating care cultures that result in improved well-being for all. The creation of effective person-centred cultures is neither easy or straightforward; it requires a common vision and goals, strategic planning, systematic approaches, supportive leadership, tenacity and dedication. In this chapter we will be sharing with you how one organsiation has developed Person-Centred Paediatric Practice as the foundation for nursing.

The practice setting

The Sydney Children's Hospitals Network (SCHN) was formed in 2010 with the amalgamation of two major paediatric hospitals (The Sydney Children's Hospital in Randwick and The Children's Hospital at Westmead) and includes Bear Cottage (hospice), NSW Newborn and Paediatric Emergency Transport Services (NETS), NSW Pregnancy and Newborn Services Network (PSN) and the Children's Court Clinic (Box 14.1). The creation of the SCHN was a result of a Special Commission of Inquiry into Acute Care Services in NSW Public hospitals (Garling 2008).

Person-Centred Practice in Nursing and Health Care: Theory and Practice, Second Edition.
Edited by Brendan McCormack and Tanya McCance.
© 2017 John Wiley & Sons, Ltd. Published 2017 by John Wiley & Sons, Ltd.

Box 14.1 Demographic information about the Sydney Children's Hospitals Network (SCHN).

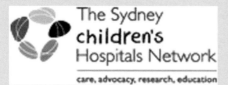

- Largest paediatric health-care organisation in Australia.
- Provides quaternery and tertiary level services.
- Over 92,000 presentations to emergency.*
- Provided over 138,000 bed days, discharging more than 50,705 patients*(more than half are younger than 5 years.)
- Over 5000 staff with a largely RN workforce.
- Provides undergraduate placements for 22 universities.

*2013/2014 data.

Prior to the amalgamation, practice development stratieges were being used to inform and support changes in both hospitals, with each hospital having a Practice Development Unit.

Models of care

The bedrock of paediatric nursing practice is the family-centred care (FCC) model (Hutchfield 1999). This model advocates a partnership approach where staff work alongside parents, taking into account that parents are strong advocates and have a unique undertsanding of their child and are therefore able to provide key information about how best to deliver care for their child. It also acknowledges that parents and indeed patients have the right to be involved in care delivery and be part of the decision-making process. Nurses have strongly held beliefs that they not only advocate for FCC, they consistently deliver this in practice everyday (Lewis et al. 2007). While nursing staff in this study (Lewis et al. 2007) could clearly articulate the principles of FCC and espouse their incorporation into everyday practice, it was evident that this was not happening consistently. This was influenced at times by what Casey (1995) describes as 'nurse-centred led care', where parents are either excluded (through lack of communication) or given permission to be part of care. The findings from the study led to a number of initiatives being undertaken that supported improvements in practice and enhanced the experience of childen, families and staff. (Hooke et al. 2008).

Developing the nursing vision

Whilst it was vital that we kept FCC principles at the heart of nursing practice there was a need to extend this to incorporate a more inclusive approach that took into account the needs of the child, the family and staff. Nurses across the organisation (undertaken at The Children's Hospital at Westmead prior to the amalgamation) were invited in 2008 to participate in a series of workshops to develop the nursing vision (**C**ollaboration). It was important that all nursing staff felt they had a role in contributing to the vision and that their perspectives were valued (**I**nclusion). This was followed by a period of consultation, and after some months the nursing vision was endorsed by nursing groups across the organisation in early 2009 (**P**articipatory). The philosophical approach to this work not only incorporated the CIP principles; it also supported working alongside and developing together, rather than working on people to get them to support the ideas put forward by a few staff. The framework (Figure 14.1) incorporates the principles of FCC and extends these to reflect the more inclusive nature of 'persons', in other words. It was about everyone in the care setting – patients, families and staff. It was important that staff were clear that to nurture, care and support the patient and family they needed to also nurture, care and support one another.

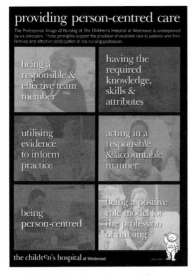

Providing Person-Centred Care
The Children's Hospital at
Westmead (2009)

(a)

**Person-centred Nursing
Framework**

(b)

Figure 14.1 (a) Providing person-centred care. **(b)** The Person-centred Nursing Framework. Source: The Children's Hospital at Westmead (2009).

You can see in this vision a strong correlation between the principles and the person-centred framework (McCormack & McCance 2010); for example, being a responsible and effective team member relates to developed interpersonal skills (prerequisites) and effective staff relationships (the care environment). There was the need to plan, implement and evaluate programmes of work that would support the realisation of this vision in everyday practice.

Once the vision was endorsed it was launched and every ward/unit received a laminated poster to display the vision. The six principles were highlighted in practice using a number of different approaches such as:

- Discussed during orientation of all nurses new to the organsation.
- Written into role descriptions and used to support/inform the recruitment process and staff appraisals.
- Used in staff meetings to discuss practice issues and support improvements.
- A reflective/education tool; i.e. 'How are you using evidence to support your practice?'

Person-centred aims and goals

A vital aspect of the work undertaken since the launch of the vision was the need to strategise and prioritise the aims and goals we hoped to achieve for patients, families, staff and the organisation. The person-centred vision and framework provided key inspiration in strategic planning and endorsement of programmes of work. This ensured that development initiatives were focused on prerequistes, the care environment and the care processes in order to achieve person-centred otucomes. Table 14.1 provides some examples of the development work and the outcomes achieved.

In the following section a number of exemplars from practice will be explored in more detail, outlining how each of these programmes or initiatives is providing further evidence of our commitment to achieving person-centred care outcomes.

Prerequisites: person-centred leadership development

Building a strong nursing leadership base to support person-centred work is essential. The Nursing Unit Manager (NUM) plays an important role in developing ideas for change: working with evidence in and from practice; improving teamwork; supporting and challenging staff through change processes; and role modelling person-centred behaviours and actions. It was therefore important to invest in a programme of work to support ongoing NUM leadership development.

The first stage in the programme was to work with NUMs to identify what aspects of person-centred leadership they wanted to focus on as well as how they wanted the programme to be structured The outcome was a programme that focused at the prerequisite level of person-centred practice with the key elements

Table 14.1 Examples of initiatives supporting the development of Person-Centred Practice (PCP)

	Initiative	Component(s) from the PCP framework	Outcomes
PR	Clinical Nurse Educator (CNE) Development Program Evidence-based programme to support CNEs to move beyond being seen as 'expert givers of knowledge' to become facilitators of work-based learning Programme run over 8 months (2/3 hours per month)	Clarity of values and beliefs Developed interpersonal skills Knowing self	Programme is now in its 5th year. Evaluation reports that CNEs have increased confidence and satisfaction in their role. Past participants now co-faciltiate the programme
CE	Let Someone Know – improving patients' and families' experiences through focusing on Clinical Bedside Handover and Multidisciplinary Ward Rounds using a Patient Journey Board (PJB)	Effective staff relationships Power sharing The physical environment	90% of multidisciplinary staff felt that the PJB has improved and streamlined communication. Observations revealed a more effective and timely handover, with an overall reduction of 20 minutes
CP	HeartBeads programme started by a few nurses was aimed at positively acknowledging what children go through as part of their stay in hospital by rewarding them with a bead for every procedure they endure. Parents were involved from the start, e.g. helping decide the types of bead and for what procedures. Each set of beads is unique to the individual child. The programme has grown since 2008 and is now embedded in practice	Working with patients' values and beliefs Having sympathetic presence Engagement	Programme has created greater awareness for staff of what each child goes through (Redshaw et al. 2011). All children with cardiac conditions have access to the HB programme (now across Australia) Parents feel their experiences are acknowledged by staff (Wilson & Chando 2014)
All	Staff survey (Person-Centred Nursing Index) is a yearly survey undertaken at the Children's Hospital at Westmead (CHW) (2008–2014) measuring a number of constructs relating to care delivery. Survey return has ranged from 38% (2008) to 59% (2012/13). Each ward receives an individual report of their results. An organisational report provides an overall picture of results	Constructs relate to overall person-centred care	A clear historical picture of many elements of person-centred care is emerging at both the organisational and individual ward levels. In 2012/13 overall satisfaction was at its highest level to date, with overall stress close to its lowest level (White & Wilson 2015)

PR, prerequisites; CE, care environment; CP, care processes.

Table 14.2 Outcomes of evaluation of a programme of work to support ongoing Nursing Unit Managers' (NUMs') leadership development

Outcomes for the NUM	Broader outcomes
• Confidence • Developing facilitation • Learning process and about myself • Feeling better about challenges • Not so hard on myself • Feeling valued • Affirmation • Connected at a deeper level with others NUMs and the organisation	• Sense of value and work in the organisation • The value of the NUM's role • Interconnectedness • Mentoring • Development and leadership • Skills • Knowledge • Attributes

of developing interpersonal skills, clarity of values and beliefs, being committed to their role, being competent in their role and becoming more self-aware. It was important to concentrate efforts on this aspect of the framework as through these elements they were then working in the care environment with care processes to ensure practice was improving.

Meeting were monthly (2–3 hours) in facilitated active learning groups; examples of the work included:

• Critical self-reflection, gathering 'evidence' about their style of leadership, including documenting three things they were proud of in terms of their leadership.
• Participating in role play (e.g. how to challenge the behaviour of a staff member).
• Using the leadership principles outlined by Kouzes and Posner (2012).
• Giving and receiving feedback (utilising challenge and support interventions with staff in a person-centred way).

The evaluation of this programme (Wilson et al. 2013) highlighted a range of outcomes, which are summarised in Table 14.2. The programme for 2015 has a focus of 'leading with compassion' and will be offered across the SCHN.

The care environment: the secret garden

A recent study examining data from almost 3000 nurses working in 46 English hospitals found that 86% of nurses were unable to perform at least one of 13 care-elements because they were too busy (Ball et al. 2014).The most commonly missed care was *comforting and talking with patients*, with 66% of nurses saying they did not have time to do this on their last shift. In supporting person-centred practice it is important to remember that these seemingly dispensable aspects of care have a huge impact for the patient, their family and for staff.

The following story emerged during the collection of stories from staff about caring with compassion. Here Christian, a nurse, is sharing his story of his encounter with one young boy with a fracture in the emergency department (SCH).

I was just trying everything I could to do you know soften him up and then try and get him laughing and talking with me and he gave me nothing ... he finally pipes up and he stopped me dead in my tracks with 'so do you cut the grass?' ...

... just out of nowhere, first thing he said to me, and I just stopped and I said, 'Sorry what was that? Do I cut the grass? What do you mean?', and then his mum explained to me that he loves his grandfather who mows the lawn and he is obsessed all about lawn mowers ... so I started talking to him about whipper snippers and he just opened up, he was a different person, he was my best friend, we were bonding over whipper snippers and lawn mowers ...

... usually when I finish with the little boys or girls I give them an ice block ... he wasn't interested so I just started telling him about my garden I had been doing at work and what we've been doing is that there is a vacant plot of land, a little courtyard where the air conditioning vents are right outside our cubicles, and when I first started here all the nurses pulled the blinds down over it because it was disgusting out there, it was just filled with weeds; apparently there were rats in there, people threw rubbish from the top of the street into the gardens, everyone was just you know condemning this place by just littering it and so the nurses would always pull the blinds down in the cubicles and kids would be stuck in cubicles for hours with these blinds closed because it was disgusting out there. So what I started to do it became like a secret project on night shift, instead of having a break I'd go out and for an hour just work, I had brought a whipper snipper in at 3.00 in the morning I snuck it through the window cause you have to climb out the window to the garden, I whipper snipped the things on the ground and brought in compost and fertiliser and a pitch fork ... everything was dead and there were no worms or anything and eventually the soil changed and we started planting sunflowers ...

... we've planted cactuses and we've put out little gnomes and bunny rabbits there's always different plants and different colours out there and now all of the sudden the nurses are pulling up the blinds in the morning and the kids are all on the window sill pointing, there's a little pig out there, pointing out the different things, and they love it. So for this little boy obsessed with lawn mowers and gardening and whipper snippers when he was finished as a reward I took him out to see the garden and we just sat there for

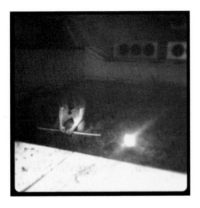

Figure 14.2 Gardening at night.

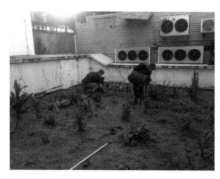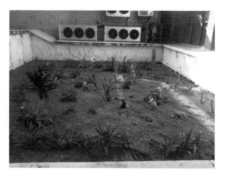

Figure 14.3 The garden comes to life.

10 minutes just pointing out everything and he was just face against the glass, dribbling down that glass just loving it all and his mum said thank you and then they left, they were great so it was kind of a win in the end.

So together we did alright in the end … everyone got involved and so we all 'own' this and everyone has a stake in it. It was something small, but it started as a condemned plot that people threw rubbish into and drew blinds on, and now it has new life!

Christian's story is a reminder that we each can make a significant contribution to the care environment that we work in and this can have positive effects for the patient, the family and for staff. The work on the secret garden demonstrates risk taking (the secret project) to improve the physical environment for children; this has had a positive and lasting impact for staff in the emergency department.

Person-centred care processes: taking just 15 steps

The staff on Hunter Baillie, a medical ward at the Children's Hospital at Westmead (CHW), volunteered to be the pilot site for a programme established in the UK called the '15 Steps Challenge' (NHS Institute n.d.). The programme originated when a mum (parent) noted that she could tell what kind of care her daughter was going to receive within 15 steps of entering the ward. This simple observation led to the establishment of a process for patient, family and staff engagement in collecting observational data that could then be used to inform changes to the care environment.

In May 2013, four staff volunteered to be internal facilitators for 15 Steps supported by the NUM and educators. Information sessions and posters/flyers were used to inform patients, families and staff about the programme. The first round of '15 steps walkabouts' was completed in June 2013 by parents, ward staff and independent observers (staff from other departments); this strategy provided opportunities to engage with stakeholders in a meaningful way and to learn through their observations. The common themes from the data were: *noisy, cluttered, busyness at the nurse's station, banging kitchen and pharmacy doors,* and *too many posters on the walls.*

The data were fed back to the staff using posters in the tea room and in a ward meeting. Over a period of 6–8 weeks staff were given the opportunity to prioritise actions by allocating a score from 1 to 5 next to the theme on the poster; whilst the response was not great, what was scored was actioned.

Completed actions were:

- Rubber seals applied to the pharmacy and kitchen door frames.
- Posters were removed for ward painting (already planned). Once completed only relevant posters were hung, i.e. parent information board opposite the entry door.
- A temporary 'pop-up' nurse's station, created due to patient requirements, resulted in reduced clutter and busyness of the main nurse's station. Feedback from staff and families was positive, and a proposal was drafted requesting a permanent second nurse's station.

A second round of 'walkabouts' was completed in May 2014, and on this occasion members of the SCHN Executive were independent observers. Themes similar to the first round in relation to clutter, noise and the nurse's station were identified. Initiatives to improve these first time round had had only a temporary impact. An alternative feedback approach (focus groups) was led by the internal facilitators, who reported experiencing more engagement from staff. Communication, staff support, smiling and being positive, and re-engaging with family-centred care in practice were identified as priorities for action. These action priorities demonstrate a strong link between families' values and beliefs about being central to caring for their child and how staff wanted the family-centred care model to lead practice on their ward.

A video, 'Small Acts of Kindness' (NSW MoH 2014), was used and the NUM said this had a powerful impact on the staff. Following this staff created a dedicated feedback board in the tea room to document positive behaviours and those that have not during each shift (Figure 14.4).

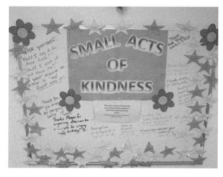
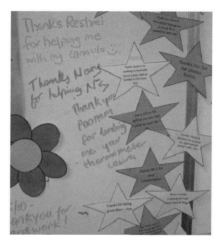

Figure 14.4 'Small Acts of Kindness' board.

To date, feedback from the NUM is that the team is more positive and engaged, the atmosphere is less tense and the noise from 'chatter' has reduced. There have been fewer complaints from parents and carers. Staff continue to write on the board each day. Evaluation of this work is ongoing.

Evaluation

It is important in undertaking this work that we were supporting staff to develop the skills required for change work; see, for example, Wales et al. (2013). In addition to this we needed to evaluate the impact in terms of achieving person-centred care in practice. We have tried to highlight in the above examples outcomes that have value for patients (e.g. the young boy's excitement of seeing the secret garden); families (e.g. increased understanding and acknowledgment of parental experience through Heart-Beads); staff (e.g. the NUMs feeling valued for their contribution to care); and for the organisation (e.g. PCNI results in 2014 indicated increased staff satisfaction and reduced stress). Systematic evaluation of this work has proven to be a vital building block in creating a person-centred culture. We have learned what has worked well, what has not, and what we can translate into different practice settings. Person-centred practice is not a one size fits all; indeed, if we were to fall into that easy trap we would be going against the very things we are trying to achieve, which is developing cultures that work for all involved, can be shaped by collective values, and have at their very core the intent of being therapeutic for all.

Moving forwards

Person-centred practice is an ongoing journey and there is a need to keep focused and to continually evolve our practice. In moving forwards in our organisation we have made a commitment to providing person-centred compassionate care. If you feel you are unable to provide care with compassion you run the risk of eroding your commitment to moral principles (Cameron & Payne 2012) that most probably drive your passion as a nurse. Providing compassionate care makes you feel good; reduces your risk of heart disease; makes you more resilient to stress; and makes you a more caring parent, a better spouse and better friend (Greater Good website). With these things in mind our person-centred development programme for 2015 includes the following examples:
- Leading with compassion (a programme for NUMs).
- The Daisy awards – a patient and family award programme that recognises the contribution of nurses.
- The Person-Centred Practice Inventory – a survey that provides staff with pertinent data to measure and benchmark person-centred care.
- The 15 Steps programme and the Small Acts of Kindness video.

- Medication safety – an action research programme that brings parents and staff together to analyse data and develop solutions aimed at improving medication administration.

As we conclude this chapter we ask you the reader to consider:

What is your role in delivering compassionate person-centred practice?

There can be a tendency to feel overwhelmed when faced with the complexity of the health-care system, and the potential barriers that may prevent you from acting. We remind you of Christian and the secret garden, and hope you feel the power you have to make a difference in the life of others.

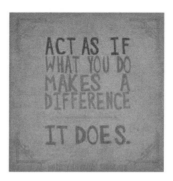

In the words of Steve Maraboli (2013):

Protect your enthusiasm from the negativity and fear of others. Never decide to do nothing just because you can only do little. Do what you can. You would be surprised at what 'little' acts have done for our world.

References

Ball, J., Murrells, T., Rafferty, A.M., Morrow, E., and Griffiths, P. (2014) 'Care left undone' during nursing shifts: associations with workload and perceived quality of care. *BMJ Quality and Safety*, **23**, 116–25.

Cameron, C.D. and Payne, B.K. (2012) The cost of callousness: Regulating compassion influences the moral self-concept. *Psychological Science*, **23**, 225–9.

Casey, A. (1995) Partnership nursing: influences on involvement of informal carers. *Journal of Advanced Nursing*, **22**, 1058–62.

Garling, P. (2008) *Final Report of the Special Commission of Inquiry Acute Care Services in NSW Public Hospitals*. State of NSW through the Special Commission of Inquiry: Acute Care Services in NSW Public Hospitals.

Greater Good website. 0000 Available at: http://greatergood.berkeley.edu/topic/compassion/definition (accessed 5 February 2016).

Hooke, N., Lewis, P., Kelly, M., Wilson, V., and Jones, S. (2008) Making something of it: one ward's application of evidence into practice. *Practice Development in Health Care*, **7** (2), 79–91.

Hutchfield, K. (1999) Family-centred care: a concept analysis. *Journal of Advanced Nursing*, **29**, 1178–87.

Kouzes, J.M. and Posner, B.Z. (2012) *The Leadership Challenge: How to Make Extraordinary Things Happen in Organisations*, 5th edn, Jossey-Bass.

Lewis, P., Kelly, M., Wilson, V., and Jones, S. (2007) What did they say? How children, families and nurses experience 'care'. *Journal of Children's and Young People's Nursing*, **1** (6), 259–66.

Maraboli, S. (2013) *Unapologetically You: Reflections on Life and the Human Experience*, A Better Today Publishing, New York.

McCormack, B. and McCance, T. (2010) *Person-Centred Nursing: Theory and Practice*, 1st edn, Wiley-Blackwell, Oxford.

NHS Institute (n.d.) *The 15 Steps Challenge*. Available at: http://www.institute.nhs.uk/ productives/15stepschallenge/15stepschallenge.html (accessed 5 February 2016).

NSW MoH (New South Wales – Ministry of Health). 0000 Small Acts of Kindness [video]. Available at: http://www.kfilms.com.au/small-acts-of-kindness/ (accessed 5 February 2016).

Redshaw, S., Wilson, V., Scarfe, G., and Dengler, K. (2011) Narratives of the Heart: telling the story of children with a cardiac condition through a bead program. *Journal of Clinical Nursing*, **20**, 2802–11.

Wales, S., Kelly, M., Wilson, V., and Crisp, J. (2013) Enhancing transformational facilitation skills for nurses seeking to support practice innovation. *Contemporary Nurse*, **44** (2), 178–88.

White, C. and Wilson, V. (2015) Longitudinal study of aspects of family centred nursing: changing practice through data translation. *Journal of Advanced Nursing*, **71** (1), 100–14.

Wilson, V. and Chando, S. (2014) Parental experiences with a hospital-based bead programme for children with congenital heart disease. *Journal of Clinical Nursing*, **24** (3-4), 439–46.

Wilson, V., Patterson, S., and Kornman, K. (2013) Leadership development: an essential ingredient in supporting nursing unit managers. *Journal of Healthcare Leadership*, **5**, 53–62.

CHAPTER 15

Meeting the challenges of person-centredness in acute care

Christine Boomer[1,2] & Tanya McCance[2]

[1] South Eastern Health and Social Care Trust, Northern Ireland, UK
[2] Ulster University, Northern Ireland, UK

Introduction

The aspiration to deliver a standard of care that reflects person-centredness has been evident in health strategy and policy planning globally for well over a decade (Department of Human Services 2003; Department of Health 2005; National Ageing Research Institute 2006; World Health Organization 2007). The challenges in delivering person-centred care in practice, however, continue to be well recognised, with hospital care often being a focus for the ongoing debate. This debate has been fuelled by high-profile inquiries and reviews suggesting that the experience of hospital care is variable and often fails to meet the expected standard (Francis 2013). These challenges are a result of the increasing complexity surrounding the provision of health care, particularly within acute care environments, and are reflected in the context, including influential components such as health and social care policy, strategic leadership and workforce developments. In response to these challenges different approaches have been promoted to improve the experience of care for both patients and staff. This chapter will provide insight into the challenges in providing a positive care experience and, using case studies, demonstrate different approaches to the development of person-centred practice within acute care.

Person-centredness within acute care

The promotion of person-centredness in acute care is well rehearsed, with a widespread acceptance of the principles that underpin such an approach. The literature, however, provides examples of experiences in acute care environments that do not always reflect these principles. Studies focusing on this area confirm acute hospitals as inherently complex environments and emphasise

Person-Centred Practice in Nursing and Health Care: Theory and Practice, Second Edition.
Edited by Brendan McCormack and Tanya McCance.
© 2017 John Wiley & Sons, Ltd. Published 2017 by John Wiley & Sons, Ltd.

the challenges in delivering person-centred care in this context. Bolster and Manias (2010) provide a good example of this in their qualitative study focusing on person-centred interactions between nurses and patients during medication activities. The key findings highlighted care that was centred on routines rather than individualised assessment and management, with little opportunity for patient participation. The two main contextual barriers identified were: (1) communication challenges with the multi-professional team such as the pharmacist and the medical team; and (2) time constraints perceived by the nurses as restricting their ability to engage with patients and to facilitate meaningful discussions about medication. The quality of engagement with patients is similarly reflected in other studies. Clisset et al. (2013) explored ways in which current approaches to care in acute settings had the potential to enhance personhood in older people with dementia, and concluded that health-care professionals were not grasping opportunities to make their care person-centred, suggesting that 'good practice appears to be in "pockets" as a result of individual practitioners rather than comprehensive and consistent across services' (p. 1502). In a more general study focusing on patients' experiences of in-hospital care, Laird et al. (2015) also highlighted the fragility of person-centred care, identifying one overriding theme of vulnerability at the junctures of systems, care processes and nurses' responses. This type of evidence provides an important foundation for engagement in a dialogue about interventions that enable practitioners working in acute care environments to engage in the effective person-centred practice.

CASE STUDY 15.1: Implementing a practice development programme within an acute care setting.

Aim

A practice development programme was implemented over a period of 2 years within an acute hospital setting, aimed at enabling nursing teams to explore the concept of person-centredness within their own clinical setting, in order to improve care delivery.

Context

The person-centred care programme was delivered in a large health and social care organisation, with approximately 20,000 staff, of which almost 6800 are nurses and midwives. The organisation serves a local population of 340,000 people but also provides regional services. The programme was undertaken at a time of unprecedented change, when services for health and social care in this region were being reorganised. The organisation in which the programme was delivered was the result of a merger with several other organisations, and at the time of commencement of the programme was less than one year established. The programme was delivered across nine acute inpatient areas covering a range of specialties including: cancer inpatient unit; mental health inpatient unit; brain injury unit; specialist and general medical inpatient wards such as chest medicine, cardiology and neurology; and eyes and ear, nose and throat theatre department.

The programme

The programme was underpinned by the Person-centred Nursing Framework, which acted as a lens to offer greater insights and understanding of person-centredness at practice level. The programme structure comprised facilitated activities in line with a practice development approach including a series of facilitated workshops ($n = 5$), with ongoing monthly support provided through a project team. Each workshop focused on key themes including: promoting an understanding of person-centredness; developing a shared vision; determining the quality of the user experience; systematically developing practice; and celebrating success. Each workshop profiled relevant activities to enable teams to engage with the processes more widely back in their own clinical areas.

Outcomes

Participation in this practice development programme produced some positive outcomes for staff.

- Staff experienced a level of engagement in person-centred practice that was characterised by positive ways of working and building relationships. There were times when there was a high level of commitment and energy, and this was reflected in the level of engagement across the participating sites. However, there were times when maintaining momentum was a challenge due to the organisational context.
- While the values that underpin person-centred care were not new to participants, the significance was in how they embraced person-centred values in practice, even in the challenging context described above. Participants acknowledged the difficulty of recognising how person-centred values are reflected in practice, both in support of best practice and in recognising aspects of practice that needed to change. There was also a fundamental shift during the programme when some participants began to recognise the meaning of 'person' in person-centred care, a central tenet of this way of working.
- Person-centredness in practice was impeded by conflicting priorities characterised by a sense of feeling pressurised, limited staffing and resources, and the challenges of an evolving context, particularly within the provision of services in acute hospitals. There was a constant tussle between conflicting priorities and the desire to live out person-centred values in everyday practice.

CASE STUDY 15.2: The Productive Ward (PW): *'Releasing time to care'*.

Aim

The Productive Ward programme aims to improve four dimensions of care: patient safety and reliability of care, patient experience, staff well-being and efficiency of care.

Context

The programme was initially implemented as part of a regional pilot, following a drive for the use of *LEAN* approaches in health and social care. Within one organisation serving a population of 345,000 over a wide geographical area with a workforce of 10,000 staff (approx. 3300 nurses and midwives), two sites were chosen to implement and test the programme: a maternity ward and a specialist surgical ward. These sites were chosen due to their contrasting cultures and contexts, thereby gaining insights for implementation across the wider organisation. Person-centredness was a core theme in the organisation's corporate and Nursing and Midwifery strategies, therefore the evaluation focused on determining the potential for the productive ward programme to influence this agenda.

The programme

Led by the ward manager, ward implementation teams undertook the three foundation modules within the Productive Ward programme. *Knowing How we are Doing* aims to assist the ward team to determine their starting position, a baseline. Activities undertaken included developing a ward vision and observations. The *Well Organised Ward* aims to enable teams to simplify their workplace, reduce waste by having everything in the right place, at the right time; and by concentrating on how areas should be improved. Activities undertaken included 'activity follow' and 'waste walk'. *Patient Status at a Glance* builds on work undertaken in the first two modules with further analysis of data from the tools used, e.g. activity follow analysis, information boards, handovers, discharge management, and availability/accessibility of information. Each module followed a six-step process: prepare, assess, diagnose, plan, treat and evaluate. Ward teams had access to a facilitator and attended training on the use of the various tools within the programme.

Outcomes

The programme captured staff motivation for improvement achieved through a number of *quick wins*. It had an impact on person-centredness, in particular on the Care Environment, especially relating to the physical environment. The often simple changes, e.g. stock availability and having equipment to hand, freed up staff time. Staff in both sites expressed feeling valued alongside a stronger sense of team, having demonstrated creativity to achieve multi-professional engagement.

Additional positive outcomes for staff included the acquisition of new skills and improved communication. Staff also felt they had more control, articulated as having taken back ownership of the ward. Managers too noted positive changes in the environment and *atmosphere* in the sites, expressed as a feeling of calmness reflected by, e.g., reduced noise levels. Staff did express anecdotal outcomes for their patients, and the staff teams were clearly excited from their participation in the programme, articulating a greater satisfaction in terms of their experience of care.

As a result of the pilot the programme was seen as a *way in,* to begin to engage staff in examining areas of practice more critically. However, an approach underpinned by practice development methodology was adopted for the ongoing implementation of the programme, with a clear intent of focusing on person-centredness, an area not explicit within the original programme.

CASE STUDY 15.3: Creating the conditions for person-centredness: a practice development programme.

Aim

The aim for this *fast-tracked* practice development programme was threefold: to enable participants to explore person-centred practice in relation to their own practice setting; to develop a vision for person-centred practice; and to demonstrate person-centred outcomes (which would link back to the organisation's nursing and midwifery strategy).

Context

In the same organisation as in Case 15.2, previous development work within the organisation had demonstrated sound systems and processes had been progressed, giving a solid foundation on which to start building. The nursing and midwifery strategy clearly articulated an expectation aimed at developing person-centred outcomes – for both users and staff. The programme involved working with teams in two units within one acute hospital (within the larger organisation) to create the conditions for the ongoing development of person-centredness within the wider innovation and experience agenda.

The programme

Underpinned by the person-centred practice and practice development frameworks, the programme aimed to work with staff teams from the two units over a 7-month timeframe. Teams engaged in four phases of activity: creating conditions for working together and developing shared understanding of person-centredness; developing a shared vision; evaluating and taking action and celebrating and ongoing planning for development work. Within all phases the participants engaged in activities including workshops, reflection and active learning, observation, analysis and feedback. Two facilitators, external to the units, worked with teams maintaining a focus on person-centredness throughout and creating capacity for its ongoing development.

Outcomes (to date)

At the time of writing this programme remains ongoing; however, process evaluation has revealed a number of outcomes and challenges that we can share. Both teams have developed their visions for person-centred practice, using this activity as a way to seek feedback and achieve real involvement of users to inform a truly shared vision for their practice. These visions are providing the foundations on which they are currently building. Staff completed the person-centred practice index (Slater et al. 2015) alongside other data sources (including patient stories, observations, audits). Analysis of the collective data has provided teams with an accurate understanding of their current practice all mapped to the person-centred framework. This mapping exercise has enabled teams to celebrate what is going well, highlight potential areas for development and also made the framework real and lived in relation to their own practice context – they clearly describe a better understanding of person-centredness.

The major challenge to date has been the ambitious timeframe – for facilitators and teams alike. While dedicated facilitators from a central nursing and midwifery team were aligned to the programme, competing pressures and priorities have made operationalising the programme a delicate balancing act. The participating teams have also had challenges associated with heavy and increasing workloads, staff sickness, maintaining momentum and internal organisational restructuring.

Exploring the case studies – understanding the key challenges

The three case studies are short snapshots of programmes that used different approaches, methods and tools to explore and develop person-centredness within acute care. Despite the approach, they all illustrate positive outcomes alongside challenges. These challenges fall into four broad themes: contextual challenges, leadership and facilitation, methodology and approaches, and demonstrating outcomes. We will now discuss these in the context of the cases and the current evidence base.

Contextual challenges

Context can be described as the environment or setting in which practice takes place (McCormack et al. 2002) and it is often described in tandem with culture. However, this can over-simplify the concept, as context is influenced by numerous factors such as organisational systems, power, relationships, environment, and culture – of which there are many in any context (Brown & McCormack 2011). The three contextual factors that pose the biggest challenge to the development of person-centredness in acute care are: organisational culture, learning environment, and the care environment itself (McCormack et al. 2011). In the cases presented, staff had to manage the push and pull, or tussle between context, aspiration and priorities; that meant living with the busyness and finding systems to maintain momentum and create a balance. These require a commitment at all levels within organisations if approaches to the development of care are to be realised.

Methodology and approaches

Case studies 15.1 and 15.3 utilised practice development, which has at its core the development of person-centred cultures and practices (see Chapter 9 for further detail). Practice development is intentional in its aspiration to achieve this cultural change by adopting systematic processes, authentic engagement and active learning (Dewing 2009) to explore values and beliefs, and change cultures, contexts and people to achieve person-centred cultures. The added value of using systematic practice development as a methodology is evident in the outcomes achieved, including those from Cases 15.1 and 15.2 presented in this chapter.

The LEAN improvement approach was adopted for Case study 15.2, which focuses on standardising, reducing waste and improving productivity (Robert et al. 2011; IHI 2015a). In contrast with practice development, improvement methodologies, while still aiming to improve care, tend to have a more process-driven and technical approach. These approaches can and often deliver on the quick wins and early outcomes, such as in Case 15.2, and it must be recognised that these appeal to individuals, teams and organisations. The emerging discipline of improvement science is practised close to where care is delivered, aiming to understand how to deliver better care by working through questions around purpose, intent and evidence and then working through small PDSA (plan, do, study, act) cycles of change (IHI 2015b; ISL 2015). Champions of this approach point to its ability to transform established ways of working, and we know that transformation is required for cultural change.

Cultural change is recognised to be a slow process, and if we are to achieve more than person-centred moments (McCormack et al. 2011) we need to be more creative in how we go about achieving this. Potentially a strategy adopting improvement science approaches, for example PDSA cycles, while underpinning the programme of work with the intent of emancipation and transformation of staff through approaches advocated within practice development, may be the way forward in the challenging acute context. One current example of such an approach is an international nursing study looking at key performance indicators and adopting PDSA cycles to develop practice (McCance & Wilson 2015). If there is a clear vision, founded through the exploration of values and beliefs, then it can become the foundation underpinned by the person-centred nursing framework on which all subsequent improvement or development work is built (such as those developed in Cases 15.1 and 15.3). Adopting such an integrated approach needs to demonstrate commitment and leadership, skilled facilitation at macro, meso and micro levels, and evaluation to demonstrate outcomes.

Leadership and facilitation

We have suggested that the cultural change required for person-centredness to flourish in challenging acute contexts requires effective strong leadership that role models person-centredness. Transformational leadership is the style promoted in the practice development literature. In acute care, leaders need to adopt strategies from a wide range of models (Boomer & McCormack 2010), with the most effective leaders demonstrating skills along a continuum; thereby they are not only leaders and managers, but also facilitators enabling the development of practice.

Facilitation at its most simplistic is the process of enabling or making things easier for others, and the PARIHS framework provides a useful analogy of facilitation along a continuum, from task to holistic (Rycroft-Malone 2013). The task approach is at its most effective when technical changes to care are required – for example, implementing a new regional early warning score observation chart. However, a facilitation approach underpinned with critical and emancipatory intent, as used in emancipatory or transformational practice development (Shaw 2013), requires a more holistic style, and also more skill. It is at this end of the continuum that the cultural change for sustainable person-centred cultures can be realised. However, approaches utilised by facilitators need to be appropriate, intentional and able to work with 'where people are at' (Meyer 2005).

Case studies 15.1 and 15.3 adopted more enabling and holistic approaches to facilitation (Shaw et al. 2008), allowing participants to reflect on experiences and their practice in relation to the person-centred framework and the various activities undertaken. In contrast, Case study 15.2 had strong leadership of the pilot project but the facilitation was technical in nature, focusing on achieving the various tasks within the productive ward modules. In the subsequent implementation of the Productive Ward (PW) a more enabling approach was adopted leading to enhanced person-centred nursing outcomes.

Demonstrating outcomes

The modern acute care context requires evidence of impact and positive experiences of care. While discussing practice development, Manley et al. (2013) contend that impact evidence can allow influencing of policy and funding. However, McCormack et al. (2013) remind us that demonstrating outcomes of person-centredness is complex. The media and patient, carer and staff stories often reflect negative experiences of care, on the receiving and giving ends; therefore outcomes need to demonstrate this breadth. McCormack et al. (2013) go on to suggest that there are four outcomes that can be achieved from the development of person-centred cultures: experience of good care, involvement with care, feeling of well-being, and creating a healthful culture. While the outcomes achieved in the case studies may not directly reflect those for the user, there is an association between person-centred care and the satisfaction of care giving for nurses in acute environments (Lehuluante et al. 2012) and staff outcomes should not be ignored. However, we need to become smarter at evaluating care if we want to evidence good quality care, using approaches linked to the four outcomes outlined by McCormack et al. (2013).

Concluding comments

Health care is becoming increasingly challenging across all sectors, for reasons including: an increasingly ageing population with associated complex needs; resource constraints; an ever-evolving (changing) context; high expectations; and an era of increased scrutiny. While these are not unique to acute care, the culture and context in this sector brings with it a unique set of challenges when trying to embed a culture of person-centredness. Through this chapter we have given you snapshots of three programmes within the sector, and explored these in terms of the challenges of developing sustainable person-centred cultures. Ultimately the development of person-centredness in acute care is not a one-person endeavour or a one size fits all, rather it requires a blending of methodologies, approaches, organisational commitment, leadership and facilitation. The poem below reflects the journey of enabling, becoming and being person-centred in acute care; it may be challenging but when we get it right it's like dancing!

24–7–365

Constant, night and day
People rushing, demands, change
Priorities?

Searching to see differently
A new perspective
Building the bedrock
To hold the constant tussle and flow

Rushing, yet calm
Nurturing, new life
Flourishing, care, happiness
It's like dancing!

References

Bolster, D. and Manias, E. (2010) Person-centred interactions between nurses and patients during medication activities in an acute hospital setting: Qualitative observation and interview study. *International Journal of Nursing Studies*, **47**, 154–65.

Boomer, C. and McCormack, B. (2010) Creating the conditions for growth: a collaborative practice development programme for clinical nurse leaders. *Journal of Nursing Management*, **18**, 633–44.

Brown D and McCormack BG. (2011) Developing the practice context to enable more effective pain management with older people: an action research approach. *Implementation Science* **6**:9. Available at: http://www.implementationscience.com/content/6/1/9 (accessed 6 February 2016).

Clisset, P., Porock, D., Harwood, R.H., and Gladman, J.R.F. (2013) The challenges of achieving person-centred care in acute hospitals: A qualitative study of people with dementia and their families. *International Journal of Nursing Studies*, **50**, 1495–503.

Department of Health (2005) *National Service Framework for Long-Term Conditions*, Department of Health, Leeds.

Department of Human Services (2003) *Improving Care for Older People: A Policy for Health Services*, DHS, Melbourne.

Dewing, J. (2009) Moments of movement: active learning and practice development. *Nurse Education in Practice*, **10**, 22–6.

Francis, R. (2013) *The Mid-Staffordshire NHS Foundation Trust Public Enquiry*, The Stationery Office, London.

IHI (Institute for Healthcare Improvement) (2015a) Available at http://www.institute.nhs.uk/quality_and_value/productivity_series/productive_ward.html (accessed 24 February 2016).

IHI (Institute for Healthcare Improvement) (2015b) *Science of Improvement: How to Improve*. Available at http://www.ihi.org/resources/Pages/HowtoImprove/ScienceofImprovement HowtoImprove.aspx (accessed 6 February 2016).

ISL (Improvement Science London) (2015) Website. Available at: http://islondon.org/what-is-improvement-science/ (accessed 6 February 2016).

Laird, E.A., McCance, T.V., McCormack, B., and Gribben, B. (2015) Patients' experiences of in-hospital care when nursing staff were engaged in a practice development programme to promote person-centredness: A narrative analysis study. *International Journal of Nursing Studies*, **52**, 1454–62.

Lehuluante, A., Nilsson, A., and Edvardsson, E. (2012) The influence of a person-centred psychosocial unit climate on satisfaction with care and work. *Journal of Nursing Management*, **20**, 319–25.

Manley, K., Titchen, A., and McCormack, B. (2013) What is practice development and what are the starting points? in *Practice Development in Nursing and Healthcare*, 2nd edn (eds B. McCormack, K. Manley, and A. Titchen), Wiley-Blackwell, Oxford, pp. 45–65.

McCance T and Wilson V. (2015) Using person-centred key performance indicators to improve paediatric services: an international venture. *International Practice Development Journal* **5**(Suppl) [8]. Available at: http://www.fons.org/Resources/Documents/Journal/Vol5Suppl/IPDJ_05%28suppl%29_08.pdf (accessed 6 Feb 2016).

McCance T, Gribben B, McCormack B, Laird E. (2013) Promoting person-centred practice within acute care: The impact of culture and context on a facilitated practice development programme. *International Practice Development Journal* **3**(1): manuscript 2.

McCormack, B., Kitson, A., Harvey, G., Rycroft-Malone, J., Titchen, A., and Seers, K. (2002) Getting evidence into practice: the meaning of 'context'. *Journal of Advanced Nursing*, **38** (1), 94–104.

McCormack B, Dewing J, McCance T. (2011) Developing person-centred care: addressing contextual challenges through practice development. *Online Journal of Issues in Nursing* **16**(2), manuscript 3. Retrieved from: http://www.nursingworld.org/MainMenuCategories/ANAMarketplace/ANAPeriodicals/OJIN/TableofContents/Vol-16-2011/No2-May-2011/Developing-Person-Centred-Care.html (accessed 6 February 2016).

McCormack, B., McCance, T., and Maben, J. (2013) Outcome evaluation in the development of person-centred practice, in *Practice Development in Nursing and Healthcare*, 2nd edn (eds B. McCormack, K. Manley, and A. Titchen), Wiley-Blackwell, Oxford, pp. 190–211.

Meyer, J. (2005) Action research in Education, Health and Social Care: sharing perspectives. Becoming connected, being caring. Keynote address given to Practitioner Research/Action Research (PRAR) 2005, in *Joint International Practitioner Research Conference and Collaborative Action research Network (CARN) Conference*, Utrecht, The Netherlands.

National Ageing Research Institute (2006) What is person-centred health care? A literature review. Available at: www2.health.vic.gov.au

Robert, G., Morrow, E., Maben, J., Griffiths, P., and Callard, L. (2011) The adoption, local implementation and assimilation into routine nursing practice of a national quality improvement programme: the Productive Ward in England. *Journal of Clinical Nursing*, **20** (7-8), 1196–207.

Rycroft-Malone, J. (2013) How you might use PARIHS to deliver safe and effective care, in *Practice Development in Nursing and Healthcare*, 2nd edn (eds B. McCormack, K. Manley, and A. Titchen), Wiley-Blackwell, Oxford, pp. 130–45.

Shaw, T. (2013) Approaches to practice development, in *Practice Development in Nursing and Healthcare*, 2nd edn (eds B. McCormack, K. Manley, and A. Titchen), Wiley-Blackwell, Oxford, pp. 66–87.

Shaw T, Dewing J, Young R, Devlin M, Boomer C, Leguis M. (2008) Enabling practice development: delving into the concept of facilitation from a practitioner perspective. In: *Manley K, McCormack B*, Wilson V. (eds), *International Practice Development in Nursing and Healthcare*. Oxford: Blackwell Publishing, chapter 9.

Slater P, McCance T, McCormack B. (2015) Exploring person-centred practice within acute hospital settings. *International Practice Development Journal* 5 (Suppl.) [09]. Available at: http://www.fons.org/Resources/Documents/Journal/Vol5Suppl/IPDJ_05%28suppl%29_09.pdf (accessed 6 February 2016).

World Health Organization (2007) *People-centred Health Care: A Policy Framework*, WHO, Geneva.

CHAPTER 16

Person-centredness, recovery and user involvement in mental health services

Marit Borg & Bengt Karlsson
The University College of South-East Norway, Drammen, Norway

Introduction

This chapter deals with the perspectives and approaches of person-centredness, recovery and user involvement, and their influences and potentials in mental health service transformation. First, we will briefly discuss major changes in mental health practices in the Western world. This is followed by an outline of the roots and perspectives of person-centredness, recovery and user involvement as we see it. Finally, we will debate some issues regarding standard approaches needed in mental health practice if we are going to claim person-centredness, recovery and user involvement.

The person in mental health contexts

Person-centredness, recovery and service user involvement in mental health practices all sound obvious and self-evident. All three approaches aim to place people at the forefront of their life projects and health and care programmes. This requires attention to who and what is to be in the actual centre. Carl Rogers (1978) claimed that person-centredness can be seen as radical in its attempts to give the person a central position and challenge bureaucracy and hierarchies in promoting egalitarian ideals of humans relating as equal persons, whatever their roles, status or positions. As we see it, the same challenges are present today, and are also inherent in the recent recovery-paradigm for mental health services. During the past decades, the concept of recovery has become familiar in mental health policy, practices and research as well as in voicing service users' experiences of mental distress and processes towards well-being and citizenship – issues taken for granted in society, but ones that people living with mental health issues find challenging. Recovery, like person-centredness, is

Person-Centred Practice in Nursing and Health Care: Theory and Practice, Second Edition.
Edited by Brendan McCormack and Tanya McCance.
© 2017 John Wiley & Sons, Ltd. Published 2017 by John Wiley & Sons, Ltd.

about the person retaining and keeping control over their life situation, helping the individual to make informed decisions and supporting real partnerships between persons, families and services.

As researchers and clinicians working in mental health settings, we have found ourselves caught between competing realities. On the one hand, our workplaces inevitably have humanistic and holistic-sounding vision statements that include valuing the whole person and focusing on the person in context rather than the health problems. On the other hand, we find ourselves in the midst of a health bureaucracy and procedures that by no means embody or develop these values. The World Health Organization (WHO 2007) as well as national policies have for some time stated that there remains a gap between rhetoric and reality in the field of mental health. First-person accounts tell us that the voices of service users are still not listened to, their knowledge is generally not recognised as valuable, and what they say to practitioners may well be interpreted within a diagnostic framework as a symptom of their illness rather than as a genuine exchange of crucial information. A young man described the following:

> The terrible thing with the psychiatry I have met, is that whatever you say you are pathologised. If I asked what the medication is good for, they generally think that you are paranoid or something like that, instead of giving you an answer. It's the total hardness and non-empathy.
>
> *Borg and Topor (2013, p. 14)*

In the following section, we would like to take a step back and reflect on some of these critical issues. We start by setting the scene of mental health services.

Setting the scene

In *The People-Centred Health Care – A Policy Framework* (WHO 2007), the World Health Organization summarised the challenges in health systems. WHO urged that health systems need to move beyond the traditional models of providing health care and of measuring health system performance. Instead it suggested that greater attention to health system design, financing mechanisms, and the focus and process of care is required. Based on a literature review and a series of stakeholder consultations in selected countries, WHO identified a number of gaps and weaknesses in current health systems, which need attention:

> 1. Health systems and services have become overly biomedical oriented, disease focused, technology driven and doctor driven. 2. Health care financing mechanisms have not been optimal, pushing provider behavior towards inadequate care, short consultations and lack of referrals. 3. Medical education has increasingly concentrated on body systems or disease conditions. 4. There is little patient and family participation in health care. 5. Specialization and weak referral systems have led to fragmentation and discontinuity of care, both within and between health care institutions, systems and other sources of care such as support groups and the community. 6. It is time to pay more attention to the demand side – patients, families, communities and society at large.
>
> *WHO (2007, p. 6)*

The named gaps became transformed into *The Mental Health Action Plan 2013-2020* (WHO 2013). The Action Plan states that '…mental health, which is conceptualized as a state of well-being in which the individual realizes his or her own abilities, can cope with the normal stresses of life, can work productively and fruitfully, and is able to make a contribution to his or her community. (p. 6). The overall goal for the Action Plan is: '…to promote mental health well-being, prevent mental disorders, provide care, enhance recovery, promote human rights and reduce mortality, morbidity and disability for persons with mental disorders' (p. 9). The Action Plan also describes the transition from social marginalisation to full citizenship, and represents a daunting challenge in public mental health services. An approach that focuses primarily on individuals is not sufficient for creating access to valued roles that those individuals will be able to occupy in community settings. Instead, public intervention and debate are required to promote and monitor the bond of citizenship that connects people to their communities. People with mental health issues, intellectual disabilities and substance use conditions can be included in the community only if the community is informed and welcoming.

Mental health services in most Western countries have undergone major changes over recent decades. The number of persons staying in mental health institutions has been drastically reduced. Models of community care and outreach approaches have been established with the ideals of drawing on the perspectives and principles of person-centredness, recovery and user involvement. These ideals can be seen as important initiatives contributing to fundamental changes in some places. However, implementation of services that are aligned with these perspectives is often met with barriers rooted in the dominant psychiatric culture, including resistance to shift from the biomedical paradigm orientation to humanistic, person-oriented and social-oriented mental health services, and from professional control to service user orientation (Karlsson et al. 2008). In the next section, we will discuss the perspectives and principles of person-centredness, recovery and user involvement, and the relationships between them.

Recovery, person-centredness and user involvement

Recovery

A central aspect of the notion of recovery is that this knowledge base is developed by and with people with lived experience of mental distress. The recovery perspectives are relatively recent, and as with many new terms, are inconsistently used and even somewhat contested. Yet some characteristics are typically mentioned (Davidson 2003; Borg 2007; Borg et al. 2013). Recovery has become increasingly important in mental health practices, service development and research over recent decades.

The nature of recovery in relation to mental health problems can be seen as a clinical outcome as well as a process. The outcome perspective traces recovery in mental distress back to the International Pilot Study of Schizophrenia of the World Health Organization beginning in the late 1960s, and to other parallel efforts examining the outcome of psychosis (Davidson e tal. 2005). With the finding of a broad heterogeneity in the outcomes, it became clear that individuals being diagnosed with schizophrenia or other psychoses can and do recover. Another outcome perspective is that of traditional treatment effect and symptom relief (Slade 2009). This sense of recovery refers to the fact that people can achieve mental health in which they no longer experience what is defined as clinical signs, symptoms or impairment associated with their given medical diagnosis (Davidson 2003). Furthermore, recovery can be understood as a personal as well as a social process (Tew 2005; Karlsson & Borg 2013).

The *personal process* is typically described in terms of regaining self-belief, self-control and moving beyond being a service user or patient. It is about reawakening hope for the future, developing a sense of meaning and purpose in life, and doing things you want to do. Taking back control over your situation and nurturing and pursuing ambitions are central. *The social process* emphasises the dynamic relationship between the person and the environment. Living conditions, feeling safe, work opportunities, community involvement, friends and families, helpful professionals, and available and accessible services are essential for peoples' recovery processes. These are all ordinary parts of everyday life that people with mental health issues often are excluded from.

Much of the recovery literature describes these life processes as dynamic and contextual and implies that regardless of one's aetiological perspectives on the nature and causes of mental distress, it is in everyday life and the community that the numerous situations and consequences need to be addressed (Repper & Perkins 2003; Beresford 2005; Borg & Davidson 2008). Recovery processes also involve 'taking back control and getting on with one's life', and managing most things most of the time. Recovery is not about cure, but about learning to live with and controlling what is distressful. The uniqueness of the recovery process is often experienced as essential, yet goes unrecognised because traditional treatment approaches tend to be standardised and based on diagnostic categories and guidelines, rather than on individual experiences and everyday life (Borg & Kristiansen 2008). A recovery orientation includes the understanding that while personal distress is sometimes overwhelming, the social consequences are even more challenging (Beresford 2005; Tew 2005).

Davidson (2003) talks about recovery as the opportunity to have a life outside mental distress and that this must be available to everyone, no matter how severe their problems are. This involves access, creating opportunities and not standing in the person's way, much like central issues identified in disability research where the focus is not on the individual as disabled and deviant but as much on the environmental deficits. Recovery is an ambiguous term with a mixture of associations that seem to be used in a great variety of contexts and for a number of implicit and explicit purposes. In this chapter, we understand recovery as a dynamic process incorporating individual and environmental perspectives and the relationships between the two.

Person-centredness

The concept of person-centredness has multi-faceted roots. Person-centred approaches as professional practices and personal and political philosophy are often associated with Carl Rogers' work from the early 1940s (Rogers 1978). Involvement in world issues and social justice has for long been a core element, together with relationship with the 'other' in a broad sense, belief in peoples' potentials and critique of individualistic approaches. The goal for a person-centred intervention is in Rogers' terms 'becoming a person'. Paulo Freire is another inspiration in the roots of person-centredness. Freire (1972) considers authenticity as an essential part of full humanness and sees it as a goal for people to become 'beings for themselves' – subjects of their own experiencing. Freire describes how human development and knowledge emerge through invention and re-invention and the continuing, hopeful inquiry that human beings pursue in the world, with the world, and with each other. In seeing person-centredness as an agenda for social change, contextual and political issues need to be included in approaches and developments. Contextual because the 'whole truth' needs to be attended to, like the person's nationality, class, gender, ideology and sexuality – in general trying to understand the person's place in the wold. Politically because working for person-centredness means a battle against dominating ideologies of evidence-carrying subjects originating in the medicalisation of mental distress (Proctor 2006). Person-centredness has also become a central philosophy in the care of older people, dementia care, for citizens with learning disabilities and in childcare, and to a rather minor extent in mental health care. In the latter it is mainly in the Tidal Model (Lafferty & Davidson 2006) that person-centredness as a philosophy and concept is used. Earlier in this book (see Chapter 2) the person-centred care process was described with five dimensions. Key approaches and perspectives are:

1 Working with the person's beliefs and values, meaning exploring and paying genuine attention to his/her values and how the person understands what is going in life.
2 Shared decision-making, meaning respecting and finding ways of supporting the individual in taking choices and determining small and big issues in the present life situation.
3 Engagement, meaning the connectedness of the practitioner with the person and others significant to him/her, determined by knowledge of the person, clarity of beliefs and values, knowledge of self and professional expertise.

4 Providing holistic care, meaning supporting and providing care and treatment processes with attention to the whole person through the integration
of psychological, sociocultural, socio-economic, physical health and spiritual
dimensions.

5 Having a sympathetic presence, meaning an emphasis on human relationships, understanding the complexity of interpersonal relationships and recognising the uniqueness and value of the person.

Prerequisites for person-centred care are professionally competent personnel
(knowledge and skills), including clear values and knowing self. Central outcomes of person-centred care processes are satisfaction with care, involvement
in care, a feeling of well-being and creating a therapeutic environment (McCormack & McCance 2010; see also Chapter 2).

In person-centred approaches, human relationships and caring are essential
parts. Martinsen (1989) describes how the term 'caring' consists of three different but equal elements: relational, practical and moral. The relational is based
upon a collective humanity where the basis is that we depend on each other.
Dependency in this context is not the opposite of independence. Dependence on
each other points to the moral universal principle: we can all be in the position
of needing help from other persons at some point in life. This principle is therefore embedded in the other element of the term caring, as a praxis. It points to
a situation where help is given unconditionally. Help and support are justified
from the condition of the one in need, not from an expected result.

User involvement

Strengthening user involvement in mental health services has been a key part of
policy-making in many countries over recent decades. Although this has been the
vision and intention in the practice of mental health care, there is evidence that
this vision remains theoretical rather than practical in many clinical settings. The
growing literature in recovery research and perspectives on helpful help from
persons with lived experiences of mental distress offers crucial contributions for
developing new services (Borg 2007; Davidson et al. 2007). User knowledge contributes to establishing and justifying knowledge in concrete human life contexts,
such as the competence and skills of dealing with voices and of living with side
effects of medicine, and techniques developed in order to keep a job or to survive
on a limited monthly budget. The systemisation of user experiences is particularly important in broadening the mental health knowledge base as well as in
developing new approaches to mental health care. One crucial result of studies
from the user perspective is the overruling of the illness paradigm by emphasising the idea that individuals experiencing or being diagnosed with mental health
problems can no longer be seen and met as having a chronic debilitating disease,
or being 'too ill' to have a voice or say (Borg et al. 2013).

People with mental health problems often describe negative and dehumanising experiences with mental health services (Borg et al. 2009). They describe

situations of being treated as disorders or diagnoses rather than as unique individuals. They have experiences of being viewed only in terms of their problems, symptoms and deficits rather than as being citizens with strengths and areas of competence. People are extracted from the context of their daily lives and viewed largely in terms of their compliance or cooperation with treatment rather than as the protagonist of their own life story (Davidson 2003). In addition to their critiques of current care, first-person accounts draw attention to everyday issues and how mental health problems affect people's lives in the 'real world' beyond boundaries of mental health services. People with mental health problems talk about work, education, God, beloved pets, and friends and lovers as much as, if not more than, their mental distress. In addition to the quality of interpersonal relationships, they may have practitioners who remain paramount in their narratives in both positive and negative terms; people describe what is helpful to them in highly specific and individualised terms. In contrast to a trust in manual-driven treatments, they value practitioners who allow them to take the lead, set the agenda and focus on the areas where they feel they need help. These areas quite frequently encompass everyday life concerns encountered in loving, learning, playing and belonging and are distinct from the conventional focus on treatment – issues like medication, symptoms and coping with problems. User knowledge is rich in what we may otherwise consider to be the trivialities of everyday life; activities and things we ordinarily take for granted (Davidson 2007).

The systematic investigation of user experiences represents an important vehicle for beginning to draw our collective attention to and to value this aspect of the lives of individuals with serious mental health challenges. While the customary view of serious mental health problems within medical settings may have been that of a chronic debilitating disease resulting inevitably in a poor outcome, the realm of everyday life appears to be a stage of recovery (Borg & Davidson 2008). It is here where people appear to figure out how to manage their problems and get on with their lives. In this regard, qualitative studies in user knowledge have generated insights about how recovery over time within the context of daily life may be helpful in suggesting directions for how practices can be more person-centered.

The person in a person-centred practice

As we have learned earlier in the book, the Person-centred Nursing Framework can be used as a lens that offers insights and understandings of the prerequisites for person-centred practice development. What needs to be attended to is the health-care context; the roles of the professional, the service user and family members; the collaborative relationships with and around the person and his/her social network; the knowledge base of the services; and the dominant discourses and the outcomes. Person-centred and collaborative practice in mental health care has been a priority issue in recent decades, and many models have been developed in attempts to address successful collaboration. The challenge seems to be placing the person, meaning the patient or service user, at the centre of the practice. In this chapter, we have offered an outline of concepts and perspectives in the literature central to discussions of the person's role and position in person-centred practice, namely recovery, user involvement and person-centredness. Although the roots and traditions seem to be different, the three concepts have some common strands.

People with mental health problems are first and foremost people. In order to understand what is going on in peoples' lives as well as being a useful helping partner, we need to be interested in and curious about the person and collaborate as partners where both have comprehensive and useful knowledge. This all sounds obvious. However, in spite of all the policy statements and service transformations over the last 50–60 years, people with mental health problems are still met as 'cases' and 'diagnoses'. If the perspectives and approaches of person-centredness, recovery and service user involvement are going to have a more real impact and contribute to real changes in people lives, then three things need to happen.

First, we need to understand the radical change involved in placing the person in the centre. In present services much of what is talked about, decided upon and done is on the premises of the service systems and professionals. The belief in and power of expertise is problematic if we are to base our practices on collaboration and dialogues. Meeting the person as an autonomous individual in her/his social and cultural context involves developing collaborative partnerships. Harlene Anderson (2012) states that the essence of collaborative dialogue is the professional's stance: a way of being 'with' the other. It includes the notions of mutual inquiry, relational and social competence, privileging the wisdom and expertise of the person and his/her network, and learning to live with uncertainty – meaning trying to avoid quick and premature decisions and letting procedures stand in the way of the person's life.

Secondly, we need to acknowledge mental health problems as personal *and* social. The individualistic biomedical knowledgebase of the dominant psychiatric community is a barrier to understanding what is going on as well as to meeting people as human beings in their local community with strengths and challenges in their lives. It is also a barrier to developing helpful help. The core problems identified may well be more related to the community than the person. WHO policies (WHO 2007, 2013) request commitment to this position with emphasis on the transition from social marginalisation to full citizenship. It states that an approach that focuses primarily on individuals is not sufficient in creating access to valued roles those individuals will be able to occupy in community settings. Instead, public intervention and debate are required to promote and monitor the bond of citizenship that connects people to their communities.

Thirdly, as Larry Davidson writes, life is not an outcome (Davidson et al. 2012). Mental health issues are about well-being and finding ways of getting on with life, and cannot easily be manualised or generalised. Recovery and person-centred approaches involve reawakening hope for the future, developing a sense of meaning and purpose in life, and doing the things you want to do. It is about taking back control over your situation and nurturing and pursuing ambitions. Therefore, we need to expand the narrow evidence base in which randomised controlled trials (RCTs) are the gold standard. We need to take practice-based evidence seriously, where the lived experience of service users, family members and practitioners is recognised. We need to take some steps forwards and move beyond tokenism and rhetoric.

References

Anderson, H. (2012) Collaborative relationships and dialogic conversations: ideas for a relationally responsive practice. *Family Process*, **51**, 8–10.

Beresford, P. (2005) Developing the theoretical basis for service user/survivor-led research and equal involvement in research. *Epidemiologia e Psichiatria Sociale*, **14**, 4–9.

Borg, M. (2007) *The nature of recovery as lived in everyday life: Perspectives of individuals recovering from severe mental health problems*. Dissertation, Norwegian University of Science and Technology, Faculty of Social Sciences and Technology Management, Department of Social Work and Health Science, Norway. Available from: http://brage.bibsys.no/xmlui/handle/11250/267630

Borg, M. and Davidson, L. (2008) Recovery as lived in everyday life experience. *Journal of Mental Health*, **17**, 129–41.

Borg, M. and Kristiansen, K. (2008) Working on the edge. Everyday life research from Norway on the meaning of work for people recovering in psychosis. *Disability & Society*, **23**, 511–23.

Borg, M. and Topor, A. (2013) Virksomme relasjoner. Bedringsprosesser ved alvorlige psykiske lidelser [Helpful relationships. Recovery in severe mental illness], Kommuneforlaget AS, Oslo.

Borg, M., Karlsson, B., and Kim, S. (2009) User involvement in mental health care services – principles and practices. *Journal of Psychiatric and Mental Health Nursing*, **16**, 285–92.

Borg M, Karlsson B, Stenhammer A. (2013) *Recoveryorienterte praksiser – en systematisk kunnskapssammenstilling*. Trondheim: NAPHA, rapport nr. 4. 2013.

Davidson, L. (2003) *Living outside mental illness: Qualitative studies of recovery in schizophrenia*, New York University, New York.

Davidson, L. (2007) Habits and other anchors of everyday life people with psychiatric disabilities may not take for granted. *Journal of Occupational Therapy Research*, **27**, 1–9.

Davidson, L., O'Connell, M., Tondora, J., Staeheli, M.R., and Evans, A.C. (2005) Recovery in serious mental illness: A new wine or just a new bottle? *Professional Psychology: Research and Practice*, **36**, 480–7.

Davidson, L., Kirk, T., Rockholz, P., Tondora, J., O'Connell, M.J., and Evans, A.C. (2007) Creating a r ecovery-oriented system of behavioral health care: Moving from concept to reality. *Journal of Psychiatric Rehabilitation*, **31**, 23–31.

Davidson, L., Tondora, J., and Ridgway, P. (2012) Life is not an "outcome": Reflections on recovery as an outcome and as a process. *Journal of Psychiatric Rehabilitation*, **13**, 1–8.

Freire, P. (1972) *Pedagogy of the Oppressed*, Penguin, Harmondsworth.

Karlsson, B. and Borg, M. (2013) *Psykisk helsearbeid som humane og sosiale perspektiver og praksiser*, Gyldendal Akademisk, Oslo.

Karlsson, B., Borg, M., and Kim, H.S. (2008) From good intentions to real life: introducing crisis resolution teams in Norway. *Nursing Inquiry*, **15** (3), 206–15.

Lafferty S and Davidson R. (2006) Person-centred care in practice: An account of the implementation of the Tidal Model in an adult acute admission ward in Glasgow. *Mental Health Today* March, pp. 31–4.

Martinsen, K. (1989) *Omsorg, sykepleie og medisin – historisk-filosofiske essays*, Universitetsforlaget, Oslo.

McCormack, B. and McCance, T. (2010) *Person-Centred Nursing : Theory and Practice*, Wiley-Blackwell, Oxford.

Proctor, G. (2006) Therapy: opium for the masses or help for those who need it? in *Politicizing the Person-centred Approach – An Agenda for Social Change* (eds G. Proctor, M. Cooper, P. Sanders, and B. Malcolm), PCCS Books, Ross-on Wye, UK, pp. 66–80.

Repper, J. and Perkins, R. (2003) *Social Inclusion and Recovery: A Model for Mental Health Practice*, Baillière Tindall.

Rogers, C.R. (1978) The foundations of the person-centered approach. *Education*, **100** (2), 98–107.

Slade, M. (2009) *Personal Recovery and Mental Illness: A Guide for Mental Health Professionals*, Cambridge University Press, Cambridge.

Tew, J. (2005) Core themes of social perspectives, in *Social Perspectives in Mental Health: Developing Social Models to Understand and Work with Mental Distress* (ed J. Tew), Jessica Kingsley Publishers, London, pp. 13–32.

WHO (2007) *The People-Centred Health Care – A Policy Framework*, World Health Organization, Geneva.

WHO (2013) *The Mental Health Action Plan 2013-2020*, World Health Organization, Geneva.

CHAPTER 17

Weathering the seasons of practice development: moving towards a person-centred culture in complex continuing care[1]

Nadine Janes[1], Barbara Cowie[2], Jennifer Haynes[2], Penney Deratnay[2], Shannon Burke[2] & Barbara Bell[2]

[1] *Ryerson University, Toronto, Canada*
[2] *West Park Healthcare Centre, Toronto, Canada*

Introduction

Evolving evidence on how to promote better practices in health care casts a spotlight on the context and culture of health-care settings as distinctly impactful. In particular, a culture of person-centredness within an organisation holds promise for creating the 'right' milieu or context for success in quality improvement work and ultimate transformations in care-giving practices. West Park Healthcare Centre ('the Centre'), a Rehabilitation and Complex Continuing Care (CCC) facility in the province of Ontario, Canada, therefore adopted the Person-centred Nursing Framework in 2009 as a signpost for its interprofessional practice improvement work. A programme of work embedded in Practice Development (PD) methodology was initiated with the ultimate aim of shifting the culture of the Centre to one that was person-centred as defined by McCormack and McCance (2010). This chapter reflects the authors' shared experiences and critical reflections on elements of the Person-centred Nursing Framework as a signpost for this difficult culture change work in the context of CCC.

The work in context

Canadian health care, a universally accessible system, is currently characterised by the ideology of managerialism with a drive for greater efficiencies and

[1]The views expressed in this chapter are those of the authors (represented by 'we') and do not necessarily represent those of West Park Healthcare Centre.

Person-Centred Practice in Nursing and Health Care: Theory and Practice, Second Edition.
Edited by Brendan McCormack and Tanya McCance.
© 2017 John Wiley & Sons, Ltd. Published 2017 by John Wiley & Sons, Ltd.

progressive waves of fiscal constraint, juxtaposed with demands for 'quality', 'excellence' and 'best practices' (Darbyshire 2008; Duncan et al. 2014). This context is not unique to our nation but rather parallels the pressures on systems across the globe.

The Centre formally took up the mandate to provide evidence-based interprofessional care in 2003 through corporate-wide processes based largely on project management strategies and best practice guideline implementation. While some practice improvement was realised over time, struggles with sustainability led us to a more critical reflection on our approach. What was revealed was our neglect of the socio-political context of our workplace (i.e. culture) in our practice improvement work. Consequently, in 2009 we selected the Person-centred Nursing Framework (McCormack & McCance 2006) to help structure our work going forwards and practice development (PD) as our methodology, appreciating its explicit focus on facilitating person-centred cultures. PD provides the theory and strategy to shift clinical practices in parallel to fostering the organisational milieu required to sustain and further build on improvements over the long term, the latter reflecting our missed opportunity during our initial practice improvement work.

Overview of the work

In 2010 we initiated an 18-month quasi-experimental study to evaluate PD as an approach to facilitating person-centred, evidence-based practice. What we present from here forwards is a mix of selected results from this study with the critical reflections of the authors, including some of what we learned about the Person-centred Nursing Framework as a guide to shifting workplace culture through PD methodology.

The practice development maple tree

Leadership for the PD work was provided by the Centre's Professional Practice Department. We initially implemented PD across our seven CCC units relying on our five Advanced Practice Nurses (APNs) as lead PD facilitators, supporting the work of 11 Registered Nurses (RNs) as unit-based PD facilitators. The RNs were selected by the APNs in collaboration with unit managers using a standardised tool comprising qualities, skills and related behaviours identified in the literature as enablers of facilitator success (McCormack & Garbett 2003). The APNs and RNs attended a 5-day Foundational PD School at the onset of the work.

The Canadian maple leaf is a strong national symbol, centralised on the Canadian flag. The Canadian maple tree is therefore a fitting metaphor to share our Canadian PD work (Figure 17.1): the growth of our Centre's person-centred culture. The trunk of the tree represents the philosophies and theories that underpin PD methodology. These include critical social theory, phenomenology, critical creativity and chaos theory (e.g. McCormack & Titchen 2006; Titchen et al. 2011), all of which give strength to the branches of the tree.

FOCUS and SAMPLE ACTIVITIES

Focus 1:
- 5-day foundational PD schools (2010, 2011, 2013)
- University of Ulster facilitator courses for APNS

Focus 2:
- Shared visioning (Wish Trees)
- Appreciative inquiry (documentation processes)
- BEET tool (food & beverage events; clinical leadership)
- Claims, Concerns, & Issues (fire incident medication administration)
- Observation of practice (shift exchange; meals)
- Context Assessment Index

Focus 3:
- Active learning workshop (Managing Relationships & Everyday Encounters)
- APN:Service Manager critical companionship
- Interprofessional Clinical Leadership program of development and evaluation

Focus 4:
- Phenomenological study of family experience in CCC
- Photovoice study of patient care experience in CCC
- After death care review and redesign
- Interprofessional Falls prevention strategy

Focus 5:
- Building the Emotionally Intelligent Team program of Learning for Recreation Therapy department
- Critical companionship (APN:nurse)
- Structured reflection for practice reviews

Focus 6:
- Culture collages (person-centred practices)
- Artifacts (leadership)
- Graffiti wall (nursing)
- Cards
- Blob cartoons

Focus 7:
- Interprofessional care delivery model program of development and evaluation
- Interprofessional active learning group

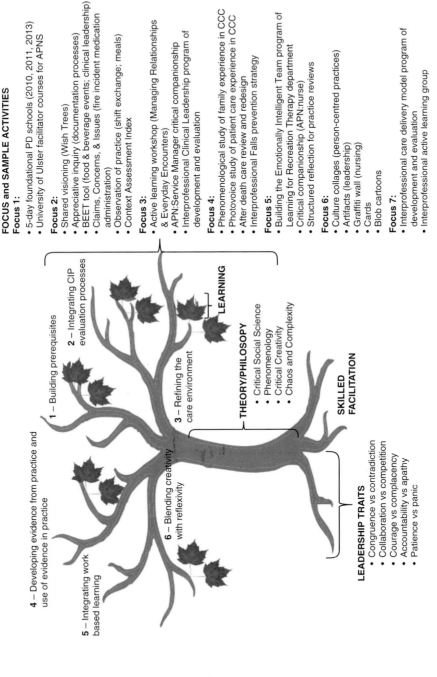

4 – Developing evidence from practice and use of evidence in practice

5 – Integrating work based learning

1 – Building prerequisites

2 – Integrating CIP evaluation processes

3 – Refining the care environment

6 – Blending creativity with reflexivity

LEARNING

THEORY/PHILOSOPY
- Critical Social Science
- Phenomenology
- Critical Creativity
- Chaos and Complexity

SKILLED FACILITATION

LEADERSHIP TRAITS
- Congruence vs contradiction
- Collaboration vs competition
- Courage vs complacency
- Accountability vs apathy
- Patience vs panic

Figure 17.1 The growth of a person-centred culture through practice development (PD). APN, Advanced Practice Nurse; CCC, Complex Continuing Care; CIP, collaborative, inclusive and participatory.

The main branches of the tree represent the main foci of our work (see 1–7 in Figure 17.1) with the smaller deviating branches representing the specific PD methods we used to meet these foci. The branches reflect our attention to building the staff prerequisites and care environment fundamental to person-centred practices as per the Person-centred Nursing Framework, and to acting on the nine PD principles described by Manley et al. (2008, p. 5). Of note is the newest and therefore smallest main branch representing our seventh focus on interprofessional collaborative practice. This branch sprouted a year into our work when our data suggested the need to actively recruit clinicians beyond nursing staff as co-facilitators to enhance team engagement in and commitment to the work.

The leaves of the tree symbolise the learning we experienced. A maple leaf begins as a bud, unfolds into a brilliant green, turns golden with the coming of autumn, and finally dries up before falling to the ground where it nurtures the soil. We took deep reflective dives into our individual and organisational practices through cycles of learning that ultimately nourished our actioning going forwards. We present two of our learning leaves in this chapter.

The roots of the tree reflect what we have come to appreciate as the leadership traits that support the work. Administrative and clinical leaders need to embody PD and move beyond superficial 'support' for 'doing PD' (congruence). This includes what we have coined 'being CIPy' in all they do to reflect the Collaborative, Inclusive and Participatory nature of PD (collaboration). They need to take risks (courage) to challenge deeply entrenched behavioural norms (accountability) and resist reactive and atheoretical approaches to leadership that fall short in enabling their staff and patients to thrive (patience). The roots draw on the soil, which provides nourishment to the tree. The soil reflects the skilled PD facilitation that feeds the work and keeps it alive.

Finally, with the changing Canadian seasons comes the changing nature of the maple tree from budding glory in spring to snow-covered dormancy in winter. Our PD work is equally dynamic in nature, ever adapting and shifting with the changing climate of our organisation and our growth as PD facilitators.

The early facilitator experience

At three points in time during our formal study of PD, all facilitators participated in focus groups and 1:1 interviews to share their experiences of PD as a process for facilitating a person-centred unit-based culture. Data analysis led in part to the following narrative of the gestalt of the experience and the enablers and obstacles along the way.

The gestalt of the facilitator experience

Four themes emerged that captured the overall gestalt of the facilitator experience: a kaleidoscope of emotions, a shouldering of responsibility, an enduring belief, and a sense of aloneness.

Kaleidoscope of emotions. The emotive experience of being a facilitator can be likened to a kaleidoscope: a patchwork of highs and lows and everything in between. In response to the good moments, facilitators described being 'happy', 'energised', 'keen', 'satisfied' and 'enthusiastic'. Conversely, when encountering the inherent challenges of their role, facilitators described experiencing PD as 'painful and messy', 'demanding', 'scary' and 'draining'.

Shouldering responsibility. Facilitators carried a weight of responsibility. There is 'lots on my shoulder' as one facilitator described, itemised by others as expectations from peers and management to 'be perfect', to 'solve problems', to 'motivate others' and to 'set an example'. These expectations were experienced by some facilitators as 'beyond my ability' at times and as a source of frustration. Conversely, other facilitators described feeling 'excited' by the responsibility they shouldered and 'getting better' at working through problems over time. The nature of the problems shouldered by facilitators ranged from histrionic, relational issues between staff that were particularly complex, to what one facilitator described as 'everything' including 'petty things' which she felt belonged in the 'garbage bin'.

Enduring belief. Across all focus group sessions facilitators demonstrated an overall belief in PD as a 'good thing', a 'phenomenally good concept'. They described it as something 'needed' and expressed belief in its ability to bring about 'positive change'. This enduring belief existed despite the 'hiccups in the process' of PD. What appeared to help sustain the facilitators' ability to 'keep going' and 'see it through' was an appreciation for 'baby steps'. Facilitators acknowledged the need to be 'flexible', 'strong' and 'confident' as 'change cannot come quickly'.

Sense of aloneness. Although infrequently mentioned, from the first focus group session through to the final sessions at the end of the study, facilitators alluded to being different as a result of their PD training and subsequent facilitator role and to feeling 'alone'. This sense of separateness was apparent when facilitators lamented the lack of opportunity they had to 'talk' to each other and to 'share' experiences, leaving one facilitator feeling 'really lost'.

Enablers and obstacles

A number of factors shaped the PD work, captured in five themes that speak to what helps move the work forwards and what serves to impede progress: time, support, engagement, inclusivity and momentum.

Time

On an operational level, finding time to implement PD strategies on their units and to engage in continuous learning to enhance their facilitator skills was a universally experienced challenge for facilitators, described by one facilitator as 'the greatest challenge' of the work. PD activities involved in creating a shared vision for a unit were experienced as 'time consuming', made more so because of shift work. Endeavouring to include as many staff from the team as possible in the visioning work meant facilitators had to find ways to engage staff across three shifts and during varied patterns of days off: 'everyone can't be there at the same time to do the activities'. In the context of day-to-day practice accountabilities, PD was experienced as an add-on to an already heavy workload by many.

Time also factored into facilitators' expressed patience waiting for positive results from the work. It is important to 'give [change] the time it needs' and 'for things to take root and to mature'. Doing otherwise may set unrealistic expectations for PD and lead to waning engagement as alluded to by facilitators.

Support

While some facilitators described the importance of support from their peers for the work, support from administrative and clinical leaders emerged as particularly influential. The consequence of a perceived lack of support led one facilitator to feeling 'discouraged' while receiving sufficient support left another facilitator feeling 'energised' with the work.

Support for facilitators manifested itself in transactional efforts like a manager being present at a unit PD activity (e.g. visioning exercise) or helping facilitators organise their workday to reserve time for PD work. For many, support was also described as something more, involving the leader as 'part of the process'. Manager and APN (aka lead facilitator) engagement was identified as useful in mitigating opposition from staff to the PD work. This effect was linked to these leaders' perceived 'authority'.

Support was also conceptualised as leader behaviours that helped mitigate a facilitator's 'shouldering of responsibility', characteristic of the gestalt of their experience. Facilitators valued managers' 'acknowledge[ment]' for 'how hard this work actually is', periodic 'checking in to see how it's [PD] going', and 'reinforce[ing]' the importance of PD and the facilitator role on the unit with staff. From APNs, facilitators valued coaching and opportunities to build confidence in their facilitation skills.

Engagement

A lack of staff engagement, at times displayed as overt opposition to PD, was consistently identified by facilitators as an obstacle to success, leaving them feeling 'disheartened', 'frustrate[ed]' and as if 'nothing will change'. Every facilitator relayed the negative influence of 'dissenters', 'naysayers' and 'bad apples': staff who are 'sceptical', 'not open to change', 'pessimistic' and 'resistant'. One facilitator lamented how such staff 'are like poison to the group'. From facilitators' perspective, a lack of staff engagement can be attributed in part to staff belief that 'it [PD] won't last'.

In contrast to disengagement, 'some of the staff welcomed [PD] with open arms and were excited'. Such staff were described by facilitators as 'open', 'positive', 'passionate' and 'engaged in the process'. One facilitator summarised this range in staff engagement as follows: 'I guess overall I have experienced both extremes of the spectrum.'

Momentum

Momentum was minimally highlighted by facilitators as an enabler of PD until the final phase of data collection. Over time 'momentum' for the work appeared to wane from facilitators' perspectives. While units completed shared visions of person-centred practice, some facilitators lamented that 'we have not done anything to change the way we are'. Not 'moving forwards' led to facilitator 'discourage[ment]', 'backward [movement] into old habits' on units, 'negative[ity]' about PD, and according to one facilitator, a 'slip' in her 'confidence'. A particularly resentful feeling was conveyed by one facilitator who spoke of 'so much effort and time' at the beginning of PD implementation but a lack of 'continuous' work: 'I think the people that started this process just dumped it on us and expect us to carry it.'

Inclusivity

The theme of inclusivity as an enabler emerged more than one year after PD was introduced. The majority of facilitators at that time agreed that having more staff 'exposed' to PD through some training would be a 'game changer'. It would 'get everyone on the same page', enhance feelings of being 'included' among staff, minimise 'tension and resistance' and build 'cohes[ion]'. This was the budding start of our interprofessional collaboration branch whereby staff from allied health professions were invited to PD facilitator training.

Despite the challenges revealed in the above narrative, PD did result in facilitators experiencing personal growth as well as changes in their approach as leaders on the unit. On a contextual level facilitators described positive changes in relational patterns amongst health-care team members, responses to unit issues and practice dilemmas, and in the emotional tone of the unit.

The current facilitator experience

Metaphorically, the early days of PD can be likened to a maple tree in spring: a time of new growth while we worked to shift our ways of working and quality improvement processes. There was an energy on the units and a hope for brighter days. The Centre's culture at the unit (micro) level made some movement towards person-centredness during the study. The spring season, however, isn't without its rainy days: the process of facilitating this shift posed emotional, intellectual and operational challenges for the facilitators. These findings parallel recent exploration into the PD facilitator experience by others (Crisp & Wilson 2011; Shaw 2012).

The RN facilitators, with the help of the APN lead facilitators, finalised shared visions on the units for person-centred practices through engagement of the interprofessional team. The process took months across the units due to the dis-ease many staff felt as we exposed the incongruencies between our espoused and real practices. Facilitators were challenged to manage a continuum of responses from staff, service users and managers, described by Haynes and Janes (2011) as dealing with relational complexities beyond anything they could have anticipated. Subsequent to the visioning work, efforts were made to action on discrete practices the unit teams wanted to shift. In parallel to the unit-based work, the primary author worked strategically to embed PD methods in organisational-level ways of working through such efforts as an interprofessional active learning group and structured departmental programmes of learning.

Our PD maple tree did begin to bloom and grow but the autumn came early. Some progress was made at the unit and corporate levels, but it was negatively impacted by multiple competing priorities in the organisation such as turnover of unit managers, preparing for accreditation, and a significant service redesign with associated nursing staff layoffs. The waning momentum identified by facilitators at the end of the study period as well as support- and time-related obstacles got worse. Our branches became bare and our maple tree settled into a winter state of dormancy as the PD work became less visible, focused and impactful. While the work has not ceased altogether, it has been a long winter. We have yet to regenerate and bloom. We continue our PD work more by stealth to give the organisation a chance to respite from the difficult journey towards person-centredness, and time for the authors to learn from that early journey and map out our work going forwards.

Reflection on using the Person-centred Nursing Framework

Facilitating person-centred practices through PD methodology is hard work given the operational context of health care (i.e. too little time, too few resources, and too many demands). This parallels a central challenge of *any* approach to changing practices and/or cultures in health care. When we reflect on our seasons with PD as described above, we propose that other challenges unique to facilitating person-centred practices as per the Person-centred Nursing Framework specifically slowed our progress. The leaves of learning we share now relate to our naivety to the complexities of developing facilitators' knowing of self (prerequisite) and of promoting a sharing of power and decision-making (the care environment) in the CCC context.

Leaf 1: the complexities of knowing self

To facilitate a person-centred culture, staff need to know self. The depth of personal knowing required and the scholarly, critical reflection needed to achieve it proved beyond the capability of the majority of our RN PD facilitators. They struggled with the *shouldering of responsibility* and finding ways to shift deeply entrenched patterns of dysfunctional behaviour to more person-centred ways amongst their peers, all the while coping with the inevitable 'failures' along the way.

The following excerpt from a reflection written by one of the APN facilitators speaks to this mindfulness and the associated vulnerabilities she experienced while accessing the requisite scholarship to enhance her effectiveness.

The facilitation of critical consciousness with unit staff in the direction of being person-centred may exact a cost for the facilitator involved. For me, this was a gut wrenching and vulnerable experience emerging from the cyclic effects of 'cognitive load' and drain as described by Pitner and Sakamoto (2005). During times of staff disengagement and criticism of PD, I heard comments that extracted a piece of my soul. I had to step back, remove my rose colored glasses to take a very deep dive into reexamining 'knowing self' and the part that I may have played in things not going well with the work. I needed to delve deeply into what the staff may be feeling and experiencing. I felt vulnerable and experienced shame. It was imperative that I viewed myself as staff saw me in the context of my helping role and I therefore drew on Schein's (2009) concepts of 'social currencies' (p. 14) and 'social theatre' (p. 21). I questioned whether staff viewed me as having higher status and felt that deference was required? In asking for help, did staff experience 'one-downness' and experience me as being 'one-up' (Schein 2009, p. 31)? In seeing myself as others do, I am consciously thinking about Schein's reflective question: 'I wonder what was going on backstage?' (p. 22). I have also used Schein's work (2013) as a guide to effective helping by cultivating 'the gentle art of asking instead of telling' and manifesting a spirit of humble inquiry.

Worried about burdening already busy and fatigued staff with expectations for facilitating beyond their individual resources, we acted on this learning by relieving our RNs from being PD facilitators after the study period. We limited the shouldering of lead facilitator responsibility to our APNs who, by virtue of their graduate level education, we felt had the advanced abilities for critical, scholarly reflexivity needed to truly 'know self'.

Leaf 2: sharing power and decision-making in context

Power sharing and shared decision-making are intricately linked as contextual factors that enable person-centredness in a health-care facility. Reflecting on our experiences, however, we have learned that shifting to these specific relational patterns at the micro-level may require a significant process of unlearning, facilitated by more support than we had anticipated. We ruminated on our facilitators' continuous cries for support and questioned why is this work so hard? Why isn't everyone jumping at the chance to take up the 'opportunity'?

We learned that the nature of caring for particular patient populations within certain interprofessional care delivery models needs careful and critical consideration in building the right care environment for person-centredness to thrive. Various configurations of shared power and decision-making evolve over time for diverse reasons in different contexts. Some contexts may require very specific facilitator strategies to move old patterns in a new direction.

The nature of relationships between clinicians and patients in CCC and their families is unique. Our patients come to live with us, many for years and most until their death. They bring with them a personal narrative of their journey with chronic illness: one that has been protracted, dynamic, and impactful on self and others. Their journey has influenced how they perceive their care needs and interrelationships with their formal and informal care providers. Alongside many of our patients comes their family or significant other: individuals who also bring a narrative of their journey supporting and caring for their loved one throughout their chronic illness trajectory. Being person-centred, including sharing power and decision-making in partnership with CCC patients and families, consequently requires deep understanding, unwavering sensitivity and artful negotiation from clinicians.

The relational challenges of CCC have received very little empirical attention (McGilton et al. 2008). The presence of unregulated care providers (UCPs) in CCC environments may pose a particular challenge to person-centred relationships requiring further study. UCPs represent a group of workers in long-term care type environments such as CCC who experience a power imbalance within health-care teams, often feeling unheard and disempowered (Janes et al. 2008; McGilton et al. 2008). Our experiences suggest that this marginalised status complicates efforts to involve them in promoting shared power and decision-making in their relations with patients and their families due largely to their own unsatisfied needs for authority. Our facilitators' cries for support related in part to these complexities.

By not doing a deep enough dive into the uniqueness of our patient population and staffing model, we wonder if we didn't set up our PD facilitators for obstacles that were ultimately beyond their ability to influence. Actioning on this learning, we are now working more systematically to better understand the relational complexities of CCC and of our particular organisation for the tough work that is PD. We initiated two formal studies to expand our understanding: a photovoice study into the care experiences of our CCC patients, and a phenomenological study into the experiences of families in CCC. We anticipate the learning from these studies will be helpful in understanding how best to translate the Person-centred Nursing Framework into effective facilitation strategies that target our particular relational context.

Conclusion

We looked to the Person-centred Nursing Framework to guide us towards a person-centred culture. Without question the Person-centred Nursing Framework makes clear *the destination*: what needs to be in place to position person-centred practices for success. What we were unsuspecting of was the nature of *the journey*: how to avoid wrong turns, if not driving off the road all together.

Naive to the road conditions, so to speak, we placed expectations on our RN PD facilitators and on ourselves as leaders of the PD work that were perhaps unfair in the context of our workplace. We therefore narrowed our selection criteria for lead facilitators to clinicians with graduate education, in recognition of the complexities of knowing self. We are also stepping back to better understand and account for the relational uniqueness of CCC to better ready ourselves to re-engage in PD. This pre-work will be critical in moving our maple tree from its current winter phase of dormancy to a spring season full of new growth for our PD work.

Acknowledgements

The authors wish to acknowledge TD Bank Group for their funding support for the Practice Development programme described in this chapter. Also, Maggie Barnes-Ahlbrand, physiotherapist at West Park Healthcare Centre, for her conceptual contributions to the Practice Development metaphor presented in this chapter.

References

Crisp, J. and Wilson, V. (2011) How do facilitators of practice development gain the expertise required to support vital transformation of practice and workplace cultures? *Nurse Education in Practice*, **11**, 173–8.

Darbyshire, P. (2008) 'Never mind the quality, feel the width': The nonsense of 'quality', 'excellence', and 'audit' in education, health and research. *Collegian*, **15**, 35–41.

Duncan, S., Rodney, P.A., and Thorne, S. (2014) Forging a strong nursing future: insights from the Canadian context. *Journal of Research in Nursing*, **19**, 621–33.

Haynes and Janes N. (2011) Visioning with service users: tensions and opportunities for a new facilitator. *International Practice Development Journal* **1**(1), art. 8.

Janes, N., Sidani, S., Cott, C., and Rappolt, S. (2008) Figuring it out in the moment: A theory of unregulated care providers' knowledge utilization in dementia care settings. *Worldviews on Evidence-Based Nursing*, **5**, 13–24.

Manley K, McCormack B, Wilson V (eds). (2008) *International Practice Development in Nursing and Healthcare*. Oxford: Blackwell Publishing Ltd.

McCormack, B. and Garbett, R. (2003) The characteristics, qualities and skills of practice developers. *Journal of Clinical Nursing*, **12**, 317–25.

McCormack, B. and McCance, T. (2006) Developing a conceptual framework for person-centred nursing. *Journal of Advanced Nursing*, **56** (5), 472–9.

McCormack, B. and McCance, T. (2010) *Person-Centred Nursing: Theory and Practice*, Wiley-Blackwell, Oxford.

McCormack, B. and Titchen, A. (2006) Critical creativity: melding, exploding, blending. *Educational Action Research*, **14** (2), 239–66.

McGilton, K., Guruge, S., Librado, R., Block, L., and Boscart, V. (2008) Healthcare aides' struggle to build and maintain relationships with families in complex continuing care settings. *Canadian Journal on Aging*, **27** (2), 135–43.

Pitner, R.O. and Sakamoto, I. (2005) The role of critical consciousness in multicultural practice: Examining how its strength becomes its limitation. *American Journal of Orthopsychiatry*, **75** (4), 684–94.

Schein, E.H. (2009) *Helping*, in *How To Offer, Give, And Receive Help*, Berrett-Koehler Publishers, Inc, San Francisco.

Schein, E.H. (2013) *Humble Inquiry, The Gentle Art of Asking Instead of Telling*, Berrett-Koehler Publishers, Inc., San Francisco.

Shaw T. (2012) Unraveling the consequences of practice development: an exploration of the experiences of healthcare practitioners. *International Practice Development Journal* **2**(2), art. 2.

Titchen A, McCormack B, Wilson V, Solman A. (2011) Human flourishing through body, creative imagination, and reflection. *International Journal of Practice Development* **1**(1), art. 1.

CHAPTER 18

Person-centred community nursing

Caroline Dickson
Queen Margaret University, Edinburgh, UK

Introduction

There is currently a political move towards implementing person-centred care as an approach to keeping people well and avoiding unnecessary hospital admissions. Community nursing (CN) plays a vital role within this agenda. The challenge set by the Health Foundation (2014) is to move from traditional approaches of 'doing for and to' to 'with', requiring a fundamental shift in the way services are delivered as well as roles and responsibilities of both staff and patients. Drawing on research into the role of Specialist Practitioner District Nurses (SPDNs), the aim of this chapter is to illustrate person-centred practice within CN in the home. However, as CN practice extends beyond the home environment to the community, I propose McCormack and McCance's (2010) Person-centred Nursing Framework can also be useful in broader population-based contexts of practice. I will begin by considering CNs' roles in achieving person-centred outcomes. I will then introduce research I have undertaken and interpret some of the findings from a person-centred perspective before broadening the debate. The chapter will close with reflections on using the Person-centred Nursing Framework.

Person-centred outcomes

Community nurses are ideally placed to deliver person-centred outcomes, working interdependently, often within patients' own homes or in non-clinical locations, with patients, families, groups and populations. Whilst models of CN, like that of Orem and Newman, promote holistic practice, resilience, independence, health and well-being within systems of family, community and the environment also feature (Fawcett & Desanto-Madeya 2013). Contemporary health visiting (HV) and school nursing (SN) practice is based on salutogenesis or health-creating models rather than on factors that cause disease (Antonovsky 1987; Cowley et al. 2015). In contemporary health care, new service models arguably augment CNs' practice values by overtly seeking to enable person-centred care. These new models are clearer about the importance

Person-Centred Practice in Nursing and Health Care: Theory and Practice, Second Edition.
Edited by Brendan McCormack and Tanya McCance.

of coordinated care, the enabling role of the professionals and strengths-based approaches aimed at tapping into and promoting social capital. The 'House of Care,' promoted by The King's Fund (http://www.kingsfund.org.uk/sites/files/kf/field/field_publication_file/delivering-better-services-for-people-with-long-term-conditions.pdf) is a model that aims to enable and empower patients with long-term conditions to take an active role in directing their own care and support through personalised care planning (Coulter et al. 2013). Central to the model is partnership working with patients, crucially, within supportive systems and processes that will make this happen. At the other end of the lifespan, contemporary Scottish HV and SN practice is based on 'Getting it Right for Every Child' (GIRFEC) (http://www.gov.scot/Topics/People/Young-People/gettingitright). This inter-agency approach focuses on improving outcomes for children, young people and their families based on a shared understanding of well-being. It is an open, transparent partnership approach between children, their families and professionals underpinned by consistent high standards of cooperation, joint working and communication. These models of co-production reflect a shift in thinking within health care as a means of addressing the inability of health and social care services to meet the demands of the changing demographics within the population. Their aim is to develop service users who are well-informed, proactive partners in care, motivated to self-manage.

Within district nursing (DN) (similar to home or home health nursing) in the UK, however, there is currently a lack of robust service models to guide practice. In England, a vision and model for DN was published in 2012 based on the 6Cs from the Framework of Compassion in Practice (NHS England 2012): care, compassion, competence, communication, courage and commitment. However, the focus on professional behaviours appears to miss the emphasis of approaches that enable self-management and co-production with patients. Enabling patient choice is included as a foundational principle, but there is no clarity about how this is achieved, nor the impact on person-centred outcomes. These aspects are, however, emphasised in the principles of DN identified by the Queens Nursing Institute (2009): 'better care, closer to home', 'patient choice', 'integrated care' and 'co-production'. Unfortunately, the most recent definition of DN according to the Department of Health (England) (2013, p. 8) reflects a more outdated, deficits model of DN practice:

> [Specialist Practitioner] DNs are qualified nurses who have undertaken a further graduate Specialist Practitioner programme. They lead and support a team to deliver care in a variety of community settings. The nature of DN has changed to meet the needs of patients in the community. Complex care once only delivered in acute settings is now being provided by DN teams in collaboration with key partners.

An exploration of 'specialisation'

My research explored specialisation as experienced by SPDNs, often referred to as qualified DNs, within one NHS Board in Scotland. Eight participants with experience ranging from 7 to 26 years engaged with the study. I used interpretive phenomenological analysis to uncover what Heidegger referred to as 'person-in-context' (Smith 2007). The strength of this approach was in identifying what Heidegger referred to as being-in-the-world, which he suggested gets lost in everydayness. This approach revealed one interpretation of what it is like to be a SPDN, by looking beyond the everyday to implicit experiences in and of practice. Its strength was the ability to uncover what worked and what did not work as well as differences in practice (Smith et al. 2009). Through semi-structured interviews and audio-journals, two supraordinate themes were revealed: *being expert* and *managing responsibility*. *Being expert* was suggestive of person-centred approaches to care, although it appeared to be constrained at times by the care environment. This theme is the focus of this chapter. In the following sections, findings have been interpreted through the lens of McCormack and McCance's Person-centred Nursing Framework.

Care processes

Participants' expertise was evidenced in their person-centred approach, not only to care, but also to team leadership. This was interpreted as being what Rogers (1961) referred to as being a skilled helper. His description was directed at therapeutic relationships between counsellor and patient, although Benner (1984) also used this concept in her attempt to identify what it means to be an expert nurse. In this study, being a skilled helper was extended to interactions with carers and the team. Participants' approach in team leadership was demonstrated in the way some participants were enabling their team to problem-solve:

> *I think sometimes we maybe staff nurses will not see the bigger picture and it's something you have to tease out of them ... well what will we do about that? And have you thought about that? ... because sometimes they will go in and follow more of a checklist approach as opposed to ... because they haven't been exposed to that higher level of assessment and thinking ... '*
>
> INTERVIEWER: So what is the bigger picture that you're talking about?
>
> *It's that patient in their house and their life ... not just what I'm going in to do, it's not that task part.*
>
> *Participant 002*

However, there were also examples where helping was more concerned with 'doing for', reflecting old ways of working. This appeared to manifest for a number of reasons, including a perception of a lack of willingness of registered nurses in the team to make autonomous decisions and the need to assure competent staff delivering care as lone workers.

With the change of orientation of health and social care services, participants described using their expertise to address patient and carer expectations, which they perceived could at times be unrealistic of what the service was able to offer. The theme mediating complexity resonated with findings in a study by Skott and Lundgren (2009). They described this concept in relation to Home

Health Nurses working with ethnic minority families in Sweden, mediating needs and expectation between patients and families. It is also reflective of the expertise literature where 'mediation' is a means of utilising theoretical and practical knowledge, or professional artistry and practical wisdom, which enables expert nurses to understand 'wholeness' or the 'bigger picture' (Hardy et al. 2009). Seeing the bigger picture allowed participants to promote person-centred outcomes. Participants' approach, evident in their interactions with patients and families, described as sympathetic presence in McCormack and McCance's framework, is also a hallmark of person-centred expertise. Demonstration of understanding and empathy extending here to carers and families in diverse situations is referred to as appreciation and attunement by Manley et al. (2005). The manner in which participants achieved this was typical of DN practice, suggestive of what Nagington et al. (2013) referred to as a discourse of friendliness, and Griffiths et al. (2010) referred to as 'therapeutic chatting'.

> *Part of it is understanding where people are coming from, so you do need a little bit of background. The boundaries that carers are working from, you know ... what to expect from families. It's about influencing families not to expect too much of themselves. I see that in palliative care all the time. You know with the family – it's not the patient that is struggling, it's the families that's struggling so it's more knowing when to influence them to access services, to accept a little bit more care*
>
> *Participant 004*

Participants' expertise in assessing patients and their home contexts, allowed them to consider and provide both in the moment and for a range of possible future outcomes. This anticipatory approach was a major theme in the study, linked to their responsibility for being proactive and prepared. Kennedy (2002) referred to this in her early work as 'making visits work'. Her more recent work also found DNs use anticipatory care, although not the view of anticipatory care held by policy makers (Kennedy et al. 2011). Concurring with the findings of my study, SPDNs have the ability to tailor interventions for individuals, maintaining their independence and a 'sense of self'. These findings suggest SPDNs contribute to avoiding unnecessary interventions and hospital admission.

The helping relationship is dependent on the 'helper' bringing part of him/herself to the relationship and the empathetic understanding demonstrated is mutually rewarding (Rogers 1961; Brownhill et al. 2013). One participant described how she worked to maintain visibility and availability within the community to encourage engagement with a particular ethnic population that had been 'hard to reach'. Another used her skills to ensure a carer received the treatment and care they needed, whilst taking the opportunity to negotiate care of her husband. She described how her approach differed from that of her social work colleague, who approached the situation efficiently but with less sensitivity to the patient and carer. The social worker was also less concerned with anticipating future care needs than the SPDN, only appearing to problem-solve in the present. Titchen and Higgs (2001, pp. 274–5) refer to this as 'using the whole self therapeutically to contact and work with the humanity of the patient'. This approach enabled participants in this study to 'negotiate space to care'.

The extent of the emotional toll felt by participants in this study could have been in part due to their person-centred approaches, perhaps for a number of reasons. There was evidence of participants going 'above and beyond' to find solutions to keep people at home. Examples were cited of 'knowing the patient' and 'knowing the family', either in the present circumstances, or because of a family member having been previously cared for too. The increasing challenges of meeting patient and family expectations may also have contributed to an emotional toll. Brownhill et al. (2013) and Redshaw et al. (2013) suggest the reciprocal nature of person-centredness helps CNs, patients and carers cope with death and dying. The study by Redshaw et al. (2013) considered the role of bereavement support visits within McCormack and McCance's Person-centred Nursing Framework. They proposed that relationships with carers, built as a consequence of caring for the patient, enabled CNs to assess how well carers might cope after death. They described 'being present' and 'being open' in their psychological support of patients and carers. They felt they were an outlet for carers following patients' deaths, being viewed as non-judgemental and a confidant, even for those participants with whom they felt rapport was not the best. The bereavement visit, not always viewed as a priority by some managers, was viewed in this study as significant in ending a relationship and of achieving mutual psychological support.

Care environment

There appears to be a disconnect between policies driving person-centred practice and the culture within health care. Organisational systems in this study were not perceived to be supportive in enabling person-centredness. Kennedy et al. (2011) highlight the lack of visibility of person-centredness in organisational criteria and in the allocation of time. Disler and Jones (2010) and Tomison and McDowell (2011) suggest 'nursing need' and 'homebound' as referral criteria hamper the ability to organise care packages, a particular issue for patients nearing the end of life. Kennedy et al. (2011) suggest the categorisation of task 'masks' the time needed for continuity of care, identifying and meeting patient/family wishes collaboratively and enabling patients and carers. Time enabled participants to be anticipatory in their approach to care, ensuring care coordination, particularly during out of hours. Jones (2001) argues that lack of time in nursing is due to the dominance of medicine, which does not commit fully to holistic practice. Carl May (2007) suggests that this is because tasks, rather than holistic care, are the means by which work is measured. He posits that this has currency within organisations, refers to this as 'legitimate work', and suggests there is a dissonance between holistic, person-centred practice and the adoption of business and process models by management to manage health care. Consequently, time and recognition are only allocated for tasks. In this study, participants feeling the need to shoulder responsibility could be a consequence of this mind-set, as could the feelings they described of not being valued by organisational management. Current approaches of safe, effective, person-centred care, advocated by policy (Scottish Government 2010; Department of Health 2014) are demonstrated throughout the analysis, but achieving this is time-dependent. If DN is to be recognised and valued by others, then this aspect of DNs' role has to become legitimate work (May 2007). Kennedy et al. (2011) assert that to increase the visibility of the role, professional discourse should be altered to reflect person-centredness rather than being focused on task.

Prerequisites

Kennedy's early work in 2002 identified the different types of knowledge that enable SPDNs to adopt different strategies to 'make visits work', but my study goes further in highlighting participants' ability to mediate complexity to 'anticipate future care needs', 'finding solutions' and 'enabling carers to care'. This was illustrated by participants' use of sophisticated communication skills, symbolised in the descriptions of 'doing the dance around', which enabled difficult conversations around current status, planned outcomes, coping, and ultimately death and dying.

> You just realise. You just pick up on wee bits and pieces – cues that they are saying to you and the way they communicate with you. Sometimes they are waiting for you – you know they drop you the hint so they can give you the cue and you can say something back and do your dance around and … I think the first thing is that I'll try and do a proper assessment first off and that I'm not just going on, oh I don't think you're managing here, so that I've got something to go on and speak to them about how she can't get out of her chair and a culmination of your experience and your knowledge and your assessment skills
>
> Participant 008

'Being a detective' was part of a quote illustrative of SPDNs' ability to pick up nuances and recognise when a patient was deteriorating, achieved by having 'my senses ablaze'. This is referred to by Watson and Rebair (2014) as therapeutic noticing, where noticing precedes verbal exchange and prompts action. Tanner (2006) suggests this leads to interpretation of the situation and is the first stage of clinical decision-making.

Participants in this study appeared to consider their expertise from what Kotzee (2014) refers to as an anti-intellectualist, 'fluent' standpoint, although my study has revealed SPDNs' ability to articulate practice that, according to Rolfe (1998), is reflective of advanced rather than specialist practice. This may be due to the increased emphasis on the art of nursing, particularly in CN (Potter & Wills 2013) and on reflective practice (Schon 1983). Reflective practice is now a fundamental skill taught in nursing education and is developed in practice. While participants emphasised the role of experience in their development of specialist expertise, they did recognise the contribution of their Specialist Practitioner Qualification (SPQ) programme (Nursing and Midwifery Council 2001). However, their perception that managers favour experience over education does appear to be consistent with the work conducted by Harris et al. (2012). It also may be a contributory factor in the current debate of whether the SPQ programme is fit for purpose. Whichever aspect has been most influential in participants' development into the role of SPDN, participants' expertise in this study reflects McCormack and McCance's person-centred practice and fits with the requirements of current policy driving care of patients within their homes. Their expertise in using strengths-based approaches to care management, balanced with an ability to manage teams to deliver care within communities, is pivotal in avoiding unnecessary hospital admissions.

A people-centred framework to promote healthy populations.

The usefulness of McCormack and McCance's (2010) Person-centred Nursing Framework in population-based contexts of CN practice has not previously been explored in the literature. Public health values, arguably person-centred, underpin the aim of public health, which is promoting healthy populations and reducing health inequalities (Marmott et al. 2010) through social and political effort (Box 18.1). As public health seeks to improve the health of populations, an adaptation of McCormack and McCance's person-centred practice to one that is 'people-centred' could offer a means of service design and of evaluation of current integrated public health practice. However, I propose that the usefulness of such a framework would require some alterations. The intended outcomes of practice would be less concerned with therapeutic cultures and 'care' and more aligned to feelings of well-being, achieving a healthy start in life, resilience-building, building social capital, accessibility of services and justice. Other aspects of the framework would also require some shaping.

Box 18.1 Public health values.

- Equity and social inclusion
- Participation, collaboration and community empowerment
- Social justice and health as a human right.

Source: Health 21 (World Health Organisation 1998)

The aim of promoting health and alliance-building between professionals and users of services reflects some of the central tenets of the care environment. The diverse physical environments of CN practice and the nature of CNs' practice, dependent on integrated service provision, is increasingly being led by social care and the third sector. Current policy driving integration highlights the need for change if, as a society, we are to continue to meet the needs of the population at a time when inequalities have never been greater (Department of Health 2014; Scottish Government 2013a, 2013b). Inter-agency working advocated by professional standards (Nursing and Midwifery Council 2001, 2004, 2010, 2015) means adopting person-centred team-working and collaborative approaches, to achieve 'people-centred' health promotion of individuals, families, groups and communities. Nicola Cotter, Voices Scotland Lead with Chest Heart & Stroke Scotland, has been instrumental in engaging and developing service users and professionals, not only to enable self-management, but to contribute to service design and delivery across Scotland. (Box 18.2).

Box 18.2 Nicola Cotter – Voices Scotland Lead, Chest Heart & Stroke Scotland.

At Chest Heart & Stroke Scotland we aim to improve the quality of life for people living with chest, heart and stroke conditions and over the past two years we have been supporting people to become champions of self-management. We want to raise the profile of self-management as the key to people living a more fulfilled life, enabling individuals to take more control but still feel supported at the same time. The Voices Scotland COSMIC programme supports the public, health and social care staff in the third and statutory sectors, to champion self-management and support people to have a clear strong voice to:
- **INFLUENCE** policy effectively to promote self-management
- **INFORM** people about self-management
- **INVOLVE** people in the development of person-centred services

  Self-management should not and cannot, be seen as something people need to 'just get on with' but through this work we are encouraging a collaborative approach between patients, their families and the professionals who support them. We believe that the COSMIC training and support can galvanise the people of Scotland and the staff who support them, to become real advocates of self-management. We aim to influence the transformational shift that is required to change the culture of a traditional patient-caregiver relationship to one of true partnership with the supporting services in place.

In a 'people-centred' framework, care processes would be concerned less about providing holistic care of the individual, but rather responding to health needs of populations. The process elements could equally be relevant to groups, thereby being used to target health needs of communities. A fundamental skill of CNs is in carrying out health needs assessments, using and analysing qualitative and quantitative data to identify and respond to the health needs of specific populations. The principle of equity, fundamental in public health practice, recognises and respects diversity and engagement. Incorporated in community development approaches, these principles are central in CN practice (Potter & Wills 2013). Community nurses' empowering role puts them in positions where they are able to dispel myths and traditions, whilst respecting and harnessing cultural values and beliefs to promote health and shape service design. Working in partnership with service users allows service users to identify their own needs and find ways of responding in a way that is appropriate for the context. During the programme, a health visitor (HV) student, Lauraine, developed an initiative to meet the needs of young parents. The health need was identified through health needs assessment:

> During my HV programme I worked in partnership with the HV team, inter- agency partners and most crucially young parents within an area of deprivation. The practice development initiative was designed to enhance the health and wellbeing of vulnerable young parents and their babies and young children, through support of other parents and practitioners in a protected group environ- ment. The young parents helped shape their parenting support service. Initial evaluation showed parents felt empowered to make decisions about their education, employment and lifestyle. I think the collaborative approach helped enable and empower all those involved, not only the young mums and dads.
>
>   Khaleelah Lauraine Duncan, Health Visitor, Lewisham and Greenwich Health Care Trust

Promoting a sense of coherence advocated by Antonovsky (1996) and the abil- ity to reach shared decision-making is reflected in a range of health-promoting approaches including behaviour change and empowering, client-centred approaches. These aim to enhance capacity through developing knowledge and skill. 'People-centred' approaches would be concerned with connecting with all members of communities, including those who may be 'hard to reach' for traditional, medically dominated services.

Utilising a 'people-centred' framework, practitioners would need to demon- strate a broad range of prerequisites. Cowley et al. (2015) emphasise the impor- tance of having an orientation to practice that is salutogenic (health-creating), to demonstrate a person-centred approach (human valuing) and to recognise the person-in-situation (human ecology) in HV practice specifically. In-depth knowledge and understanding of the community, gained through population, neighbourhood and community health needs assessments, would be prerequi- sites in CN. Ensuring visibility of services, key to being accessible, and using innovative means to reach out into the community, are evident in CN practice. Some examples are: the use of mobile units in the form of buses and lorries car- rying out health promotion and prevention; being available in communities in shops, community houses and walk-in centres; and health promoting schools, workplaces and cities. Winters et al. (2007) note the importance of having skills of facilitating change.

Reflection on using the Person-centred Nursing Framework

In this chapter I have argued that person-centredness is embedded within CN practice at individual, family, group and populations levels. It is this embedded- ness that enables CNs to play a central role in keeping people well and avoid- ing unnecessary hospital admissions. It is also this embeddedness that has left them feeling that their contribution to health care and promoting health and well-being is invisible (Low & Hesketh 2002; Haycock-Stuart & Kean 2012a, 2012b). Whilst that may be true, McCormack and McCance's person-centred model offers a framework to be able to articulate their contribution and their strengths as practitioners. Research into the appropriateness and usefulness of a 'people-centred' framework may contribute to the ongoing service redesign that places CN at the heart of contemporary, integrated health and social care.

Acknowledgements

I would like to gratefully acknowledge the contributions of the participants in my study, and also those of Nicola Cotter – Voices Scotland Lead, Chest Heart and Stroke Scotland – and Khaleelah Lauraine Duncan, Health Visitor, Lewisham and Greenwich Health Care Trust.

References

Antonovsky, A. (1987) *Unraveling the Mystery of Health: How People Manage Stress and Stay Well*, Jossey-Bass, San Francisco.

Antonovsky, A. (1996) The salutogenic model as a theory to guide health promotion. *Health Promotion International*, **11**, 11–18.

Benner, P. (1984) *From Novice to Expert : Excellence and Power in Clinical Nursing Practice*, Addison-Wesley, Menlo Park, CA.

Brownhill, S., Chang, E., Bidewell, J., and Johnson, A. (2013) A decision model for community nurses providing bereavement care. *British Journal of Community Nursing*, **18** (3), 133–9.

Coulter, A., Roberts, S., and Dixon, A. (2013) Delivering better services for people with long-term conditions. *Building the house of care. London: The King's Fund.*

Cowley, S., Whittaker, K., Malone, M., Donetto, S., Grigulis, A., and Maben, J. (2015) Why health visiting? Examining the potential public health benefits from health visiting practice within a universal service: A narrative review of the literature. *International Journal of Nursing Studies*, **52**, 465–80.

Department of Health (2013) Care in local communities: a new vision and model for district nursing. Available at: https://www.gov.uk/government/uploads/system/uploads/attachment_data/file/213363/vision-district-nursing-04012013.pdf (accessed 8 February 2016).

Department of Health (2014) Adult social care outcomes framework 2015 to 2016. Available at: https://www.gov.uk/government/publications/adult-social-care-outcomes-framework-ascof-2015-to-2016 (accessed 8 February 2016]

Disler, R. and Jones, A. (2010) District nurse role in end-stage COPD: a review. *British Journal of Community Nursing*, **15** (9), 428–33.

England, N.H.S. (2012) *Framework of Compassion in Practice*, NHS England, London.

Fawcett, J. and Desanto-Madeya, S. (2013) *Contemporary Nursing Knowledge: Analysis and Evaluation of Nursing Models and Theories*, 3rd edn, F.A. Davis Co., Philadelphia, PA.

Foundation, H. (2014) *Person-centred care: from ideas to action*, The Health Foundation, London.

Griffiths, J., Ewing, G., and Rogers, M. (2010) "Moving swiftly on." Psychological support provided by district nurses to patients with palliative care needs. *Cancer Nursing*, **33** (5), 390–7.

Hardy, S., Titchen, A., Mccormack, B., and Manley, K. (eds) (2009) *Revealing Nursing Expertise Through Practitioner Inquiry*, Wiley-Blackwell, Oxford.

Harris J, Nimmo S, Cantrell J. (2012) *District nursing skills requirements and options for future education provision: Discussion Paper*. Scottish Government.

Haycock-Stuart, E. and Kean, S. (2012a) Contrasting perceptions about the delivery of care in the community. *Nursing Management – UK*, **18** (10), 26–9.

Haycock-Stuart, E. and Kean, S. (2012b) Does nursing leadership affect the quality of care in the community setting? *Journal of Nursing Management*, **20**, 372–81.

Haycock-Stuart, E., Jarvis, A., and Daniel, K. (2008) A ward without walls? District nurses' perspectives of their workload management priorities and job satisfaction. *Journal of Clinical Nursing*, **17**, 3012–20.

Institute, Q.'s.N. (2009) *2020 Vision. Focusing on the Future of District Nursing. London: Queen's Nursing Institute.*

Jones, A.R. (2001) Time to think: temporal considerations in nursing practice and research. *Journal of Advanced Nursing*, **33** (2), 150–8.

Kennedy, C. (2002) The decision-making process in a district nurse assessment. *British Journal of Community Nursing*, **7**, 505–13.

Kennedy, C., Harbison, J., Mahoney, C., Jarvis, A., and Veitch, L. (2011) Investigating the contribution of community nurses to anticipatory care: a qualitative exploratory study. *Journal of Advanced Nursing*, **67**, 1558–67.

Kotzee, B. (2014) Expertise, fluency and social realism about professional knowledge. *Journal of Education and Work*, **27** (2), 161–78.

Labonte, R. (2001) Capacity building in health promotion, Part 1: For whom? And for what purpose? *Critical Public Health*, **11** (2), 111–27.

Low, H. and Hesketh, J. (2002) *District nursing: the invisible workforce*, The Queen's Nursing Institute, London.

Manley, K., Hardy, S., Titchen, A., Garbett, R., and McCormack, B. (2005) *Changing Patients' Worlds Through Nursing Practice Expertise*, Royal College of Nursing, London.

Marmott M, Allen J, Goldblatt P et al. (2010) *Fair Society, Healthy Lives: Strategic Review of Health Inequalities in England Post-2010. The Marmot Review*. Available at: http://www.instituteofhealthequity.org/projects/fair-society-healthy-lives-the-marmot-review (accessed 9 February 2016).

May, C. (2007) The clinical encounter and the problem of context. *Sociology*, **41**, 29–45.

McCormack, B. and McCance, T. (2010) *Person-Centred Nursing: Theory and Practice*, Wiley-Blackwell, Oxford.

Nagington, M., Luker, K., and Walshe, C. (2013) 'Busyness' and the preclusion of quality palliative district nursing care. *Nursing Ethics*, **20**, 893–903.

Nursing and Midwifery Council (2001) *Standards of Specialist Education and Practice*. London: UKCC.

Nursing and Midwifery Council (2004) *The Code: Standards of conduct, performance and ethics for nurses and midwives*. London: NMC.

Nursing and Midwifery Council (2010) *Standards for Pre-registration Nursing*. London: NMC.

Nursing and Midwifery Council (2015) *The Code for nurses and midwives*. London: NMC. Available at: https://www.nmc.org.uk/standards/code/ (accessed 22 February 2016).

Potter, K. and Wills, J. (2013) Community development and building capacity, in *Sines D, Aldridge-Bent S, Fanning A, Farrelly P* (ed W.J. Potter), *Community and Public Health Nursing*. Oxford, Wiley-Blackwell, pp. 22–36.

Redshaw, S., Harrison, K., Johnson, A., and Chang, E. (2013) Community nurses' perceptions of providing bereavement care. *International Journal of Nursing Practice*, **19**, 344–50.

Rogers, C. (1961) *On Becoming a Person: A Therapist's View of Psychotherapy*, Constable, London.

Rolfe, G. (1998) Beyond expertise: theory, practice and the reflexive practitioner. *Journal of Clinical Nursing*, **6**, 93–7.

Schon, D.A. (1983) *The Reflexive Practitioner*, Temple Smith, London.

Scottish Government. Getting It Right For Every Child (GIRFEC). Available at: http://www.gov .scot/topics/people/young-people/gettingitright (accessed 9 February 2016).

Scottish Government (2010) *The Healthcare Quality Strategy for NHS Scotland*, Scottish Government, Edinburgh.

Scottish Government (2013a) *A route map to the 2020 vision for health and social care*, Scottish Government, Edinburgh.

Scottish Government (2013b) *Everyone Matters: 2020 Workforce Vision*, Scottish Government, Edinburgh.

Skott, C. and Lundgren, S.M. (2009) Complexity and contradiction: home care in a multicultural area. *Nursing Inquiry*, **16** (3), 223–31.

Smith, J.A. (2007) *Qualitative Psychology: A Practical Guide to Research Methods*, Sage, London.

Smith, J., Flowers, P., and Larkin, M. (2009) *Interpretive Phenomenological Analysis: Theory, Method and Research*, Sage, London.

Tanner, C.A. (2006) Thinking like a nurse: a research-based model of clinical judgment in nursing. *Journal of Nursing Education*, **45** (6), 204–11.

Titchen, A. and Higgs, J. (2001) A dynamic framework for the enhancement of health professional practice in an uncertain world: The practice-knowledge interface, in *Practice Knowledge and Expertise in the Health Professions* (eds J. Higgs and A. Titchen), Butterworth Heinemann, Oxford, pp. 215–25.

Tomison, G. and McDowell, J.R.S. (2011) Nurses' needs in delivering palliative care for long-term conditions. *British Journal of Community Nursing*, **16** (6), 274–81.

Watson, F. and Rebair, A. (2014) The art of noticing: essential to nursing practice. *British Journal of Nursing*, **23**, 514–17.

Weeks, J., Scriven, A., and Sayer, L. (2005) The health promoting role of health visitors: adjunct or synergy? in *Health Promoting Practice* (ed A. Scriven), Palgrave Macmillan, London.

Wilhelmsson, S. and Lindberg, M. (2009) Health promotion: Facilitators and barriers perceived by district nurses. *International Journal of Nursing Practice*, **15** (3), 156–63.

Winters, L., Gordon, U., Atherton, J., and Scott-Samuel, A. (2007) Developing public health nursing: barriers perceived by community nurses. *Public Health*, **121** (8), 623–33.

World Health Organization (1998) *Health 21 – Health for all in the 21st century*. European Health For All Series No. 5. Copenhagen: World Health Organization.

CHAPTER 19

Person-centredness in palliative care

Antonia Lannie[1] & Lorna Peelo-Kilroe[2]
[1] *University of Dundee, Scotland, UK*
[2] *Office of the Nursing and Midwifery Services Director, Dublin, Republic of Ireland*

Introduction

This chapter will review palliative care in the context of key elements of the McCormack and McCance (2010) Person-centred Nursing Framework that have particular significance for palliative care assessment and provision. Although palliative care is sometimes seen as a specialty domain, this chapter is appropriate to all health and social care professionals providing palliative care at all levels and in diverse settings. We will discuss areas of significance when developing skills in palliative care that relate to the Person-centred Nursing Framework.

The World Health Organization (2002) defines palliative care as:

> an approach that improves the quality of life of individuals and their families facing the problem associated with life-threatening illness, through the prevention and relief of suffering by means of early identification and impeccable assessment and treatment of pain and other problems, physical, psychosocial and spiritual.

The importance of a person-centred approach in health care is advocated internationally by the World Health Organization (2007, 2013, 2015), and in palliative and end-of-life care within national policy and direction both in the UK (Department of Health 2008, 2010; Scottish Government 2008, 2011) and in Ireland (Health Information and Quality Authority 2012; Health Service Executive 2014; Ryan et al. 2014). The words of Cicely Saunders, founder of the modern hospice movement, perhaps encapsulate the importance of person-centred care in palliative care:

> You matter because you are you, and matter to the end of your life. We will do all we can not only to help you die peacefully, but also to live until you die.

Cultures of person-centred palliative care

Palliative care is guided by health and social care professionals who recognise the inevitability of death, and provide opportunities for individuals, and their families should they so wish, to make decisions and set goals about their care (Health Service Executive 2014). Palliative care delivery requires enhanced emotional awareness and developed interpersonal skills (Bolton 2000). Effective interpersonal ability is linked to emotional intelligence and knowing self, identified as prerequisites to managing the care environment and providing person-centred care in the to Person-centred Nursing Framework.

When interpretations of person-centredness are not clarified there is a risk that the care and culture will be task focused. Manley et al. (2013) maintain that culture is about social contexts and not necessarily about the individual. Individual efforts to provide person–centred care will have limited effect on the overall care experience of service users and their families in the absence of a collective team approach. Developing person-centred cultures requires a focus on change that can maximise the potential for growth, development and human flourishing (Titchen & McCormack 2010). As human beings we need to have an ethical dimension as well as a technical one in order for us to flourish and feel satisfied (Hinchliffe 2004). Maximising potential requires us to engage our whole selves in the provision of care, including our valued competencies, wisdom, knowledge, experience and emotions.

Emotion work in palliative care

Supporting individuals at times of great emotion proves to be a challenge for health-care professionals as they often do not know what to say (Wilkinson et al. 2008). Palliative care involves having 'difficult conversations', which includes sharing sad, bad and difficult news, and dealing with difficult questions including talking about prognosis and dying. It is important that information is shared sympathetically at a pace and depth that enables the person to retain a sense of control and be there in the moment (Schofield et al. 2008; Wilkinson et al. 2008; McCormack & McCance 2010). Honest disclosure of information can have an effect on patient outcomes including anxiety and depression. However, it is also important to have a *sympathetic presence* as well as good communication skills.

Enabling well-being and human flourishing in palliative care

Well-being is a major consideration in palliative care assessment and places equal focus on four domains, namely physical well-being, social well-being, emotional well-being and spiritual well-being (Health Service Executive 2014). There is growing realisation that staff well-being impacts on care experiences and is a necessary consideration when developing cultures of person-centredness. The connection to positive care outcomes for service users becomes obvious when the right decisions are made and acted upon, and Titchen and McCormack (2010) uphold that individuals can recognise and flourish through the expertise of a particular nurse or health-care professional. Perhaps the account of flourishing by Senge et al. (2005) may explain this in part, when they say that there is an effortless transition from inner knowing to right action that is embodied when we flourish.

Feeling valued as a person enables us to flourish and requires us to engage in and nurture relationships with others that make us feel valued (Gaffney 2011). Creating environments where flourishing can take place requires a focus on transforming practice that releases creative positive energy with the purpose of seeing possibilities for change and where this energy is felt by individuals and their families (Titchen et al. 2011). According to McCormack and Titchen (2006) and Titchen and McCormack (2010), when we engage in transformational practice development we also engage our creative, ethical and spiritual senses, making it possible for us to be attuned to our personal attributes and see ourselves and others as whole human beings.

Emotional engagement

This chapter will now consider one of the components of the Person-centred Nursing Framework in relation to emotional engagement – having a sympathetic presence, knowing self, and clarity of values and beliefs. Having a sympathetic presence means 'an engagement that recognises the uniqueness and value of the individual, and reflects the quality of the nurse-patient relationship' (McCormack & McCance 2010, p. 37). An example of how this is carried out in practice is through the use of the following statements from health-care professionals while speaking with older patients with palliative care needs (Lannie 2014). These data were taken from a qualitative study comparing care delivery in two ward settings.

Levels of emotional engagement
Professionals engaged with the person's emotions in three ways: superficial, reflective and authentic engagement. These will be discussed in turn.

Superficial engagement
Superficial engagement is engagement that appears to be acted out to comply with the remit of the professional's role, rather than their personhood:

We are like clowns and change our faces as to what patients want from us.

Staff Nurse Krise, specialist ward

The quotation from Staff Nurse Krise expresses the notion of superficial emotions when engaging with patients. The patient (Jinty), who was a nurse on the same specialist ward for 15 years in which she is now a patient, comments:

> *Her vibes ... I don't know how to word this to be sociable. My vibes are the very same. I don't know how to take her, and I don't know how she takes to me but she's a very funny person. I want to be sociable with everybody, but she is a very* funny *[researcher's emphasis]* lassie. *You can see it in her. I don't know if she likes me and, to be honest with you, and she doesn't like me why does she not tell me, then maybe get it out of the blue. But she can be a funny person. I can be funny as well, but not like that*

> *Jinty, diagnosed with breast cancer with metastases*

This tension between clinical and social perspectives demonstrates that this professional is strange or confusing to the patient. Reflecting on the quotation, it appeared the patient was relating to the nurse's moral agency. Moral agency is an individual's ability to make moral judgments based on some commonly held notion of right and wrong and to be held accountable for those actions (McCormack & McCance 2010).The patient has an idea that her expectations are being breached.

Reflective engagement

Reflective engagement is where professionals emulate emotions by looking at the past such as their personal experience of cancer or that of loved ones in addition to their professional role:

> *I think it is harder if they get a diagnosis that you, because you are nursing them, and you don't think that their condition is that bad, because they are masking it to a certain degree, as older people tend to hide their pain ... and if they get a diagnosis of cancer, then that's very hard because you think, 'My God, how can that be?'*

> *Staff Nurse Krise, medical ward*

From the above quotation it could be argued that Staff Nurse Krise is reflecting on her own emotions and feelings for the patient. She also is recognising the fact that older people may mask pain due to stoicism. This is also exemplified in the quotation from Staff Nurse Jenkins:

> *If you've experienced, as you say, a loved one with cancer as well, that informs how you care for a patient.*

Authentic engagement

Authentic engagement is where professionals' conveyed expressions are unconditionally given from the person rather than perceived totally within the remit of their role:

> *And it's listening to them, keeping them ... safe is not the word, it's their emotions, because it is a death sentence you've just given them and they know that so it is quite hard for them to talk to you .... Even your emotions get involved because it could be your family; it could be mine, it could be anybody's. It is quite difficult.*

> *Staff Nurse Jenkins, medical ward*

Staff Nurse Jenkins focuses on her own emotions in order to show sympathetic presence through being in touch with her inner feelings and knowing self. She also reveals the dual role of professional and personal empathy and how it helps her to form a relationship with patients. Staff Nurse Krise also relates to the context of the specialist ward, stating that having patients for longer combined with being older makes 'one' more professional:

> Here [specialist ward] it is different because you are forming different relationships with your patients. Maybe it is because I am getting older as well, I am a bit more emotional as I get older.

There was another dimension to being authentic and knowing self. On the one hand, some nurses and other professionals are focused on the patient's response, as represented in the quotations from Staff Nurse Jenkins and Staff Nurse Krise. However, there is an aspect of being authentic in the need for professionals to protect themselves from the patient's suffering.

Discussion

It is recognised that for people with advanced and life-limiting illness there are significant levels of distress, including anxiety and depression, that can be left unaddressed (Rayner et al. 2010). The multiple influences on communication between patients and health-care professionals include fears, attitudes, beliefs and values. Communication can be ineffective when health-care professionals 'distance' themselves from the person's concerns. Research has focused on the importance of communication in identifying patients' concerns and having a sympathetic presence (Wilkinson et al. 2008).

It is recognised that emotional management in the stages of palliative care is more complex than a commercial industry, such as the work of flight attendants, discussed in the seminal work of Hochschild (1983), who first explored 'emotion work'. Bolton (2000) critiqued the nature of emotional engagement and stated that nurses played a special role through providing a 'gift' for patients, which was caring through unconditional giving. Fawcett and McQueen (2010) also note how nursing emphasises a holistic relationship between nurse and patient. Holman (2014) stresses the importance of looking after oneself when dealing with sensitive issues in palliative care. However, implementing person-centred relationships in the absence of a guiding framework can make this more of a belief than a reality.

Caring for individuals in palliative care requires the development of effective, sensitive and facilitative interpersonal relationship skills ensuring sympathetic presence. Thorne et al. (2005) reviewed research that addressed the impact of poor communication in cancer care and found that it had a reduced impact on psychosocial experience, treatment decisions and quality of life. Good communication skills are necessary to establish rapport with patients and their families, to elicit and respond to concerns, to undertake holistic assessments and to

Table 19.1 Key points regarding effective communication in palliative care.

Effective communication is:	Effective communication is based on:
• Non judgmental • Empathetic • Genuine and enabling	• Active listening • Reflection and authentic engagement • Legitimisation of persons' views, valuing the knowledge and experience of their needs
• Open and honest • Collaborative • Supportive • Person-centred	• Demonstrating respect for the person and their need for truth • Partnership and inclusiveness • Demonstration of sympathetic presence • Respectful and supportive interaction with and about the person, his/her family and colleagues, recognising all as whole human beings that can flourish

provide information appropriately (Department of Health 2014). There is a balance between emotional engagement as part of person-centred processes and developed interpersonal skills. The two can be articulated through a sympathetic presence.

Providing palliative care requires continuous development of skills and self-awareness (knowing self) to respond to difficult issues that living with and dying from advanced illness can raise for people and their families (Becker 2000). This includes being able to attend to the individual's meaning of death and dying and the associated losses, concerns and fears (Bolton & Murray 2010). Because good palliative care must be person-centred, practice development approaches need to be able to address cultures of care with the aim of transforming workplaces where human flourishing is possible for all.

In the UK and Ireland competence documents have been developed to support palliative and end-of-life care (Department of Health 2008, 2014; National Health Service 2013; Ryan et al. 2014). Communication is of central importance in all competence documents and reflects an understanding of the individual's values and beliefs. Table 19.1 highlights some key points regarding effective communication in palliative care.

Palliative care and the Person-centred Nursing Framework

We recognise that all the elements within McCormack and McCance's (2010) Person-centred Nursing Framework are of equal importance to the development of person-centred palliative care practice and cultures, and we have highlighted five key areas of particular importance that 'speak to' a palliative care approach and principles. We have linked these five areas to the Person-centred Nursing Framework, demonstrated visually in Figure 19.1.

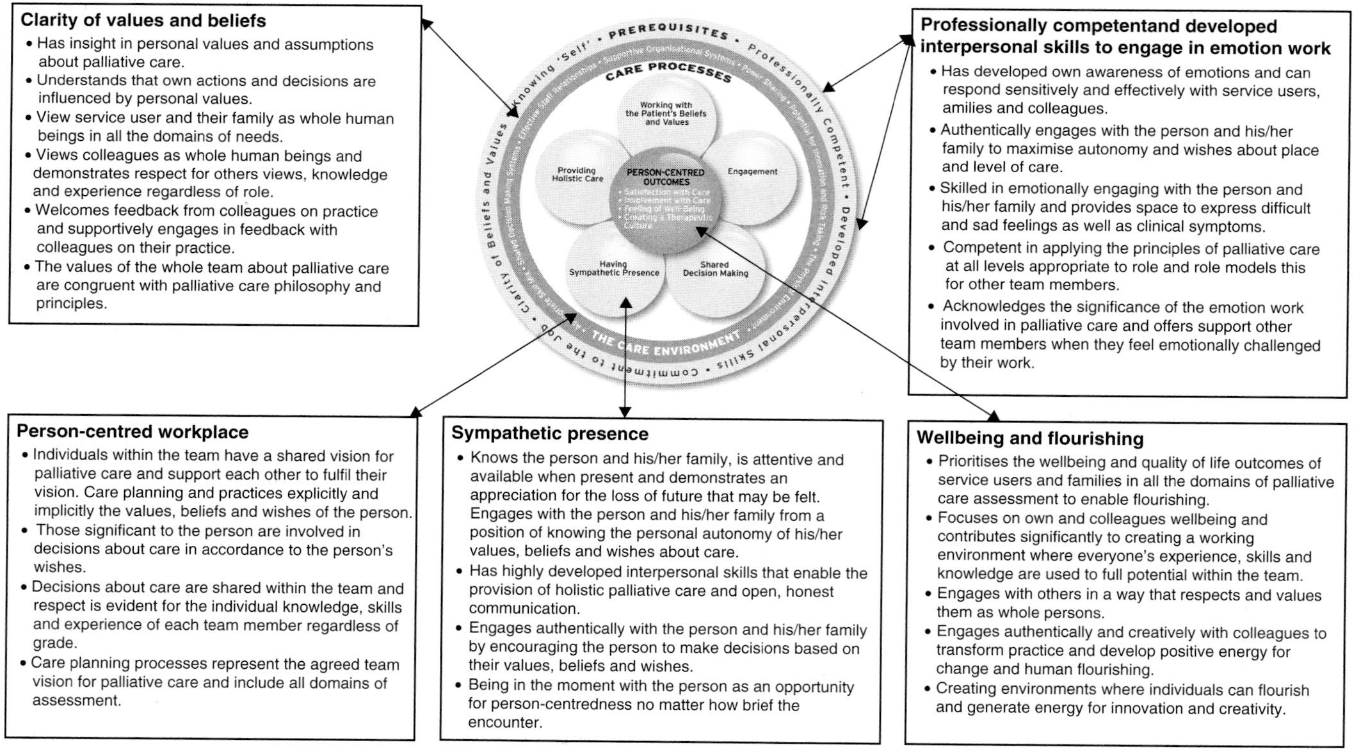
Clarity of values and beliefs
• Has insight in personal values and assumptions about palliative care.
• Understands that own actions and decisions are influenced by personal values.
• View service user and their family as whole human beings in all the domains of needs.
• Views colleagues as whole human beings and demonstrates respect for others views, knowledge and experience regardless of role.
• Welcomes feedback from colleagues on practice and supportively engages in feedback with colleagues on their practice.
• The values of the whole team about palliative care are congruent with palliative care philosophy and principles.
PREREQUISITES
Knowing 'Self' • Professionally Competent • Developed Interpersonal Skills • Commitment to the Job • Clarity of Beliefs and Values
CARE PROCESSES
Working with the Patient's Beliefs and Values
Providing Holistic Care
Engagement
PERSON-CENTRED OUTCOMES
Having Sympathetic Presence
Shared Decision Making
THE CARE ENVIRONMENT
Professionally competentand developed interpersonal skills to engage in emotion work
• Has developed own awareness of emotions and can respond sensitively and effectively with service users, amilies and colleagues.
• Authentically engages with the person and his/her family to maximise autonomy and wishes about place and level of care.
• Skilled in emotionally engaging with the person and his/her family and provides space to express difficult and sad feelings as well as clinical symptoms.
• Competent in applying the principles of palliative care at all levels appropriate to role and role models this for other team members.
• Acknowledges the significance of the emotion work involved in palliative care and offers support other team members when they feel emotionally challenged by their work.
Person-centred workplace
• Individuals within the team have a shared vision for palliative care and support each other to fulfil their vision. Care planning and practices explicitly and implicitly the values, beliefs and wishes of the person.
• Those significant to the person are involved in decisions about care in accordance to the person's wishes.
• Decisions about care are shared within the team and respect is evident for the individual knowledge, skills and experience of each team member regardless of grade.
• Care planning processes represent the agreed team vision for palliative care and include all domains of assessment.
Sympathetic presence
• Knows the person and his/her family, is attentive and available when present and demonstrates an appreciation for the loss of future that may be felt. Engages with the person and his/her family from a position of knowing the personal autonomy of his/her values, beliefs and wishes about care.
• Has highly developed interpersonal skills that enable the provision of holistic palliative care and open, honest communication.
• Engages authentically with the person and his/her family by encouraging the person to make decisions based on their values, beliefs and wishes.
• Being in the moment with the person as an opportunity for person-centredness no matter how brief the encounter.
Wellbeing and flourishing
• Prioritises the wellbeing and quality of life outcomes of service users and families in all the domains of palliative care assessment to enable flourishing.
• Focuses on own and colleagues wellbeing and contributes significantly to creating a working environment where everyone's experience, skills and knowledge are used to full potential within the team.
• Engages with others in a way that respects and values them as whole persons.
• Engages authentically and creatively with colleagues to transform practice and develop positive energy for change and human flourishing.
• Creating environments where individuals can flourish and generate energy for innovation and creativity.

Figure 19.1 Visual translation of the Person-centred Nursing Framework into a palliative care context.

Professionally competent and developed interpersonal skills to engage in emotion work

McCormack and McCance (2010) maintain that person-centredness requires a strong interpersonal skill base. In previous work (McCormack & McCance, 2006, p. 475) describe developed interpersonal skills as 'the ability of the nurse to communicate at a variety of levels', and in palliative care this includes an awareness and sensitivity particularly at times of heightened emotions both for the person and their family and also for members of the team. The Person-centred Nursing Framework identifies prerequisites relating to professional competence encompassing knowledge skills and attitudes demonstrated when staff incorporate palliative care principles in care planning and care practices.

Well-being and flourishing

Person–centred outcomes in palliative care relate to maximising quality of life and well-being for individuals and their families as a priority (Health Service Executive 2014). The centre section of the Person-centred Nursing Framework. Which applies to service users and staff, promotes the focus of positive care experiences that engender feelings of well-being and being valued. By generating an appetite for innovation and possibilities for development and change using our valued competencies, it increases opportunities for human flourishing for all (Titchen & McCormack 2010).

Sympathetic presence

The Person-centred Nursing Framework identifies sympathetic presence as an integral element in developing person-centred practice, and having sympathetic presence emphasises the uniqueness and worth of the individual and ultimately the quality of the nurse-patient relationship. The focus on *being with* rather than *doing to* in that moment of interaction where there is an opportunity to be person-centred, reflects the philosophy of palliative care and is a way for staff to demonstrate their togetherness with their patients and families (Person-centred Nursing Framework).

Person-centred workplace

The context of the care environment according to the Person-centred Nursing Framework is the supporting structures that enable person-centred practice to take place, including the quality of the leadership, the culture of the workplace, and how care is evaluated. In the absence of supporting structures palliative care will be task focused and concerned mainly with physical needs rather than the needs of the person as a whole.

Clarity of values and beliefs

Clarity of values and beliefs enables practitioners to practise, behave and communicate effectively in the care environment. McCormack and McCance assert that values, beliefs and assumptions should be observable in the behaviours of the team, with concerns arising when espoused values do not match behaviours. Palliative care principles (World Health Organization 2002) outline how care ought to be, starting with knowing own values and beliefs.

Summary

We have attempted to demonstrate the relevance and usefulness of the PCNF when planning and providing person-centred palliative care. The communication processes involved in creating a therapeutic presence to ensure a person's well-being are central. Human flourishing is achieved when staff feel a sense of satisfaction and fulfilment with their work, and have a sense of well-being and positive growth. When staff engage emotionally and authentically in palliative care they can feel fulfilled and valued. All health and social care professionals have a duty to reflect on their skills when communicating, assessing care and ultimately in understanding the importance of authentic engagement.

In summary, this chapter has reinforced the importance of shared values and beliefs to ensure staff are professionally competent and emotionally responsive. Person-centred outcomes have reinforced the importance of empowering cultures that encourage supportive spaces and places where individuals feel valued and heard beyond their disease.

References

Becker, R. (2000) Competency assessment in palliative nursing. *European Journal of Palliative Care*, **7** (3), 88–91.

Bolton, S. (2000) Who cares? Offering emotion work as a 'gift' in the nursing labour process. *Journal of Advanced Nursing*, **32** (3), 580–6.

Boyd, K. and Murray, S. (2010) Recognising and managing key transitions in end of life care. *British Medical Journal*, **341**, 649–52.

Department of Health (2008) *End of life care strategy. Promoting high quality care for all adults at the end of life*. London, Department of Health.

Department of Health (2010) *Personalisation through person centred planning*, Department of Health, London.

Department of Health (2014) Common core competences and principles for health and social care workers working with adults at the end of life (Skills for Care, Skills for Health). Department of Health and NHS End of Life Programme. Retrieved from: www.skillsforcare.org.uk/Skills/End-of-life-care/End-of-life-care.aspx (accessed 9 February 2016).

Fawcett, T. and McQueen, A. (2010) *Perspectives on Cancer Care*, Wiley-Blackwell, Oxford.

Gaffney, M. (2011) *Flourishing*, Penguin Books, London.

Health Information and Quality Authority (2012) *National Standards for Safer Better Healthcare.* Retrieved from: www.hiqa.ie (accessed 9 February 2016).

Health Service Executive (2014) *Palliative Care Needs Assessment Guidance.* Retrieved from: www.hse.ie/palliativecareprogramme (accessed 9 February 2016).

Hinchliffe, G. (2004) Work and human flourishing. *Educational Philosophy and Theory,* **36,** 535–47.

Hochschild, A.R. (1983) *The Managed Heart: The Commercialization of Human Feeling,* University of California Press, Berkeley, CA.

Holman, D. (2014) The emotional labour of caring for patients at the end of life. *End of Life Journal,* **4.** doi: 10.1136/eoljnl-04-01.4

Lannie A. (2014) Experiences of the older person with cancer: a qualitative study of medical and specialist ward settings. PhD thesis, University of Dundee.

Manley, K., Solman, A., and Jackson, C. (2013) Working towards a culture of effectiveness in the workplace, in *Practice Development in Nursing and Healthcare,* 2nd edn (eds B. McCormack, K. Manley, and A. Titchen), Wiley-Blackwell, Oxford, pp. 146–68.

McCormack, B. and McCance, T. (2006) Developing a conceptual framework for person-centred nursing. *Journal of Advanced Nursing,* **56** (5), 472–9.

McCormack, B. and McCance, T. (2010) *Person-Centred Nursing: Theory and Practice,* Wiley-Blackwell, Oxford.

McCormack, B. and Titchen, A. (2006) Critical creativity: Melding, exploding, blending. *Educational Action Research,* **14** (2), 239–66.

National Health Service (2013) *National End of Life Care Programme.* Retrieved from: http://webarchive.nationalarchives.gov.uk/20130718121128/http:/endoflifecare.nhs.uk (accessed 9 February 2016).

Rayner, L., Higginson, I.J., and Price, A. (2010) *The Management of Depression in Palliative Care: European Clinical Guidelines,* Department of Palliative Care, Policy & Rehabilitation/European Palliative Care Research Collaborative, London.

Ryan, K., Connolly, M., Charnley, K. *et al.* (2014) *Palliative Care Competence Framework,* Health Service Executive, Dublin.

Schofield, N., Green, C., and Creed, F. (2008) Communication skills of healthcare professionals working in oncology – can they be improved? *European Journal of Oncology Nursing,* **12,** 4–13.

Scottish Government (2008) *Living and Dying Well: An Action Plan for Palliative and End of Life Care,* Scottish Government, Edinburgh.

Scottish Government (2011) *Living and Dying Well, Building on Progress,* Edinburgh, Scottish Government.

Senge, P., Scharmer, C.O., Jaworski, J., and Flowers, B. (2005) Presence: Exploring Profound Change in People, Organisations and Society, Nicholas Brealey Publishing, London.

Thorne SE, Bultz BD, Baile WF, SCRN Communication Team. (2005) Is there a cost to poor communication in cancer care? A critical review of the literature.*Psychooncology* **14**(10):875–84; discussion 885–6.

Titchen, A. and McCormack, B. (2010) Dancing with stones: critical creativity and methodology for human flourishing. *Education Action Research,* **18,** 531–54.

Titchen A, McCormack B, Wilson V, Solman A. (2011) Response to Commentary. Human flourishing through body, creative imagination and reflection. *International Practice Development Journal* **1**(1) [1].

Wilkinson, S., Perry, R., Blanchard, K., and Linsell, L. (2008) Communication skills training for nurses: working with patients with heart disease. *British Journal of Cardiac Nursing,* **3,** 475–81.

World Health Organization (2002) *WHO Definition of Palliative Care.* Retrieved from: http://www.who.int/cancer/palliative/definition/en/ (accessed 9 February 2016).

World Health Organization (2007) *People-Centred Health Care: A policy framework.* Western Pacific Region: WHO Library Cataloguing in Publication Data. Available at: http://www.wpro.who .int/health_services/people_at_the_centre_of_care/documents/ENG-PCIPolicyFramework .pdf

World Health Organization (2013) *Towards People-centred health care systems: An innovative approach to better health outcomes. World Health Organization Europe.* Available from: http://www.euro .who.int/healthsystems

World health Organisation (2015) *People-centred and integrated health services: an overview of the evidence.* Interim Report. Geneva: WHO Document Production Services. Available at: http://www.who.int/servicedeliverysafety/areas/people-centred-care/evidence-overview/ en/ (accessed 22 February 2016).

CHAPTER 20

A considered reflection and re-presenting the Person-centred Practice Framework

Tanya McCance[1] & Brendan McCormack[2]

[1] *Ulster University, Northern Ireland, UK*
[2] *Queen Margaret University, Edinburgh, UK*

Introduction

In this book we have attempted to tell the story of the Person-centred Practice Framework – its underpinning principles, how it evolved over time, its relevance to key policy strategic directions, its centrality to practice development as an approach to developing person-centred cultures, and finally, how it has been used to shape developments that impact on practice. Reflecting on the chapters presented, we would like to conclude by synthesising what the book offers in advancing knowledge and understanding of person-centred practice in contemporary health and social care services.

Validation of the Framework

The contributions so willingly offered in this book by colleagues across the globe, first and foremost, confirm the applicability of the Person-centred Practice Framework in a range of different contexts. In Section 2 we hear of the Person-centred Practice Framework being used to guide and influence research, inform curriculum developments, and influence at strategic and policy levels through leadership that holds true to the underpinning principles of person-centredness. Section 3 positions the Framework as central to developing person-centred cultures through practice development, illustrating its significant contribution in this field. Finally Section 4 illustrates use of the Framework in practice, validating the underpinning rationale for its original development – to provide a means of operationalising person-centredness in practice in order to effect improvements in care. There are accounts that describe and critique the use of the Framework within mental health (Marit Borg and Bengt Karlsson, Chapter 16), community nursing (Caroline Dickson, Chapter 18), care at end

Person-Centred Practice in Nursing and Health Care: Theory and Practice, Second Edition.
Edited by Brendan McCormack and Tanya McCance.
© 2017 John Wiley & Sons, Ltd. Published 2017 by John Wiley & Sons, Ltd.

of life (Antonia Lannie and Lorna Peelo-Kilroe, Chapter 19), and paediatrics (Val Wilson and Annette Solman, Chapter 14). Furthermore, the Person-centred Practice Framework as presented and discussed within this new edition of the book highlights its relevance within a wider multidisciplinary and multiprofessional health-care context. Several contributions within the book are beginning to provide evidence of its value within multiprofessional teams. This heralds an exciting new period in the life of the Framework where we anticipate its use more broadly outside of the professional boundaries of nursing. The fact that the Person-centred Practice Framework has remained relatively stable over time is heartening, but the widespread use of the Framework as evidenced in this book provides crucial feedback and critique that informs an ongoing critical dialogue about the validity of the Framework moving into the future.

Developing the workforce

The Person-centred Practice Framework articulates a set of desirable attributes for professional practice and presents the relationship between these attributes and the ability of health-care staff to manage the care environment in order to engage in effective person-centred processes. In Chapter 7, Deirdre O'Donnell and colleagues provide an excellent and innovative example of how we can embed person-centredness into the early learning experience for students. Ongoing development of competence and professional expertise, however, is a lifelong journey, but we are still challenged to develop and implement supportive models within health care that can develop the workforce taking account of the organisational context and the wider political agenda. In Section 3 we are provided with examples of approaches underpinned by practice development that focus on the development of the health-care workforce and on creating conditions that enable human flourishing – the desired outcome of person-centredness. Angie Titchen and Karen Hammond in Chapter 11 discuss their experience of using a critical companionship model as a means of achieving human flourishing at a practitioner level, while in Chapter 10 Jan Dewing and Brendan McCormack describe the characteristics of a flourishing organisation. Emergence of differing workforce models is discussed in the context of skill mix in Chapter 3, and is a central political agenda in developing person-centredness into the future particularly within a multiprofessional context.

Influence of culture and context (practice, organisational and political)

Practice development is celebrated in this book as a robust approach to developing workplace cultures that are person-centred. As illustrated by Kim Manley in Chapter 9, practice development focuses on workplace culture, recognised as the most immediate culture experienced and/or perceived by staff, patients, users and other key stakeholders. This is the culture that impacts directly on the delivery of care, and both influences and is influenced by organisational culture. There is an increasing recognition, however, of the need to consider whole systems, and whilst practice development works at a micro systems level, there are barriers in the wider system that stymie growth and development. This requires practice developers to be strategic and political and to consider factors that are significant within the wider system in order to identify ways to reduce barriers to change.

A whole systems approach to service redesign is presented by Annette Solman and Val Wilson in Chapter 5, with person-centredness as the core organising principle. Their rationale for organisational change is a message echoed through many chapters within this book, and that is the requirement for 'staff to think and behave differently in the way they engage with their work, each other and the patient'. The processes used are underpinned by strategic leadership that enables staff engagement in the delivery of an organisational strategy through ongoing capability development of the workforce and the continued focus on person-centredness in everyday practice. Shaun Cardiff in Chapter 6 also reaffirms a model of leadership that is based on humanistic values aligned to person-centredness. Strategic leadership is a crucial ingredient in health and social care systems if we are to create the conditions that will enable the development of person-centred systems that in turn support effective workplace cultures.

What is interesting about the articulation of person-centred leadership offered by Shaun Cardiff is the influence of context, described as that which includes: organisational culture; differing stakeholder needs; safe critical and creative spaces; and systems of evaluation. This is a theme throughout the book, where we see contributors discussing the impact of context on the development of person-centred cultures. For example, in Chapter 17, Nadine Janes and colleagues discuss the enablers and obstacles in the context of moving towards person-centred cultures within an organisation delivering complex continuing care; these include: time, support, engagement and momentum. Not surprisingly, this is very similar to the issues highlighted by Christine Boomer and Tanya McCance in Chapter 15, in relation to meeting the challenges of person-centredness across acute care settings. The role of expert facilitation in such challenging contexts is an old message, but reaffirmed by several accounts in this book. Famke van Lieshout and Nadine Janes both provide insights into the challenges in relation to person-centred facilitation and the strategies being developed to build capacity for facilitation that can overcome these challenges in practice.

Demonstrating outcomes

The passion and commitment to develop person-centred practice characterise the chapters presented in this book. We read of initiatives and developments that push the boundaries of practice to drive forwards improvements and innovations, the desire being to provide a good care experience for both patients and staff. We hear consistent messages from our contributors that reflect the approaches required and the outcomes that are possible. For example, Catherine Buckley describes a narrative approach to person-centredness with older people in residential care, and identifies positive outcomes that enhance our understanding of: how people respond to change (knowing); the development of a shared understanding (being); and intentional action (doing). Outcomes reported in this book are in contrast to the experiences reported in the media reflecting a poor care experience. Recent care scandals, particularly within the UK, are often used to argue the point for more compassionate care. There is, however, a need to reframe this, moving the critical dialogue towards addressing the issue at a systems level and how a set of conditions can be created that influence behavior and cultural norms. Jon Glasby offers a refreshing critique in relation to this and brings the reader back to the idea of emotional labour, and the need for practitioners to view their resilience in terms of an emotional bank account that becomes depleted from caring work, which needs to be 'topped up'. This again places the outcome of human flourishing, as discussed by Jan Dewing and Brendan McCormack in Chapter 10, at the centre of person-centred practice and emphasises the importance of creating workplaces that enable flourishing for all.

Being political and strategic

A thread throughout this book is the importance of strategic and political directions and their influence in the development of person-centred practice. Chapter 1 provides a detailed critique of this landscape globally. The relationship between the political agenda and organisational strategy is an important one and provides the impetus and drivers that facilitate developments in practice. Whilst political and strategic frameworks are important they are not the full answer. Translating political will into action is more easily said than done, an argument clearly articulated by Jon Glasby in Chapter 4. He presents an insightful critique of the policy perspectives that aim to promote person-centred approaches, identifying complexity and fragmentation as the underlying problems. He further levels well-placed critique at the Person-centred Practice Framework, suggesting that whilst it is extremely helpful it does not fully take account of an environment that is influenced by the organisational and policy context. We cannot underestimate the power of political will and the impetus this can bring to bear on transforming health care. Without supportive policy and strategic direction it will always feel at best like swimming against the tide, or at worst drowning in a sea of competing and changing priorities.

The Framework re-presented

Key learning over the last decade has on one level informed specific changes within constructs of the Framework, which are described in this book. At another level, however, we have become aware of other factors that are strategic and political in nature that influence the use of the Framework in practice and the implementation of initiatives that are aimed at developing person-centred cultures. From critique and critical reflection of the contributions offered in this book and our ongoing experience of using the Framework, we have become aware of the influence of what we would describe as the macro context. We have identified four components of the macro context, within which the Person-centred Practice Framework sits, including:

1 Health and social care policy
2 Strategic frameworks
3 Workforce developments
4 Strategic leadership.

Application of the Framework without taking account of the macro context is somewhat naive, and if not taken account of, will influence the extent to which person-centred outcomes can be achieved. Figure 20.1 presents the current Framework, suggesting that it sits within a macro context that influences how the Framework is used within practice, education, research and policy.

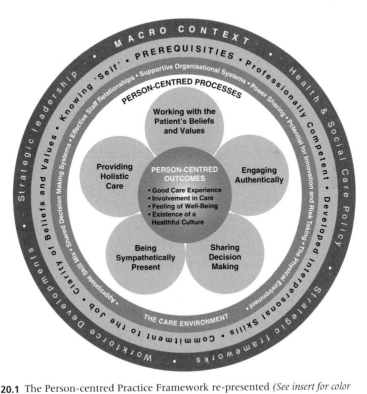

Figure 20.1 The Person-centred Practice Framework re-presented *(See insert for color representation of the figure).*

Final note

It was our intention within this book to take the reader on a journey to enhance their understanding of person-centred practice using the Framework, and to provide insights that challenge accepted norms and ways of working, thus generating an appetite for developing practice for the benefit of all. We chart the evolution of the Framework over nearly a decade and close this book by presenting it in its current form as a theoretical model that can:

- influence the practice of multiprofessional teams;
- inform curriculum developments impacting on education provision;
- underpin research and development studies;
- influence the policy and strategic directions within health care.

We very much hope that the next decade continues to validate the usefulness of the Framework and produces ever more robust evidence that demonstrates the impact of the Framework to the wider health-care agenda.

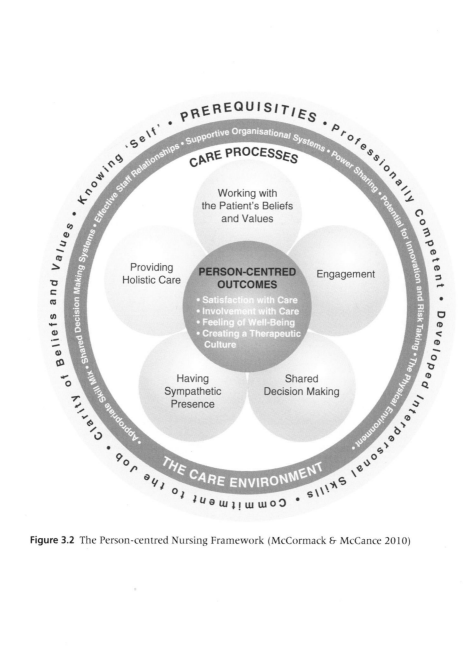

Figure 3.2 The Person-centred Nursing Framework (McCormack & McCance 2010)

Person-Centred Practice in Nursing and Health Care: Theory and Practice, Second Edition.
Edited by Brendan McCormack and Tanya McCance.
© 2017 John Wiley & Sons, Ltd. Published 2017 by John Wiley & Sons, Ltd.

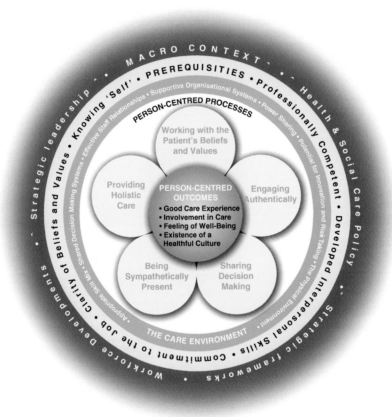

Figure 20.1 The Person-centred Practice Framework re-presented.

Index

Person-Centred Practice in Nursing and Health Care: Theory and Practice, Second Edition.
Edited by Brendan McCormack and Tanya McCance.
© 2017 John Wiley & Sons, Ltd. Published 2017 by John Wiley & Sons, Ltd.